Multiple True False Questions for the Final FFICM

Multiple True False Questions for the Final FFICM

Emma Bellchambers BMedSci, BMBS, MRCP, FRCA
Specialty Trainee in Anaesthesia and Intensive Care Medicine, Severn Deanery, Bristol, UK

Keith Davies MA, MBBS, FRCA, FFICM
Specialty Trainee in Anaesthesia and Intensive Care Medicine, Severn Deanery, Bristol, UK

Abigail Ford BSc (Med Sci), MBChB, MRCP, FRCA
Specialty Trainee in Anaesthesia and Intensive Care Medicine, Severn Deanery, Bristol, UK

Benjamin Walton MBChB, MRCP, FRCA, FFICM
Consultant in Critical Care and Anaesthesia, North Bristol NHS Trust, Bristol, UK

CAMBRIDGE
UNIVERSITY PRESS

CAMBRIDGE
UNIVERSITY PRESS

University Printing House, Cambridge CB2 8BS, United Kingdom

One Liberty Plaza, 20th Floor, New York, NY 10006, USA

477 Williamstown Road, Port Melbourne, VIC 3207, Australia

4843/24, 2nd Floor, Ansari Road, Daryaganj, Delhi - 110002, India

79 Anson Road, #06-04/06, Singapore 079906

Cambridge University Press is part of the University of Cambridge.

It furthers the University's mission by disseminating knowledge in the pursuit of education, learning and research at the highest international levels of excellence.

www.cambridge.org
Information on this title: www.cambridge.org/9781107655317

© Emma Bellchambers, Keith Davies, Abigail Ford, Benjamin Walton 2015

This publication is in copyright. Subject to statutory exception and to the provisions of relevant collective licensing agreements, no reproduction of any part may take place without the written permission of Cambridge University Press.

First published 2015

A catalogue record for this publication is available from the British Library

Library of Congress Cataloging in Publication data
Bellchambers, Emma, 1983– author.
Multiple true false questions for the final FFICM / Emma Bellchambers,
Keith Davies, Abigail Ford, Benjamin Walton.
p. ; cm.
Multiple true false questions for the final Faculty of Intensive Care Medicine
Examination
Includes bibliographical references and index.
ISBN 978-1-107-65531-7 (pbk : alk. paper)
I. Davies, Keith (Specialty trainee in anaesthesia and intensive care medicine),
author. II. Ford, Abigail, author. III. Walton, Benjamin, author. IV. Title.
V. Title: Multiple true false questions for the final Faculty of Intensive Care
Medicine Examination. [DNLM: 1. Intensive Care – Great Britain – Examination
Questions. WX 18.2]
RC86.9
616.02′8076 – dc23 2014020935

ISBN 978-1-107-65531-7 Paperback

Cambridge University Press has no responsibility for the persistence or accuracy of URLs for external or third-party internet websites referred to in this publication, and does not guarantee that any content on such websites is, or will remain, accurate or appropriate.

Every effort has been made in preparing this book to provide accurate and up-to-date information which is in accord with accepted standards and practice at the time of publication. Although case histories are drawn from actual cases, every effort has been made to disguise the identities of the individuals involved. Nevertheless, the authors, editors and publishers can make no warranties that the information contained herein is totally free from error, not least because clinical standards are constantly changing through research and regulation. The authors, editors and publishers therefore disclaim all liability for direct or consequential damages resulting from the use of material contained in this book. Readers are strongly advised to pay careful attention to information provided by the manufacturer of any drugs or equipment that they plan to use.

Contents

Introduction

In the United Kingdom, successful completion of the examinations for both the Primary and Final Fellowship of the Faculty of Intensive Care Medicine (FFICM) is now an integral part of the assessment for a Certificate of Completion of Training (CCT) in Intensive Care Medicine (ICM). Currently, a pass in the Primary examination of one of the relevant UK medical colleges – MRCP (UK), MCEM or FRCA Primary – allows candidates to sit the Final FFICM exam. Discussions are under way on the introduction of a FFICM Primary examination in its own right.

The Final FFICM exam comprises three sections: a multiple choice question examination (MCQ), an objective structured oral examination (OSCE) and a structured oral examination (SOE). From July 2014, the MCQ part of the exam has consisted of 90 questions, 60 of the multiple true false (MTF) type and 30 of the single best answer (SBA) type. While this book will be useful for all three components of the exam, it is best placed as a revision aid for the MTF part of the MCQ exam. The three 90-question papers contained in the book have been designed to encompass the 13 sections that make up the current syllabus for a CCT in ICM. This syllabus is broadly similar to the CoBaTrICE syllabus developed under the auspices of the European Society of Intensive Care Medicine, so the questions will be of direct relevance to those candidates undertaking this exam as well.

Each question has an answer and then both short and long explanations. The former will provide a quick revision refresher, while the long explanation gives the candidate further information on the question topic, along with one or more references for further reading.

All exams require a certain element of luck to pass, but we believe that detailed revision – including attempting a number of relevant MCQ questions – will improve a candidate's chances of success.

Exam A: Questions

Question A1

The 2012 Berlin definition of acute respiratory distress syndrome (ARDS):

A. Requires PEEP/CPAP of 10 cmH_2O to calculate the P/F ratio
B. Does not require a plain chest radiograph (CXR) for diagnosis
C. Specifies that a diagnosis of ARDS can only be made in intubated patients
D. Includes a factor that corrects for altitude
E. Defines severe ARDS as a P/F ratio of $\leq$ 100 kPa

Question A2

Regarding the timing of defibrillation during cardiopulmonary resuscitation:

A. It should be delayed until after 2 minutes of good-quality CPR
B. Epinephrine should be given after the second shock for refractory VF/VT
C. Three shocks can be given before CPR for a witnessed, monitored arrest
D. A 10-second pulse check should be performed after each shock
E. Defibrillation should be delayed until the patient's core temperature is > 30 °C

Question A3

With regards to the management of patients who have tricyclic antidepressant (TCA) toxicity, which of the following are correct?

A. Cardiac function is affected late or at high plasma levels compared to other tissues in the body
B. TCAs competitively inhibit sodium channels in the heart, leading to slowed conduction
C. Life-threatening effects are most likely to be seen after at least 12 hours following ingestion of high doses
D. Seizures are usually preceded by significant change in mental status or other neurological changes
E. Increasing the plasma pH to achieve alkalosis reduces the free fraction of TCA by up to 20%

Question A4

Regarding synchronised intermittent mandatory ventilation (SIMV):

A. Set tidal volume should be 6 ml/kg actual body weight
B. It may be useful for patients with raised intracranial pressure
C. It is a form of volume-controlled ventilation
D. Inspiratory flow decreases exponentially
E. It may lead to an increase in intrinsic positive end-expiratory pressure (iPEEP)

Question A5

The APACHE II severity of illness score includes the following variables:

A. Age
B. Serum lactate
C. PaO_2/FiO_2 ratio
D. Glasgow Coma Scale
E. $PaCO_2$

Question A6

Regarding treatment for acute coronary syndromes (ACS):

A. Aspirin and clopidogrel should be offered to all ACS patients
B. β-Blockers are contraindicated in asthma, pulmonary oedema and atrioventricular block
C. Unfractionated heparin should be used in preference to low-molecular-weight heparin (LMWH) in renal impairment
D. STEMI patients should be transferred for primary PCI if available within 90 minutes
E. Thrombolysis is contraindicated in patients taking warfarin

Question A7

With regards to the assessment and management of patients with acute upper gastrointestinal bleeding, which of the following are correct?

A. The Blatchford scoring system should be used in all patients at first assessment
B. The full Rockall scoring system should be used following endoscopy
C. Proton-pump inhibitors should be commenced in all patients at presentation
D. Terlipressin should be commenced only once variceal bleeding is confirmed
E. Aspirin should not be recommenced once haemostasis is achieved

Question A8

According to the Surviving Sepsis guidelines (2012), the following supportive therapies are recommended for all patients with severe sepsis:

A. Selenium
B. Sodium bicarbonate to improve haemodynamics in lactic acidaemia ($pH \geq 7.15$)
C. Glucose control between 4.5 and 6.0 mmol/l (80–110 mg/dl)
D. Unfractionated heparin (UFH) if creatinine clearance is < 30 ml/min
E. Stress ulcer prophylaxis

Question A9

Which of the following statements concerning cardiac output (CO) monitors using pulse contour analysis (PCA) are true?

A. They calculate SV and CO using the arterial pressure waveform, compliance and SVR
B. They may be calibrated using indicator dilution CO measurements
C. Demographic and physical data may be used to estimate arterial compliance
D. Accuracy is largely unaffected by damping of the arterial trace
E. Choice of arterial site may affect data quality

Question A10

Regarding the investigation and management of primary and secondary spontaneous pneumothorax (PSP and SSP):

A. Expiratory chest radiographs are preferred to inspiratory chest radiographs
B. A large pneumothorax is defined as a visible rim of air > 3 cm at the level of the hilum
C. Patients with large pneumothoraces should be admitted to hospital
D. Patients with secondary spontaneous pneumothorax should always be admitted to hospital
E. A large pneumothorax should be treated with an intercostal drain

Question A11

With regards to thermoregulation, which of the following are correct?

A. Rectal temperature is an accurate way to assess core temperature
B. Heat stroke can be life-threatening
C. Genetic factors predispose to heat stroke
D. Heat stroke is rare in elderly patients, as they are more susceptible to hypothermia
E. The hypothalamus is not involved in temperature regulation in patients with heat stroke

Question A12

In the treatment of shock:

A. Colloids are better than crystalloids for treating hypovolaemia
B. Intra-aortic balloon pumps reduce afterload and improve coronary perfusion
C. Treatment should start with fluid boluses, then vasoconstrictors, followed by inotropes
D. Treatment should focus on restoring pre-morbid blood pressure
E. Fluid resuscitation should be guided by measures such as CVP, stroke volume variation or central venous oxygen saturation

Question A13

Hypernatraemia:

A. Is a recognised cause of subarachnoid haemorrhage

B. Should be treated with 0.9% sodium chloride if the plasma sodium is > 160 mmol/l
C. Should be reduced by no more than 10 mmol/l/day
D. If caused by diabetes mellitus should be treated with desmopressin
E. Is caused by treatment with intravenous ciprofloxacin

Question A14

Inotropic drugs:

A. Cause increased force of contraction of the heart
B. Usually increase intracellular calcium levels by increasing cAMP levels
C. Act on cell-surface receptors
D. Increase myocardial work and oxygen demand
E. Need to be given with a vasoconstrictor to offset vasodilatation

Question A15

With regards to parenteral nutrition, which of the following are correct?

A. Soybean oil is commonly used as a source of essential fatty acids and lipid
B. Carbohydrate is usually supplied as fructose
C. Glutamine supplementation improves patient outcome
D. Protein is given as amino acid mixes and acts as an energy substrate
E. Trace elements such as selenium are added separately, for stability reasons

Question A16

Regarding the management of acute asthma, which of the following are correct?

A. Mortality is higher in patients with adverse psychosocial factors
B. A single dose of intravenous magnesium sulphate should be administered to patients with life-threatening asthma
C. Intravenous aminophylline is no longer recommended for any patients
D. Heliox is recommended as a treatment for near-fatal asthma in patients who are admitted to intensive care
E. Non-invasive ventilation has no place in the treatment of acute asthma in adults

Question A17

Regarding the causes of hypotension, which of the following are correct?

A. Anaphylaxis is accompanied by tachycardia
B. Bradycardia and hypotension are seen in neurogenic shock
C. Hypotension is commonly a late sign in hypovolaemic shock due to haemorrhage
D. Sepsis causes tachycardia, hypotension and reduced cardiac output
E. Cardiogenic shock is accompanied by hypotension

Question A18

The following are sources of inaccuracy in pulse oximetry monitoring of oxygen saturations:

A. Arterial oxygen saturations below 70%
B. Movement
C. Cyanide poisoning
D. Methaemoglobinaemia
E. Carbon monoxide poisoning

Question A19

Concerning the causes of acute seizures:

A. Multiple sclerosis causes acute seizures in 2% of patients with the disease
B. Hypernatraemia can cause seizures
C. Patients must have two or more seizures to be diagnosed with epilepsy
D. Non-epileptic seizures usually involve incontinence
E. Febrile convulsions lead to epilepsy in most patients

Question A20

With respect to the cleaning of medical equipment:

A. Hydrogen peroxide treatment will sterilise an object
B. Pasteurisation is the removal of all viable microorganisms and infectious agents from an object
C. Sterilisation will effectively remove prions
D. Autoclaving an object will sterilise it
E. 2% glutaraldehyde will disinfect an object

Question A21

Regarding the anterior triangle of the neck:

A. The common carotid artery divides at the level of the cricoid cartilage
B. The internal jugular vein travels in the carotid sheath lateral to the carotid artery
C. The vagus nerve travels posterior to the carotid sheath
D. The internal jugular vein is valveless
E. The carotid body contains baroreceptors and is found above the carotid bifurcation

Question A22

The following are absolute indications for tracheal intubation and ventilatory support:

A. $PaO_2 < 8$ kPa (60 mmHg)
B. $PaCO_2 > 8$ kPa (60 mmHg)
C. GCS < 8
D. Septic shock with a severe metabolic acidosis
E. Ventilatory insufficiency from fractured ribs

Question A23

With respect to the measurement of venous blood gases:

A. Mixed venous oxygen saturation is normally 70%
B. Central venous saturations are generally 5% lower than mixed venous oxygen saturations
C. Mixed venous oxygen saturation is decreased by shunt in septic shock
D. Venous bicarbonate is usually 3–4 mmol/l higher in venous blood than in arterial
E. Venous pH is usually 0.03–0.05 pH units lower than arterial pH

Question A24

Chest compressions during cardiopulmonary resuscitation:

A. Should be at a rate of 100–120/minute
B. Increase the likelihood of VF being successfully defibrillated
C. Provide a circulation to the brain and heart that is at best 25% of normal
D. Should be continuous if a supraglottic airway has been inserted
E. Should be continued while the defibrillator is charging

Question A25

Regarding the intraosseous (IO) route of drug administration, which of the following are correct?

A. It is a good alternative to central venous access for children requiring long-term antibiotic therapy
B. It should always be considered in the paediatric resuscitation scenario, where obtaining intravenous access is likely to be challenging
C. The iliac crest is the preferred location for access, because of its proximity to the skin
D. The incidence of serious complications such as skin necrosis or osteomyelitis is around 5%
E. The speed of drug onset following administration is likely to be slower than following intravenous administration

Question A26

Transfusion-related acute lung injury (TRALI):

A. Is more common if blood is donated by a multiparous woman
B. Is most common after red cell transfusion
C. Is a complication of intravenous immunoglobulin therapy
D. Is usually seen between 12 and 24 hours after transfusion
E. Is associated with high pulmonary artery wedge pressures

Question A27

Ventilatory modes useful in weaning a patient from mechanical ventilation include:

A. Synchronised intermittent mandatory ventilation (SIMV) with pressure support
B. Bilevel ventilation (BIPAP) with pressure support
C. Non-invasive ventilation (NIV)

D. Airway pressure-release ventilation (APRV)
E. Pressure-support ventilation without automatic tube compensation

Question A28

Regarding the Glasgow Coma Scale (GCS):

A. It is a three-part scoring system giving a score of 0–15
B. The motor score is the most useful discriminator
C. It should only be applied to patients with head injuries
D. A score of ≤ 8 defines severe head injury and mandates intubation
E. It can be modified for use in children

Question A29

In the treatment of drowning victims:

A. Chest compressions should be started immediately in the presence of cardiac arrest
B. Cervical spine injury is common in drowning victims
C. Salt-water drowning causes more severe acute respiratory distress syndrome (ARDS) than fresh-water drowning
D. Antibiotics should be started after open-water drowning
E. Non-fatal fresh-water drowning is characterised by a dilutional hyponatraemia

Question A30

Regarding skin disinfection:

A. 0.5% chlorhexidine has a concentration below the minimal inhibitory concentration (MIC) for most nosocomial bacteria
B. 2% chlorhexidine in 70% alcohol is recommended for skin disinfection prior to insertion of a central venous catheter
C. Aqueous 0.5% chlorhexidine is recommended for skin disinfection prior to insertion of an epidural catheter
D. 10% povidone–iodine has a similar efficacy to 2% chlorhexidine in preventing catheter-related bloodstream infections (CRBSI)
E. The use of acetone to remove skin lipids prior to insertion of a central venous catheter reduces CRBSI

Question A31

Concerning ventilator-associated pneumonia (VAP):

A. VAP is associated with increased mortality and length of stay
B. VAP is defined as a pneumonia occurring after 48 hours of ventilation
C. Lung-protective ventilation (6 ml/kg IBW) reduces rates of VAP
D. Gastric ulcer prophylaxis with proton-pump inhibitors increases VAP rates
E. Selective decontamination of the digestive tract (SDD) reduces VAP rates

Question A32

Which of the following drug assays are routinely available to measure plasma levels?

A. Phenytoin
B. Tacrolimus

C. Flecainide
D. Digoxin
E. Sodium valproate

Question A33

Which of these statements about pulmonary function tests are correct?

A. FEV_1 is normal or increased in restrictive lung disease
B. Gas transfer of CO measures V/Q matching
C. PEFR monitoring can be used to predict exacerbations of asthma
D. Spirometry gives values for FEV_1, FVC, FRC and tidal volume
E. FEV_1/FVC ratio of < 70% is consistent with an obstructive lung disease

Question A34

With regards to smoke inhalation, which of the following are correct?

A. Early bronchoscopy and washout can be helpful
B. Upper airway swelling occurs rapidly, and intubation should be performed pre-hospital
C. Cut endotracheal tubes are preferred
D. Hoarseness is a common sign and does not signify airway compromise
E. Burns to the face, lips and eyebrows are a worrying sign

Question A35

Regarding the monitoring of cardiac output (CO):

A. Thermodilution with a pulmonary artery (PA) catheter is the gold standard
B. Pulse contour analysis (PCA) requires calibration with indicator studies
C. CO monitors use the Fick principle to calculate CO
D. The ability to accurately measure CO is more important than tracking changes
E. Fluid responsiveness is reflected by an observed increase in stroke volume (SV) after a fluid bolus

Question A36

With respect to mast-cell tryptase sampling after anaphylaxis:

A. A-tryptase is measured to ascertain if a reaction is anaphylaxis
B. The volume of intravenous resuscitation fluid should be taken into account
C. The assay has a high sensitivity
D. Samples taken more than 12 hours post mortem are unreliable
E. Tryptase levels are likely to be raised by myocardial infarction

Question A37

Regarding lumbar puncture (LP):

A. Blood-stained CSF is not diagnostic of subarachnoid haemorrhage (SAH)

B. Post-dural puncture headache (PDPH) is prevented by the use of a 25G pencil-point needle
C. Absolute contraindications include coagulopathy, patient refusal and local infection
D. LP should not be performed in patients with raised intracranial pressure
E. LP can be performed at any lumbar level

Question A38

Regarding antibiotic resistance:

A. Free bacterial DNA is commonly found in the blood of intensive care patients
B. Genetic mutation is the most common mechanism of acquisition of resistance
C. Plasmids move independently of bacteria to spread resistance
D. Intrinsic resistance occurs as a result of genetic mutation
E. Transposons may insert DNA into either the bacterial chromosome or a plasmid to confer resistance

Question A39

The following physiological changes contribute to stress hyperglycaemia:

A. Increased cortisol levels
B. Reduced corticotrophin-releasing hormone (CRH) levels
C. Insulin resistance
D. Increased glycogenesis
E. Increased norepinephrine levels

Question A40

Following return of spontaneous circulation (ROSC) from out-of-hospital cardiac arrest (OHCA), the following are useful indicators of neurological outcome:

A. Fixed dilated pupils on admission
B. Isoelectric EEG
C. Post-arrest myoclonic status epilepticus
D. Absent somatosensory evoked potentials (SSEPs)
E. Loss of grey–white distinction on CT brain

Question A41

Appropriate immediate management of acute cardiogenic pulmonary oedema includes:

A. Intravenous opiates
B. Norepinephrine
C. Haemofiltration
D. ACE inhibitors
E. Intra-aortic balloon pump (IABP)

Question A42

The following ECG changes are characteristic of hypokalaemia:

A. Bradycardia more commonly than tachycardia
B. Delta waves
C. T-wave inversion
D. ST depression
E. U waves

Question A43

With respect to antifungal agents used in critical care:

A. Echinocandins have the best side-effect profile of the antifungal agents
B. Fluconazole should be first line for invasive aspergillosis
C. Amphotericin B is fungistatic
D. Oral fluconazole is 100% bioavailable
E. Amphotericin B exhibits dose-limiting nephrotoxicity

Question A44

The following sites allow accurate measures of core temperature:

A. Tympanic membrane
B. Nasopharynx
C. Bladder
D. Groin
E. Forehead

Question A45

Chronic obstructive pulmonary disease (COPD):

A. Is classified for severity on the basis of forced expiratory volume in 1 second (FEV_1) measurements
B. Requiring ICU admission confers a 50% 1-year mortality
C. Is responsible for approximately 40% of patients admitted in type 2 respiratory failure
D. Treated with long-term oxygen therapy has improved mortality
E. Should be treated with non-invasive ventilation as a first-line therapy for $PaCO_2$ > 6 kPa

Question A46

Regarding the differences between partial- and full-thickness burns, which of the following are correct?

A. Partial-thickness burns are usually painless
B. Full-thickness burns are usually more extensive than partial-thickness burns
C. Full-thickness burns can include loss of hair follicles and nerve endings
D. A white and rubbery appearance indicates a full-thickness burn
E. Partial-thickness burns often require escharotomy

Question A47

When planning extracorporeal membrane oxygenation (ECMO) treatment:

A. Patients with cardiorespiratory failure are suitable for venovenous ECMO
B. Patients should have a reversible cause or be on a transplant list
C. Venoarterial ECMO can be used as a bridging device prior to insertion of a ventricular assist device
D. Arteriovenous ECMO is useful to increase blood oxygenation
E. Carbon dioxide clearance is more efficient than oxygenation

Question A48

Regarding delayed cerebral ischaemia (DCI) following subarachnoid haemorrhage (SAH):

A. DCI may be effectively prevented with oral nimodipine
B. Digital subtraction angiography (DSA) is the best investigation for vasospasm
C. Maintenance of euvolaemia is as effective as hypervolaemia in treating DCI
D. Haemodilution is only effective in patients with high haematocrits
E. DCI in patients with unsecured aneurysms can still be treated with hypertension

Question A49

Meropenem:

A. Does not require dose reduction in acute kidney injury
B. Is a β-lactam antibiotic
C. Is contraindicated in patients with a penicillin allergy
D. Is effective against methicillin-resistant *Staphylococcus aureus* (MRSA) infections
E. Is ineffective against extended-spectrum β-lactamase (ESBL) Enterobacteriaceae

Question A50

Specific ECG changes are characteristically associated with certain conditions. Which of the following associations are correct?

A. COPD – P mitrale
B. Paracetamol overdose – prolonged QT interval
C. Hypothermia – U waves
D. Hyperchloraemia – widened QRS complex
E. High digoxin levels – concave ST elevation in chest leads

Question A51

With regards to the assessment of delirium, which of the following are correct?

A. The CAM-ICU assessment tool can be performed on patients who are intubated
B. The DSM-IV criteria can only be used by psychiatrists in the identification of delirium
C. The Intensive Care Delirium Screening Checklist (ICDSC) requires a qualified doctor to carry out the assessment
D. The CAM-ICU assessment tool cannot be used if a patient is sedated
E. The CAM-ICU assessment and ICDSC have been shown to have high sensitivity in identifying patients with delirium

Question A52

Causes of bacterial meningitis include:

A. *Haemophilus influenzae*
B. *Staphylococcus aureus*
C. *Listeria monocytogenes*
D. *Streptococcus pneumoniae*
E. *Staphylococcus epidermidis*

Question A53

Risk factors for pulmonary embolus include:

A. Renal replacement therapy on ICU
B. Lightning strike
C. Factor V Leiden mutation
D. Rheumatoid arthritis
E. Cardiac failure

Question A54

The following are evidence-based criteria for discontinuation of renal replacement therapy (RRT):

A. pH > 7.30
B. Serum urea < 10 mmol/l
C. Serum potassium < 5 mmol/l
D. Urine output > 450 ml/day
E. Serum creatinine < 200 μmol/l

Question A55

Following diagnosis of brain death:

A. Myocardial damage often occurs
B. There is commonly hypotension followed by hypertension
C. Patients are at greater risk of hypothermia
D. Diabetes insipidus is a common feature
E. Patients commonly develop an active inflammatory response and/or disseminated intravascular coagulation (DIC)

Question A56

With regards to patients who are intoxicated with ethanol, which of the following are correct?

A. Outcome following traumatic brain injury is worse if the patient is intoxicated at time of injury compared with a similar injury in a sober patient
B. A metabolic alkalosis is the commonest acid–base derangement seen
C. Insulin and dextrose infusion is recommended in patients with alcoholic ketoacidosis
D. Outcome following major burns is worse in intoxicated than in non-intoxicated patients

E. Alcoholic ketoacidosis is most commonly seen in patients with chronic alcohol dependence

Question A57

Stress ulcer prophylaxis in ICU:

A. Should be given to all ventilated patients
B. Increases the risk of *Clostridium difficile* infection
C. Reduces ICU mortality
D. Leads to the side effect of interstitial nephritis more commonly with proton-pump inhibitors (PPIs) than with histamine H_2 receptor antagonists (H_2RAs)
E. Is associated with lower rates of ventilator-associated pneumonia (VAP) when PPIs are used, compared with H_2RAs

Question A58

With regards to the intra-aortic balloon pump (IABP) which of the following are correct?

A. The balloon inflates during systole to improve cardiac output
B. Cardiac output is improved by up to 20%
C. Post-acute MI ventricular septal defect is an indication for use
D. Aortic stenosis is a contraindication to its use
E. The balloon should be left in situ for 6 hours once it has been weaned off in case of deterioration

Question A59

The following are recognised causes of rhabdomyolysis:

A. Statins
B. Diabetic ketoacidosis (DKA)
C. Epilepsy
D. Isoflurane
E. Gentle exercise

Question A60

With regards to the assessment and management of a patient with diabetic ketoacidosis (DKA), which of the following are correct?

A. DKA most commonly occurs in patients without a previous diagnosis of diabetes mellitus
B. Hyperglycaemia commonly causes a falsely elevated measured plasma sodium concentration
C. The cause of DKA is often not found
D. An elevated anion gap metabolic acidosis is a key feature of DKA
E. An elevated white cell count is often seen in DKA even in the absence of infection

Question A61

In the case of a general surgical patient with severe sepsis:

A. The patient should be operated on within 6 hours unless resuscitation is required
B. The mortality rate is < 10%
C. A predicted mortality score of ≥ 5% indicates a high-risk patient
D. In septic shock, a delay to surgery of > 12 hours increases mortality rates to 60%
E. All patients with predicted mortality ≥ 10% should receive postoperative care on HDU or ICU

Question A62

With regards to severe eclampsia, which of the following are correct?

A. It is the commonest reason for maternal admission to the intensive care unit
B. High-resistance uterine spiral arteries persist due to deficient placental implantation
C. Seizures are due to ischaemia caused by cerebral vasoconstriction
D. Because of volume depletion, aggressive fluid resuscitation should be commenced without delay
E. Phenytoin loading should be started after two seizures

Question A63

The following treatments have been shown to reduce mortality in systolic heart failure (heart failure with left ventricular ejection fraction < 40%)

A. Loop diuretics
B. Mineralocorticoid receptor antagonists (MRAs)
C. β-adrenergic receptor antagonists
D. Statins
E. Non-dihydropyridine calcium-channel blockers

Question A64

Regarding myasthenia gravis (MG):

A. MG affects central more than peripheral muscles
B. The Tensilon (edrophonium) test is the most sensitive and specific diagnostic test for MG
C. Almost all patients have autoantibodies to postsynaptic acetylcholine receptors
D. Vital capacity (VC) < 15 ml/kg is an indication for intubation
E. Plasma exchange is the most effective treatment for myasthenic crisis

Question A65

Diagnosis of death:

A. Is made by a doctor
B. Can be determined by somatic, cardiorespiratory or neurological criteria
C. Requires demonstration of the loss of consciousness and loss of cardiac output
D. Takes 5 minutes using cardiorespiratory criteria in the UK
E. Is impossible to determine neurologically in massive craniofacial injuries

Question A66

Regarding acute liver failure:

A. Coagulopathy, jaundice and encephalopathy must be present to make the diagnosis
B. It may be diagnosed if encephalopathy follows jaundice within 6 months
C. The commonest cause worldwide is paracetamol toxicity
D. Clinical examination commonly reveals signs of chronic liver disease
E. It is often caused by hepatitis B and C viruses

Question A67

The following structures will be traversed during a midline lumbar puncture (LP):

A. Interspinous ligament
B. Pia mater
C. Supraspinous ligament
D. Arachnoid mater
E. Ligamentum flavum

Question A68

In a case of neutropenic sepsis:

A. It is defined as fever (> 38 °C) in a patient with neutrophil count < 1.0×10^9/l
B. Broad-spectrum antibiotics should be started within 8 hours
C. Antibiotics should not be delayed for taking of blood and other samples for culture
D. Empirical therapy should include antibacterial and antifungal agents
E. Tunnelled lines may be safely left in situ in neutropenic patients with bacteraemia

Question A69

With regards to short bowel syndrome, which of the following are correct?

A. Intestinal remnant length is the primary determinant of outcome in patients with short bowel syndrome
B. Short bowel syndrome will develop in most patients once 50% of the small intestine is lost
C. Bile salt malabsorption is unusual in patients with large terminal ileum resections
D. Iron deficiency is common in patients who have had significant ileal resections
E. Cholelithiasis is a common problem and has a higher incidence in patients receiving total parenteral nutrition (TPN)

Question A70

Necrotising fasciitis:

A. Is most commonly polymicrobial
B. Is rarely caused by fungal infection
C. Spreads between the dermis and superficial fascia

D. Should not be treated with clindamycin as first-line unless the patient has a penicillin allergy
E. Is a cause of hypocalcaemia

Question A71

Causes of adrenal insufficiency in critically ill patients include:

A. Heparin-induced thrombocytopenia (HIT)
B. Sepsis
C. HIV
D. Addison's disease
E. Asthma

Question A72

With regards to the measurement of cerebral blood flow, which of the following are correct?

A. There is good-quality evidence that measurement of cerebral oxygenation ($PbrO_2$) can guide treatment and improve outcome in traumatic brain injury
B. If cerebrovascular autoregulation is lost the CPP target value should be between 50 and 70 mmHg
C. Cerebral oxygenation ($PbrO_2$) measured using a miniaturised Clark electrode correlates well with regional cerebral blood flow
D. It is recommended that patients with a severe but potentially survivable traumatic brain injury and an abnormal CT scan have ICP monitoring
E. Microdialysis catheters allow measurement of non-ischaemic forms of brain tissue hypoxia

Question A73

Clearance of solutes during renal replacement therapy depends on:

A. Haemofiltration flow rate
B. Dialysis flow rate
C. Vascular access device properties
D. Solute molecular size
E. Membrane sieving coefficient

Question A74

Regarding platelet transfusions:

A. Platelets should be stored at 37 °C
B. Platelet transfusions should be ABO-compatible
C. Nearly one-third of transfused platelets will be sequestered in the spleen
D. One unit of platelet concentrate increases the platelet count by 10×10^9/l per m^2 body surface area
E. The shelf-life of platelets is 5 days

Question A75

Physiological effects of a metabolic acidosis include:

A. Increased myocardial contractility
B. Tachycardia
C. Increased serum ionised calcium concentration
D. Shift of the oxyhaemoglobin dissociation curve to the left
E. Renal vasoconstiction

Question A76

With regards to the management of patients with paracetamol (acetaminophen) overdose, which of the following are correct?

A. The toxic metabolite of paracetamol which causes liver damage is glutathione
B. The antidote *N*-acetyl-cysteine is a sulphydryl donor
C. *N*-acetyl-cysteine should not be administered to patients presenting with staggered overdose
D. Most patients should be considered to be on the low-risk line of the nomogram
E. Liver transplantation should be considered in patients with high lactate at admission

Question A77

Weaning methods for a patient with a temporary tracheostomy include:

A. Cuff deflation
B. Use of a 'Swedish nose'
C. Removal of heat and moisture exchange (HME) filter from a T-piece to reduce work of breathing
D. Downsizing to a minitracheostomy
E. Reducing the tracheostomy tube size

Question A78

With regards to refeeding syndrome, which of the following are correct?

A. The hallmark biochemical feature is hyperphosphataemia
B. During starvation, plasma electrolytes are usually maintained in the normal range
C. Refeeding syndrome does not usually occur if starvation has been less than 14 days
D. Refeeding syndrome does not occur if patients receive total parenteral nutrition
E. Patients with anorexia nervosa and alcohol dependence are at high risk of refeeding syndrome

Question A79

Pleural effusions are usually transudates in the following conditions:

A. Hypoalbuminaemia
B. Pneumonia

C. Squamous cell lung cancer
D. Right ventricular failure
E. Pulmonary tuberculosis

Question A80

Levosimendan:

A. Is a synthetic catecholamine
B. Causes inotropy and vasodilatation
C. Antagonises intracellular calcium
D. Increases myocardial oxygen demand
E. Is not affected by concomitant β-blocker use

Question A81

Concerning the effects of oxygen therapy, which of the following are correct?

A. Acute tracheobronchitis is a late sign of oxygen toxicity
B. Central nervous system oxygen toxicity occurs with hyperbaric oxygen therapy
C. Acute tracheobronchitis is unusual in patients receiving normobaric oxygen therapy
D. Oxygen-induced diffuse alveolar damage is pathologically similar to ARDS
E. Acute tracheobronchitis and CNS oxygen toxicity are usually reversible complications

Question A82

With regards to the management of arrhythmias on the intensive care unit, which of the following are correct?

A. Excessive bradycardia can lead to torsades de pointes
B. Sotalol can precipitate life-threatening ventricular arrhythmias due to QT interval shortening
C. Magnesium should be administered for treatment of torsades de pointes only when the plasma level is low
D. Procainamide is useful for the treatment of all types of ventricular tachycardias
E. Atropine can be administered to prevent polymorphic ventricular tachycardia

Question A83

Regarding the diagnosis and management of the syndrome of inappropriate antidiuretic hormone secretion (SIADH), which of the following are correct?

A. Patients are usually hypovolaemic
B. Urine osmolality is inappropriately high
C. Demeclocycline can be administered
D. Urinary sodium is usually > 40 mmol/l
E. Plasma uric acid levels are usually high

Question A84

With regards to leaving a patient with an open abdomen, which of the following are correct?

A. A Bogota bag allows active drainage of fluid out of the abdomen
B. Negative-pressure devices have been shown to be superior to a Bogota bag
C. Complications of leaving a patient with an open abdomen include the development of ventral hernias and intestinal fistulas
D. An open-abdomen technique is recommended in patients with acute pancreatitis and high intra-abdominal pressure
E. Abdominal compartment syndrome can recur in patients who have undergone decompressive laparotomy and have an open abdomen

Question A85

Which of the following statements about the management of aspirin overdose are correct?

A. Plasma levels should be measured 4 hours or more after ingestion
B. Plasma levels > 300 mg/l indicate severe toxicity and are likely to require haemodialysis
C. Tinnitus is a late sign of overdose and indicates severe toxicity
D. During urine alkalinisation plasma pH should not exceed 7.65
E. Urinary alkalinisation should be continued even if haemodialysis is commenced

Question A86

With regards to heparin-induced thrombocytopenia (HIT), which of the following are correct?

A. A reduction in the platelet count of > 25% after day 14 of heparin exposure strongly suggests HIT
B. Severe thrombocytopenia (platelet count $< 15 \times 10^9/l$) is common in HIT
C. New arterial or venous thrombosis may occur before thrombocytopenia in patients with HIT
D. The presence of anti-PF4/heparin antibodies is diagnostic for HIT
E. The platelet count will generally recover within 2 weeks once heparin is discontinued

Question A87

Mechanisms of drug-induced nephrotoxicity include:

A. Cyclosporin, constriction of efferent arteriole
B. Non-steroidal anti-inflammatory drugs (NSAIDs), crystal formation
C. Aminoglycosides, renal cell toxicity
D. Rifampicin, rhabdomyolysis
E. Radiocontrast dye, renal cell toxicity

Question A88

Which of the following statements about MDMA are correct?

A. It is a Class A drug in the UK

B. Intake can lead to a clinical syndrome similar to malignant hyperthermia
C. Inhibition of ADH can result in water overload and hyponatraemia
D. Peak core body temperature > 39 °C usually results in development of rhabdomyolysis
E. Serotonin, norepinephrine and dopamine reuptake inhibition in the central nervous system results in euphoria

Question A89

Which of the following investigations can be used to diagnose or predict cerebral vasospasm following subarachnoid haemorrhage?

A. Digital subtraction angiography (DSA)
B. CT angiography (CTA)
C. CT perfusion imaging (CTP)
D. Transcranial Doppler ultrasonography (TCD)
E. Intracortical EEG

Question A90

With regards to ionising radiation:

A. 1 gray (Gy) is equivalent to 1 sievert (Sv) when comparing radiation dose from alpha particles
B. Haematopoietic dysfunction is the first manifestation of acute radiation syndrome
C. The risk of malignancy is dependent on the dose
D. Ultraviolet light is an example of non-ionising radiation
E. The dose rate for radiation decreases as the square of the distance from the source

Exam A: Answers

Question A1: Acute respiratory distress syndrome

The 2012 Berlin definition of acute respiratory distress syndrome (ARDS):

A. Requires PEEP/CPAP of 10 cmH_2O to calculate the P/F ratio
B. Does not require a plain chest radiograph (CXR) for diagnosis
C. Specifies that a diagnosis of ARDS can only be made in intubated patients
D. Includes a factor that corrects for altitude
E. Defines severe ARDS as a P/F ratio of ≤100 kPa

Answer: FTFTF

Short explanation

There are four aspects to a diagnosis of ARDS: timing within 1 week of known insult or worsening symptoms; chest imaging (CXR or CT) showing bilateral infiltrates; oedema not explicable by cardiac failure or fluid overload; P/F ratio (ratio of arterial oxygen concentration to the fraction of inspired oxygen), calculated with ≥ 5 cmH_2O PEEP or CPAP (does not require intubation). Mild ARDS is defined as a P/F ratio > 200–300 mmHg; moderate > 100–200 mmHg; and severe ≤ 100 mmHg, corrected for altitude if > 1000 m.

Long explanation

The Berlin definition of ARDS was an update of the original definition from 1994 in response to numerous criticisms relating to complexity, applicability and predictive value. The important changes included:

- abolition of the term 'acute lung injury', to leave three severity levels of ARDS: mild, moderate and severe
- recognition of the importance of PEEP/CPAP for PO_2 measurement
- clarification of chest radiography criteria
- removal of requirement for pulmonary capillary wedge pressure (PCWP) measurement

A draft definition was drawn up by a worldwide consensus process. The draft definition was then used to categorise cohorts of patients into three levels of severity of ARDS. Predictive value for mortality and ventilator-free days was then tested against the old definition and found to be superior.

There are four aspects to a diagnosis of ARDS:

(1) Timing: onset within 1 week of known insult or new/worsening symptoms.
(2) Chest imaging (CXR or CT) showing bilateral infiltrates, not fully explainable by effusions, collapse or nodules.
(3) Oedema not explainable by cardiac failure or fluid overload. May require echocardiography.
(4) P/F ratio, calculated with ≥ 5 cmH_2O PEEP or CPAP (i.e. a diagnosis may be made in a non-intubated patient on non-invasive CPAP).

The P/F ratio is used to stratify ARDS into mild, moderate and severe. Mild ARDS is defined as a P/F ratio > 200 and ≤ 300 mmHg. Moderate ARDS is defined as a P/F ratio > 100 and ≤ 200 mmHg. Severe ARDS is defined as a P/F ratio of ≤ 100 mmHg. If measured at altitude (> 1000 m), a corrected calculation is as follows:

$$P/F \text{ ratio} = (PaO_2/FiO_2) \times (\text{barometric pressure}/760)$$

Ranieri VM, Rubenfeld GD, Thompson BT, *et al.* Acute respiratory distress syndrome: the Berlin definition. *JAMA* 2012; 307: 2526–33.

Question A2: Defibrillation during CPR

Regarding the timing of defibrillation during cardiopulmonary resuscitation:

A. It should be delayed until after 2 minutes of good-quality CPR
B. Epinephrine should be given after the second shock for refractory VF/VT
C. Three shocks can be given before CPR for a witnessed, monitored arrest
D. A 10-second pulse check should be performed after each shock
E. Defibrillation should be delayed until the patient's core temperature is > 30 °C

Answer: FFTFF

Short explanation

Early defibrillation improves outcome in VF and pulseless VT, and should take place as soon as the defibrillator becomes available. Compressions should be commenced immediately following shock delivery in the absence of signs of life. Three shocks may be given with a core temperature < 30 °C. If unsuccessful, further defibrillation should not be attempted until the temperature is > 30 °C. Epinephrine should be given after the third shock for refractory VF/VT.

Long explanation

Defibrillation involves passing an electric current across the myocardium with sufficient amplitude to depolarise the cardiac muscle simultaneously, allowing the natural pacemaker cells to resume their function. Early defibrillation improves outcome in VF and pulseless VT and should take place as soon as the defibrillator becomes available. In the absence of CPR, mortality increases by 10–12% for each minute that passes between onset of VF/VT and defibrillation. CPR should be started while the defibrillator is brought to the patient, but an immediate rhythm check should take place, with defibrillation as necessary. There is no benefit in delaying the first shock for CPR.

In witnessed, monitored arrests (e.g. in the cardiac catheter laboratory), three stacked shocks may be given before commencing compressions. Compressions should be commenced immediately following shock delivery in the absence of signs of life. This is because an unsuccessful shock usually means the myocardium requires greater perfusion to restore natural rhythmicity after defibrillation. Good-quality CPR will increase the chance of successful defibrillation with the second shock. If a perfusing rhythm has been restored with defibrillation, then a pulse is unlikely to be palpable immediately and delays reduce brain and myocardial perfusion further. CPR will not increase the chance of VF recurring. Epinephrine and amiodarone are used after the third shock in refractory VF/VT. In the case of a patient with hypothermia and a shockable rhythm, three shocks may be given with a core temperature < 30 °C. If this is unsuccessful, further defibrillation should not be attempted until the temperature is > 30 °C.

Davey AJ, Diba A. *Ward's Anaesthetic Equipment*, 5th edn. Philadephia, PA: Elsevier Saunders, 2005; pp. 474–7.
Resuscitation Council (UK). Defibrillation. In *Advanced Life Support*, 6th edn. London: Resuscitation Council, 2011; Chapter 9.

Question A3: Tricyclic antidepressant toxicity

With regards to the management of patients who have tricyclic antidepressant (TCA) toxicity, which of the following are correct?

A. Cardiac function is affected late or at high plasma levels compared to other tissues in the body
B. TCAs competitively inhibit sodium channels in the heart, leading to slowed conduction
C. Life-threatening effects are most likely to be seen after at least 12 hours following ingestion of high doses
D. Seizures are usually preceded by significant change in mental status or other neurological changes
E. Increasing the plasma pH to achieve alkalosis reduces the free fraction of TCA by up to 20%

Answer: FTFFT

Short explanation

Tricyclic antidepressants have a predilection for cardiac muscle cells, and the heart is affected early in overdose. Life-threatening effects are often seen soon after overdose and are most pronounced between 2 and 6 hours following ingestion. Seizures are common and may occur with no preceding neurological changes.

Long explanation

Tricyclic antidepressants (TCAs) are one of the most commonly prescribed medications for depression in both primary and secondary care. Some TCAs (such as amitriptyline and nortriptyline) are also used in patients with chronic pain syndromes, migraines and peripheral neuropathy. TCAs are toxic in overdose and are one of the commonest causes of overdose fatalities. Effects are usually seen within 2 hours of ingestion, and peak effects are not usually seen later than 6 hours following ingestion.

TCAs inhibit the reuptake of excitatory neurotransmitters such as norepinephrine and serotonin. In addition, they have variable anticholinergic effects, which can lead to delayed gastric emptying in overdose, and so effects are occasionally seen later than 6 hours following ingestion.

Clinical features of overdose include tachycardia, dry mouth, dilated pupils, urinary retention, ataxia and drowsiness. Coma can occur with myoclonus, hyperreflexia, increased muscle tone and divergent squint. Respiratory depression may occur, requiring mechanical ventilation. Convulsions can occur in 10% of patients and may precipitate cardiac effects due to lactic acidosis.

The cardiovascular system is commonly affected, with initial tachycardia, followed by increased PR interval and QRS interval, ventricular arrhythmias and then bradycardia. α-Adrenergic receptors are inhibited peripherally, leading to vasodilatation and hypotension.

Oral activated charcoal can be administered within 1 hour of ingestion but is probably not useful after this time. General supportive measures such an intravenous fluids and vasopressors should be given to all patients with haemodynamic instability. Sodium-channel blockade can be reversed by large concentration of extracellular sodium, and some would advise the administration of hypertonic saline if arrhythmias are refractory to supportive treatment. The toxic effects of TCAs are worse if there is an acidosis present, and sodium bicarbonate should be administered in acidotic patients or those with arrhythmias. In addition, all patients with a QTc of > 430 ms should receive sodium bicarbonate, regardless of arterial pH. An increase in pH from 7.38 to 7.5 can reduce the free drug concentration by around 20%. If patients have ECG monitoring for 6 hours and it remains normal, then they can be discharged from ICU care.

Kerr G, McGuffie A, Wilkie S. Tricylic antidepressant overdose: a review. *Emerg Med J* 2001; 18: 236–41.

Question A4: SIMV

Regarding synchronised intermittent mandatory ventilation (SIMV):

A. Set tidal volume should be 6 ml/kg actual body weight
B. It may be useful for patients with raised intracranial pressure
C. It is a form of volume-controlled ventilation
D. Inspiratory flow decreases exponentially
E. It may lead to an increase in intrinsic positive end-expiratory pressure (iPEEP)

Answer: FTTFT

Short explanation

Lung-protection ventilation strategies aim for tidal volumes no more than 6 ml/kg ideal body weight. SIMV is useful to control CO_2 (essential in raised intracranial pressure) but should be used with carefully set peak pressure limits to reduce the risk of ventilator-induced lung injury. During SIMV, inspiratory flow remains constant.

Long explanation

SIMV is a form of volume-controlled ventilation. It will deliver a set tidal volume and respiratory rate to the patient, although if the patient takes a spontaneous breath within a set time window the ventilator will synchronise the mandatory breath to the patient's. Outside of this time window any spontaneous breaths will be either unsupported or pressure-supported, depending on the settings. SIMV is usually time-cycled. This means that if the tidal volume is delivered in less than the time allotted for inspiration there will be an inspiratory pause. SIMV may also be volume-cycled, where the ventilator switches to expiration as soon as the set tidal volume is delivered. Any pressure-supported breaths are flow-cycled.

The pressure waveform in SIMV shows a linear pressure increase to a peak, with an exponential decrease in expiration representing constant inspiratory flow. The speed at which the tidal volume is delivered is determined by the inspiratory flow rate. This should be kept at low as possible to minimise heterogenic ventilation of lung units with different time constants and to reduce peak pressures.

The main advantage of SIMV is the ability to set a known tidal volume and therefore minute volume. Minute volume is the main variable controlling carbon dioxide levels, making SIMV an attractive option in patients with raised intracranial pressure, where carbon dioxide control is of paramount importance. However, there is a greater risk of high airway pressures with consequent barotrauma, there is little ability to wean ventilatory support, and the ventilator will not compensate for leaks. Equally, the ventilator takes no account of the volume of air in the lungs at the start of inspiration. It is therefore possible in a patient with a long expiratory time, e.g. a patient with asthma, to have gas trapping and an increase in intrinsic PEEP.

The ARDSNet study showed that any ventilation should be tailored to a volume of 6 ml/kg ideal body weight. This is important, as obese patients would be at serious risk of volutrauma and barotrauma were actual body weight to be used.

ARDSNet (Acute Respiratory Distress Syndrome Network). Ventilation with lower tidal volumes as compared with traditional tidal volumes for acute lung injury and acute respiratory distress syndrome. *N Engl J Med* 2000; 342: 1301–8.

Gould T, de Beer JMA. Principles of artificial ventilation. *Anaesth Intensive Care Med* 2007; 8: 91–101.

Waldmann C, Soni N, Rhodes A. *Oxford Desk Reference: Critical Care*. Oxford: Oxford University Press, 2008; pp. 8–9.

Question A5: APACHE II

The APACHE II severity of illness score includes the following variables:

A. Age
B. Serum lactate
C. PaO_2/FiO_2 ratio
D. Glasgow Coma Scale
E. $PaCO_2$

Answer: TFTTF

Short explanation

APACHE II includes the following: age; chronic disease; observations (HR, MAP, RR, GCS, temperature); investigations (pH, Na^+, K^+, creatinine, haematocrit, WBC, A–a gradient). Each parameter has a weighted score. Total score is from 0 to 71; a higher score indicates higher hospital mortality.

Long explanation

The APACHE (Acute Physiology and Chronic Health Evaluation) II scoring system, first described in 1985, is a revision of the original APACHE score (1981). It is the most widely used ICU severity of illness score worldwide. It combines a 12-parameter acute physiology score, a chronic health score and an age score.

To determine the acute physiology score, the worst values for each clinical parameter in the first 24 hours following ICU admission are recorded and each value is given a score. The physiological variables are five clinical observations and seven investigation results, as follows:

Observations
Heart rate Mean arterial pressure Respiratory rate Glasgow Coma Scale Temperature
Investigations
Arterial pH Sodium Potassium Creatinine Haematocrit White blood cell count A–a gradient (if $FiO_2 < 0.5$, then use PaO_2)

The acute physiology score is added to scores for age and the presence of acute kidney injury, immunocompromise or 'severe organ system insufficiency' of hepatic, cardiovascular, renal or respiratory systems to give a number between 0 and 71.

Higher scores indicate a higher risk of mortality. To determine predicted mortality, a multiplication factor is used based on the reason for ICU admission, out of a possible 53 admission diagnoses. Predicted mortality figures can be used in audit or studies, but they are not validated for use as a prognostic tool for individual patients.

Knaus W, Draper E. APACHE II: a severity of disease classification system. *Crit Care Med* 1985; 13: 818–29.

Palazzo M. Severity of illness and likely outcome from critical illness. In Bersten AD, Soni N. *Oh's Intensive Care Manual*, 6th edn. Edinburgh: Butterworth-Heinemann, 2009, pp. 17–30.

Question A6: Treatment of acute coronary syndromes

Regarding treatment for acute coronary syndromes (ACS):

A. Aspirin and clopidogrel should be offered to all ACS patients
B. β-Blockers are contraindicated in asthma, pulmonary oedema and atrioventricular block
C. Unfractionated heparin should be used in preference to low-molecular-weight heparin (LMWH) in renal impairment
D. STEMI patients should be transferred for primary PCI if available within 90 minutes
E. Thrombolysis is contraindicated in patients taking warfarin

Answer: FTTFT

Short explanation

Aspirin should be offered to all patients; clopidogrel in intermediate or high-risk patients only. β-Blockers are contraindicated in asthma, pulmonary oedema and AV block. Unfractionated heparin should be used in renal impairment. STEMI patients should be transferred for primary PCI if available within 120 minutes, or thrombolysed if not. Oral anticoagulant therapy is a relative contraindication to thrombolysis.

Long explanation

Acute coronary syndromes (ACS) include unstable angina (UA), non-ST-elevation myocardial infarction (NSTEMI) and ST-elevation myocardial infarction (STEMI). In UA, there is myocardial ischaemia but no infarction and hence no release of cardiac enzymes. Diagnosis is made from clinical history, examination, ECG and cardiac enzymes. All ACS patients should have risk stratification using either the TIMI or GRACE scoring systems. TIMI (Thrombolysis In Myocardial Infarction) gives a 14-day risk of mortality, MI or severe ischaemia; GRACE (Global Registry of Acute Coronary Events) score gives a 6-month mortality or repeat MI score.

Unless contraindicated due to allergy or drug intolerance, all patients should be offered aspirin. Clopidogrel 300 mg should be used in intermediate and high-risk patients only (6-month mortality 3% or higher). Other antiplatelet drugs should also be considered in these patients: tirofiban or eptifibatide if percutaneous coronary intervention (PCI) will not occur within 24 hours; abciximab if it will. Fondaparinux is the antithrombin therapy of choice, unless PCI is to occur within 24 hours or in patients with renal disease or bleeding disorders, in whom unfractionated heparin should be used.

Other early therapies include: opiates (analgesia, vasodilatation); nitrates (vasodilatation); β-blockers (reduce myocardial oxygen demand); statins (plaque stabilisation); and ACE inhibitors (improve vascular and myocardial remodelling). β-Blockers are contraindicated in asthma, pulmonary oedema and atrioventricular (AV) block.

STEMI patients should be identified and triaged rapidly. In addition to oxygen, aspirin, nitrates, opiates and β-blockers if appropriate, early coronary revascularisation should be attempted. Primary PCI is the optimal method, and if it is available within 120 minutes of the onset of symptoms, patients should be given tirofiban or abciximab and transferred to a PCI centre. If primary PCI is not available within 120 minutes, thrombolysis with reteplase or tenecteplase should be administered.

Absolute contraindications to thrombolysis include:

- intracranial malignancy
- intracranial vascular lesion
- previous intracerebral haemorrhage
- closed head injury within 3 months
- ischaemic stroke within 3 months
- active bleeding (excluding menses)
- bleeding diathesis
- aortic dissection

Kumar P, Clark ML. *Clinical Medicine*, 8th edn. Edinburgh: Saunders Elsevier, 2012.
National Institute for Health and Care Excellence. *CG95: Chest Pain of Recent Onset: Assessment and Diagnosis of Recent Onset Chest Pain or Discomfort of Suspected Cardiac Origin*. London: NICE, 2010 (revised 2013). http://www.nice.org.uk/cg95 (accessed June 2014).

Question A7: Upper gastrointestinal bleeding

With regards to the assessment and management of patients with acute upper gastrointestinal bleeding, which of the following are correct?

A. The Blatchford scoring system should be used in all patients at first assessment
B. The full Rockall scoring system should be used following endoscopy
C. Proton-pump inhibitors should be commenced in all patients at presentation

D. Terlipressin should be commenced only once variceal bleeding is confirmed
E. Aspirin should not be recommenced once haemostasis is achieved

Answer: TTFFF

Short explanation

Current recommendations state that acid-suppressing medication should not be offered until after endoscopy has confirmed recent non-variceal bleeding. Terlipressin should be commenced in patients with suspected variceal bleeding at presentation. Aspirin can be recommenced once haemostasis is achieved in patients taking low-dose aspirin for the secondary prevention of vascular events.

Long explanation

Acute upper gastrointestinal bleeding remains a common medical emergency. The availability of emergency endoscopy over the past decade has improved, and these patients are often managed without the involvement of critical care services. Referral to critical care is often triggered by massive haemorrhage, persistent haemodynamic instability or concurrent illness such as decompensated chronic liver disease or acute kidney injury. The patients can be divided into two categories: those with suspected or confirmed variceal bleeding and those with non-variceal bleeding. Both can be equally serious, and management is broadly similar, though with subtle differences.

Scoring systems should be used to predict outcome in all patients at presentation. The recommended system is the Glasgow–Blatchford scoring system. This allocates a range of scores based on certain physiological and laboratory parameters including urea, haemoglobin, systolic blood pressure and pulse, as well as the presence or absence of cardiac failure, hepatic disease, melaena or syncope. A score of 6 or more strongly predicts the need for intervention. Endoscopy should be performed within 24 hours in all patients, and immediately following resuscitation in those who are unstable. Following this, the Rockall scoring system should be used to predict the risk of mortality. This assigns a score based on a number of parameters including age, the presence of shock, comorbidities, the diagnosis, and whether there was evidence of bleeding at endoscopy.

Current recommendations state that acid-suppressant medication such as proton-pump inhibitors should only be commenced after endoscopy once varices are excluded and there is evidence of recent bleeding. Terlipressin is a vasopressin analogue which acts to reduce portal blood pressure. It should be commenced in patients with suspected or confirmed variceal bleeding and continued for no more than 5 days, or less if haemostasis is achieved.

Dworzynski K, Pollit V, Kelsey A, Higgins B, Palmer K. Management of acute upper gastrointestinal bleeding: summary of NICE guidance. *BMJ* 2012: 344: e 3412.

Question A8: Surviving Sepsis guidelines

According to the Surviving Sepsis guidelines (2012), the following supportive therapies are recommended for all patients with severe sepsis:

A. Selenium
B. Sodium bicarbonate to improve haemodynamics in lactic acidaemia ($pH \geq 7.15$)
C. Glucose control between 4.5 and 6.0 mmol/l (80–110 mg/dl)
D. Unfractionated heparin (UFH) if creatinine clearance is < 30 ml/min
E. Stress ulcer prophylaxis

Answer: FFFFF

Short explanation

Selenium has not been shown to improve outcomes and is not recommended in sepsis. Sodium bicarbonate does not improve haemodynamic stability in lactic acidaemia with pH ≥ 7.15 and is not recommended. Glucose levels should be controlled at 6–10 mmol/l (110–180 mg/dl). Low-molecular-weight heparins are recommended for all patients (if creatinine clearance is < 30 ml/min). Only patients with bleeding risk factors should receive stress ulcer prophylaxis.

Long explanation

The third edition of the Surviving Sepsis guidelines were issued in 2012. The guidelines are a part of a wider Surviving Sepsis Campaign (SSC) to reduce deaths from sepsis across the globe. Strategies include increasing awareness, improving diagnosis, and the introduction of bundles of care to improve management. Guidance covers initial resuscitation, early management of infection, cardiovascular support, ventilator management and adjuvant therapies. Many adjuvant supportive therapies are listed, but most are not recommended.

Selenium levels are known to be low in sepsis. Replacement of selenium, however, has not been shown to reduce mortality, length of stay or rates of complications and is not recommended. Other interventions which are not recommended owing to a lack of clear evidence of benefit include immunoglobulins, recombinant human activated protein C, renal-dose dopamine and corticosteroids in the absence of refractory septic shock.

Sodium bicarbonate has not been shown to improve haemodynamic status in lactic acidaemia with pH ≥ 7.15 and is not recommended owing to risks of hypernatraemia, fluid overload, hyperlactataemia and hypocalcaemia. It has not been studied in patients with severe acidaemia (pH < 7.15).

Glucose control should be instigated if a patient's blood glucose rises above 10 mmol/l (180 mg/dl). Glucose levels should be maintained between 6 and 10 mmol/l (110–180 mg/dl). 'Tight' glucose control (4.5–6.0 mmol/l, 80–110 mg/dl) has been shown to increase mortality in the NICE-SUGAR trial.

Low-molecular-weight heparin (LMWH) is recommended for deep venus thrombosis (DVT) prophylaxis in all patients, as it has been found to be superior to twice-daily UFH at preventing subclinical pulmonary emboli. Patients with reduced renal function (creatinine clearance < 30 ml/min) should receive a LMWH with low renal metabolism (e.g. dalteparin).

Stress ulcer prophylaxis should only be administered to patients with a risk of bleeding (e.g. coagulopathy, corticosteroids, ventilation for > 48 hours), as they increase the risk of ventilator-associated pneumonia. Proton-pump inhibitors are recommended over H_2 antagonists such as ranitidine.

Dellinger RP, Levy MM, Rhodes A, *et al.* Surviving Sepsis Campaign. International guidelines for management of severe sepsis and septic shock: 2012. *Crit Care Med* 2013; 41: 580–637.

Question A9: Cardiac output monitors

Which of the following statements concerning cardiac output (CO) monitors using pulse contour analysis (PCA) are true?

A. They calculate SV and CO using the arterial pressure waveform, compliance and SVR

B. They may be calibrated using indicator dilution CO measurements

C. Demographic and physical data may be used to estimate arterial compliance
D. Accuracy is largely unaffected by damping of the arterial trace
E. Choice of arterial site may affect data quality

Answer: TTTFT

Short explanation

Calculating stroke volume (SV) and cardiac output (CO) requires measurement of blood pressure, compliance and systemic vascular resistance (SVR). These may be calculated with indicator dilution measures of CO, or estimated based on demographic data and waveform analysis. Accuracy can be affected by arterial catheter site (central is more accurate) and damping of the arterial waveform.

Long explanation

Pulse contour analysis (PCA) cardiac output monitors use information from the waveform of the arterial pressure trace to calculate stroke volume (SV), cardiac output (CO) and other parameters. Different monitors use different mathematical models to derive these values. Some are calibrated with indicator dilution methods, others use demographic data, and others are entirely uncalibrated.

Calculation of SV and CO from the arterial waveform requires knowledge of arterial compliance and systemic vascular resistance (SVR). Calibrated PCA monitors calculate these during calibration, and so become less accurate over time as patient or iatrogenic changes in volume status and vasoconstriction occur. Less invasive PCA monitors are not calibrated, but use demographic and physical data along with continuous waveform analysis to derive compliance and SVR. This method is less accurate, but less susceptible to inaccuracy following clinical changes. Methods involving pure PCA also exist, with less reliable results.

Another source of error in PCA cardiac output monitoring relates to the arterial site chosen for monitoring. Peripheral arteries are more affected by clinical conditions such as sepsis, high levels of vasoconstrictors and reperfusion than central arteries, which may lead to significant inaccuracies. PCA is dependent on a high-quality arterial pressure signal, and so any damping or problems with the arterial cannula can lead to underestimation of CO and insensitivity to clinical changes.

Comparison studies of PCA cardiac output monitors with each other and the gold standard (PA catheter thermodilution) have shown very good accuracy of PiCCO and LiDCO systems and good accuracy of later iterations of the FloTrac system. A trade-off may be made between accuracy and invasiveness of the monitor; most manufacturers have less invasive, less accurate monitors based on PCA alone (e.g. LiDCO rapid, FloTrac),with the option of increased accuracy from invasive calibration (PiCCO, FloTrac Volume View).

Marik PE. Noninvasive cardiac output monitors: a state-of-the-art review. *J Cardiothorac Vasc Anaesth* 2013; 27: 121–34.

Question A10: Spontaneous pneumothorax

Regarding the investigation and management of primary and secondary spontaneous pneumothorax (PSP and SSP):

A. Expiratory chest radiographs are preferred to inspiratory chest radiographs
B. A large pneumothorax is defined as a visible rim of air > 3 cm at the level of the hilum
C. Patients with large pneumothoraces should be admitted to hospital

D. Patients with secondary spontaneous pneumothorax should always be admitted to hospital
E. A large pneumothorax should be treated with an intercostal drain

Answer: FFFTF

Short explanation

Expiratory chest radiographs give no more information than standard PA inspiratory films and are not recommended. A rim of air > 2 cm at the level of the hilum indicates a large pneumothorax. Patients with large PSP may be discharged home following needle aspiration. Patients with SSP should always be admitted to hospital. Suction is not recommended for routine use, but may be useful in persistent air leak, after discussion with respiratory physicians or thoracic surgeons.

Long explanation

Spontaneous pneumothorax may occur in people with otherwise healthy lungs (primary spontaneous pneumothorax, PSP) or in the presence of underlying lung disease (secondary spontaneous pneumothorax, SSP). SSP is more difficult to treat and has a higher mortality than PSP. Any pneumothorax in a patient over 50 with significant smoking history should be treated as an SSP.

Symptoms of pneumothorax are typically chest pain and dyspnoea. These may be absent even in large PSPs, whereas small SSPs tend to be symptomatic. Significant dyspnoea, distress and cardiovascular compromise may indicate a tension pneumothorax. The degree of dyspnoea or compromise, rather than the size of the pneumothorax, will dictate the urgency and modality of treatment.

The recommended primary investigation is a PA inspiratory chest radiograph. Lateral, expiratory, supine and decubitus radiographs are not recommended as they rarely yield further important information. Ultrasound may be of use but has a degree of operator-dependency. CT scans are excellent for identifying and measuring small pneumothoraces, but usually impractical as an initial investigation. A large pneumothorax is diagnosed by a finding of a rim of air exceeding 2 cm at the level of the hilum on a PA chest radiograph.

Management of a PSP should be conservative (discharge with follow-up in respiratory clinic) if it is small and the patient is not breathless. Large PSPs should be aspirated with a 16G cannula, as should smaller PSPs in breathless patients. If the pneumothorax resolves, the patient may be discharged and followed up in clinic. If the pneumothorax fails to resolve, a chest drain should be placed and the patient admitted to hospital. Bilateral or tension pneumothoraces should always be treated with chest drains and hospital admission.

Patients with SSP should always be admitted to hospital. If the pneumothorax is small and the patient is not breathless, aspiration with a 16G cannula may be sufficient treatment, but the patient should be admitted for 24 hours of oxygen therapy and observation. Larger or non-resolving pneumothoraces should be treated with a chest drain and admission, as should breathless patients with small SSPs.

Chest drains should not be placed under suction in the first instance, because of the risk of re-expansion pulmonary oedema, but suction may be appropriate in patients with a persistent air leak after 48 hours or so. Such cases should be discussed with respiratory physicians or thoracic surgeons.

MacDuff A, Arnold A, Harvey J. Management of spontaneous pneumothorax: British Thoracic Society Pleural Disease Guideline 2010. *Thorax* 2010; 65 Suppl 2(D): ii18–31.

Question A11: Thermoregulation

With regards to thermoregulation, which of the following are correct?

A. Rectal temperature is an accurate way to assess core temperature
B. Heat stroke can be life-threatening
C. Genetic factors predispose to heat stroke
D. Heat stroke is rare in elderly patients, as they are more susceptible to hypothermia
E. The hypothalamus is not involved in temperature regulation in patients with heat stroke

Answer: FTTFF

Short explanation

Rectal temperature is usually around 0.4 °C higher than oral or core temperature. Classic heat stroke is commonest in the elderly and in small children. The hypothalamus is activated during heat stress, leading to a peripheral acute phase response.

Long explanation

Temperature regulation is mediated via peripheral thermal sensing, central regulation and efferent responses. The primary thermoregulatory control area is in the preoptic and posterior regions of the hypothalamus. Body temperature is maintained in a tight range, with the core temperature between 36.1 and 37 °C. The temperature of the skin and extremities can vary much more than this.

Fever is classed as an endogenous heat disorder where the body temperature rises above its normal daily variation. The set point appears to be reset. Infections, malignancy, autoimmune disorders and some drugs can all cause fever. Endogenous release of pyrogens such as IL-6, IL-8 and TNF-α leads to activation of the hypothalamus, which releases PGE_2. Release of cAMP in the central nervous system leads to the elevated set point, which brings about heat conservation and production, leading to fever.

Heat collapse, heat exhaustion and heat stroke are disorders on a spectrum which also includes malignant hyperthermia and neuroleptic malignant syndrome. The first three hyperthermic disorders are commoner in hot climates and in patients who are obese or have other comorbidities, such as congestive cardiac failure and neurological conditions. The former have a lower ability to direct cardiac output from the core to the skin, as cardiac output is generally reduced; they also often have higher heat production anyway due to increased respiratory rate. Those with neurological disorders such as Parkinson's disease may have failure of the thermoregulatory centre in the brain.

The main problem is a failure of heat dissipation leading to hyperthermia. The pathogenesis of heat stroke includes the cytotoxic effect of heat upon the thermoregulatory centre. This activates an inappropriate inflammatory and coagulation response, which can result in multi-organ failure.

Grogan H, Hopkins PM. Heat stroke: implications for critical care and anaesthesia. *Br J Anaesth* 2002; 88: 700–7.

Lefrant JY, Muller L, de La Coussaye JE, *et al*. Temperature measurement in intensive care patients: comparison of urinary bladder, oesophageal, rectal, axillary, and inguinal methods versus pulmonary artery core method. *Intensive Care Med* 2003; 29: 414–18.

Question A12: Treatment of shock

In the treatment of shock:

A. Colloids are better than crystalloids for treating hypovolaemia
B. Intra-aortic balloon pumps reduce afterload and improve coronary perfusion
C. Treatment should start with fluid boluses, then vasoconstrictors, followed by inotropes
D. Treatment should focus on restoring pre-morbid blood pressure
E. Fluid resuscitation should be guided by measures such as CVP, stroke volume variation or central venous oxygen saturation

Answer: FTFFT

Short explanation

Different types of shock require different approaches to improve oxygen delivery. Normotension does not necessarily signify adequate oxygen delivery, and sometimes permissive hypotension may be appropriate. Restoration of circulating volume requires fluids, but fluids may not always be needed. Therapy should be guided by measures of filling. Colloids have not been shown to improve outcome, and may cause harm. Treatment should not be predetermined, but goal-directed and guided by the clinical condition of the individual patient.

Long explanation

Shock is a condition of inadequate oxygen delivery to meet the demands of tissues. There are three main types of shock: hypovolaemic shock, distributive shock (e.g. septic and anaphylactic) and cardiogenic shock. The treatment of shock includes some aspects common to all subtypes (e.g. oxygen therapy), and some condition-specific management. Treatment should not be predetermined, but goal-directed and guided by the clinical condition of the individual patient.

Fluid therapy restores circulating volume and cardiac preload to optimise cardiac output. Treatment of hypovolaemic and distributive shock usually requires large amounts of fluid, guided by measures of circulating volume such as central venous pressure (CVP), stroke volume variation (SVV) or central venous oxygen saturation ($ScvO_2$). The choice of fluid is a matter of current debate. Colloids are thought to remain in the circulation longer than crystalloids, but no outcome benefit has been shown, and they may in fact cause harm. Balanced crystalloids are thought to be better than saline, and dextrose solutions should be avoided. Hypovolaemic shock secondary to haemorrhage should be treated with transfusion of blood products, guided by haemoglobin levels and coagulation studies. Cardiogenic and obstructive shock may also require cautious fluid therapy, guided by the patient's response to fluid challenges.

Inotropic support is vital in cardiogenic shock and may be required in septic shock. Other types of shock may require inotropic support as a holding measure while definitive treatment is awaited (e.g. pulmonary embolectomy), but this should be applied with caution and guided by clinical findings. Pharmacological agents are first-line treatment (e.g. catecholamines, phosphodiesterase inhibitors, levosimendan), with mechanical devices (intra-aortic balloon pumps, ventricular assist devices) used in refractory cases. Correctly placed in the descending aorta, an IABP increases myocardial perfusion by inflating in diastole and reduces afterload by deflating in systole.

Vasoconstrictors are commonly required in distributive shock and may be required to offset vasodilatation from other therapy. Vasoconstrictor use is often guided by blood pressure, but caution is required, as normotension does not signify adequate oxygen delivery, which depends on cardiac output and oxygen content.

In all cases, treatment of the underlying cause is the key to successful management. This may include antibiotics, surgery, pericardiocentesis, pulmonary embolectomy or coronary angioplasty.

Waldmann C, Soni N, Rhodes A. *Oxford Desk Reference: Critical Care.* Oxford: Oxford University Press, 2008.

Question A13: Hypernatraemia

Hypernatraemia:

A. Is a recognised cause of subarachnoid haemorrhage
B. Should be treated with 0.9% sodium chloride if the plasma sodium is > 160 mmol/l
C. Should be reduced by no more than 10 mmol/l/day
D. If caused by diabetes mellitus should be treated with desmopressin
E. Is caused by treatment with intravenous ciprofloxacin

Answer: TFTTT

Short explanation

In the absence of hypovolaemia with cardiovascular instability, only hypotonic fluids should be used to treat hypernatraemia. This is because of the risk of volume overload with 0.9% sodium chloride given in sufficient quantities to reduce plasma sodium. Desmopressin would be treatment of choice in hypernatraemia caused by diabetes insipidus.

Long explanation

Hypernatraemia is defined as a serum sodium concentration > 145 mmol/l. As sodium does not cross cell membranes by simple osmosis it acts as a functionally impermeable solute, contributing to tonicity. Therefore hypernatraemia leads to hypertonic hyperosmolality and cellular dehydration. Hypernatraemia may occur due to net water loss or hypertonic sodium gain and will only be severe when thirst or the ability to drink is impaired. Common causes on intensive care include insensible fluid losses, diabetes insipidus, the 'polyuric' phase of acute kidney injury and administration of hypertonic saline, sodium bicarbonate or antibiotic solutions containing large amounts of sodium.

As with other electrolyte abnormalities, symptoms depend on the severity and rate of change of the sodium concentration. Symptoms are uncommon unless the sodium concentration is higher than 155–160 mmol/l. Symptoms include pyrexia, hyperventilation, muscle cramps, drowsiness, seizures and coma. Severe brain shrinkage may result in vascular rupture leading to intracerebral or subarachnoid haemorrhage. Symptoms may also result from hypovolaemia. Compensatory mechanisms for brain shrinkage allow the brain to restore lost volume if the hypernatraemia develops slowly. The brain cells remain hypertonic, and therefore rapid administration of hypotonic fluids should be avoided, as it may lead to cerebral oedema and death.

Management of hypernatraemia is of the underlying cause to prevent further sodium acquisition or water loss (e.g. desmopressin for diabetes insipidus) and correction of the hypernatraemia itself. Acute hypernatraemia (over hours) may be corrected at a rate of 1 mmol/l/hour, but more chronic or hypernatraemia of unknown duration should be corrected at 0.5 mmol/l/hour, and by no more than 10 mmol/l/day. Ideally, fluids should be administered enterally, but many patients will require intravenous replacement. Ongoing fluid losses should be replaced, and unless there is hypovolaemia with cardiovascular instability, only hypotonic fluids (e.g. 5% dextrose or 0.45% sodium chloride) should be used. This is because of the risk of volume overload, with the quantities of 0.9% sodium chloride sufficient to reduce plasma sodium. In a patient with fluid overload and renal failure, haemodialysis or haemofiltration should be used, although caution should be exercised to ensure that the serum sodium is not corrected too rapidly on institution of renal replacement therapy.

Adrogue HJ, Madias NE. Primary care: hypernatraemia. *N Engl J Med* 2000; 342: 1493–9.

Question A14: Inotropic drugs

Inotropic drugs:

A. Cause increased force of contraction of the heart
B. Usually increase intracellular calcium levels by increasing cAMP levels
C. Act on cell-surface receptors
D. Increase myocardial work and oxygen demand
E. Need to be given with a vasoconstrictor to offset vasodilatation

Answer: TTFTF

Short explanation

Inotropes by definition increase the force of myocardial contraction, and usually increase work and oxygen demand as a corollary. The majority increase calcium levels via effects on cAMP, but only catecholamines act on cell-surface receptors. Vasodilatation is an often beneficial side effect of many inotropes, which opposes the increase in myocardial work.

Long explanation

The majority of inotropic drugs act to increase intracellular levels of cyclic adenosine monophosphate (cAMP) in the myocardium. Increased cAMP levels lead to a cascade of protein phosphorylations and eventually to increased intracellular calcium levels. Calcium ions bind to troponin C, which changes shape to uncover the myosin binding sites on actin, allowing contraction. Greater numbers of calcium ions bind to more troponin C, uncovering more myosin binding sites, leading to increased numbers of cross-bridges and hence increased force of contraction.

Increased force of contraction inevitably increases myocardial work and hence oxygen demand, but may be offset by reductions in preload caused by peripheral vasodilatation. This vasodilatation may be beneficial or problematic depending on the clinical condition of the patient, and therefore additional vasopressors may be required for haemodynamic stability.

There are two mechanisms by which inotropes increase cAMP: catecholamines act on β-adrenergic cell-surface receptors, whereas drugs such as enoximone inhibit phosphodiesterase, the enzyme which breaks down cAMP. Some other inotropes have different mechanisms of action altogether: for example, levosimendan increases troponin's affinity for calcium, and digoxin increases calcium levels by inhibiting Na/K-ATPase.

The choice of inotrope often remains a matter of personal or professional preference. Evidence supporting the use of one or another drug is lacking, and patient groups are so heterogeneous, that choice of drug is probably best made on a patient-by-patient basis. The use of multiple agents may be better than a single drug in high dose, to reduce the risk of side effects: for example, adding vasopressin to norepinephrine in severe septic shock.

Bersten AD, Soni N. *Oh's Intensive Care Manual*, 6th edn. Edinburgh: Butterworth-Heinemann, 2009.

Rang HP, Dale M, Henderson G, Ritter JM, Flower RJ. *Rang and Dale's Pharmacology*, 7th edn. Edinburgh: Elsevier Churchill Livingstone, 2012.

Question A15: Parenteral nutrition

With regards to parenteral nutrition, which of the following are correct?

A. Soybean oil is commonly used as a source of essential fatty acids and lipid
B. Carbohydrate is usually supplied as fructose
C. Glutamine supplementation improves patient outcome
D. Protein is given as amino acid mixes and acts as an energy substrate
E. Trace elements such as selenium are added separately, for stability reasons

Answer: TFFFT

Short explanation

Carbohydrate is supplied as glucose. The benefit of glutamine supplementation is a controversial subject, and as things stand the evidence for improved patient outcome is weak. Protein is supplied as amino acid mixes to replace nitrogen losses and not as an energy substrate.

Long explanation

Total parenteral nutrition (TPN) is frequently administered on the intensive care unit for those patients who are unable to receive adequate enteral nutrition. Some of the underlying conditions which lead to the requirement for TPN include inflammatory bowel disease (mainly Crohn's disease), short bowel syndrome secondary to surgical resection, mucositis secondary to chemotherapy and acute pancreatitis.

Nowadays, there are a number of commercially available generic all-in-one bag preparations that can be given to most patients. There are also special preparations to take account of specific deficiencies and fluid balance requirements.

The components of a 24-hour TPN prescription for an adult patient are relatively standardised. Patients should receive 25 kcal/kg/day. The minimum amount of carbohydrate is around 2 g of glucose per kg body weight per day. As a result, many patients will become hyperglycaemic, requiring control with intravenous insulin infusions according to local protocol. Lipid emulsions are recommended to ensure provision of essential fatty acids and to provide energy. 1–2 g/kg/day of lipid should be administered. A balanced amino acid mixture should be infused at a rate of 1.3–1.5 g/kg ideal body weight per day. This ensures that precursors for protein synthesis are available. This is particularly important in critically ill patients who are in a catabolic state, to prevent skeletal muscle breakdown. All TPN prescriptions should also contain a daily dose of micronutrients such as vitamins and trace elements. These include thiamine, ascorbic acid, copper, selenium, zinc, chromium and iron.

Singer P, Berger M, Van den Berghe G, *et al.* ESPEN guidelines on parenteral nutrition: intensive care. *Clin Nutr* 2009; 28: 387–400.

Question A16: Acute asthma management

Regarding the management of acute asthma, which of the following are correct?

A. Mortality is higher in patients with adverse psychosocial factors
B. A single dose of intravenous magnesium sulphate should be administered to patients with life-threatening asthma
C. Intravenous aminophylline is no longer recommended for any patients
D. Heliox is recommended as a treatment for near-fatal asthma in patients who are admitted to intensive care
E. Non-invasive ventilation has no place in the treatment of acute asthma in adults

Answer: TTFFF

Short explanation

Intravenous aminophylline has a place in the management of acute asthma but should be reserved for specific cases with poor response to initial bronchodilator therapy and administered after consultation with a specialist. Heliox has not been shown to be beneficial in the treatment of acute asthma. Non-invasive ventilation may have a place in the treatment of patients with acute asthma on the intensive care unit, but more trials are needed.

Long explanation

Asthma remains a potentially fatal condition in adults and children in the UK. Fatal and near-fatal asthma appears to be increased in patients with adverse psychosocial factors such as psychosis, depression, deliberate self-harm, alcohol or drug abuse, obesity, social isolation, employment problems and financial hardship. This is usually on a background of 'severe' asthma, categorised by the presence of indicators such as previous hospital or critical care admission, heavy use of β_2-agonists, 'brittle' asthma, repeated ED attendances or requiring three or more classes of asthma medication.

At presentation all patients should be assessed for severity of asthma, to be divided into near-fatal asthma, life-threatening asthma, acute severe asthma or moderate asthma exacerbation. Most critical care physicians will only be referred patients in the first three categories. Treatment should begin with oxygen, nebulised β_2-agonists (oxygen driven) and oral or intravenous steroids. Patients should receive ipratropium bromide nebulisers, particularly if there is a poor initial response to β_2-agonist therapy. A single dose of intravenous magnesium sulphate should be considered in patients with acute severe asthma who do not have a good initial response to β_2-agonist therapy, and to all patients with near-fatal or life-threatening asthma. Senior medical staff should be involved in this decision if they are not already present. The optimal route, frequency and dose of magnesium therapy is not fully determined, but a dose of 1.2–2 g given over 20 minutes is currently recommended.

Intravenous aminophylline is probably beneficial in a small number of patients, but the groups concerned have not been identified in meta-analyses. Side effects such as arrhythmias and vomiting are increased by aminophylline, and it should be administered only after advice from senior medical staff. Heliox has not been shown to be beneficial in the treatment of asthma and is only recommended for use within clinical trials. Non-invasive ventilation (NIV) has been used for many years in the treatment of chronic obstructive pulmonary disease (COPD), and there has been recent interest in the treatment of asthma. For patients with asthma, NIV should be used only in the critical care environment, and larger trials are needed to determine whether it is beneficial for these patients.

British Thoracic Society, Scottish Intercollegiate Guidelines Network. *British Guideline on the Management of Asthma: A National Clinical Guideline.* May 2008, revised January 2012. Edinburgh & London: BTS & SIGN, 2012.

Question A17: Causes of hypotension

Regarding the causes of hypotension, which of the following are correct?

A. Anaphylaxis is accompanied by tachycardia
B. Bradycardia and hypotension are seen in neurogenic shock
C. Hypotension is commonly a late sign in hypovolaemic shock due to haemorrhage
D. Sepsis causes tachycardia, hypotension and reduced cardiac output
E. Cardiogenic shock is accompanied by hypotension

Answer: FTTFF

Short explanation

Anaphylaxis can lead to hypoxia very quickly, and bradycardia may be seen immediately before cardiac arrest. Sepsis usually results in an increased cardiac output; hypotension is due to peripheral vasodilatation and relative hypovolaemia. Cardiogenic shock can be accompanied by hypertension, hypotension or normotension.

Long explanation

Shock is commonly defined as a failure of perfusion and therefore oxygenation to vital organs, leading to anaerobic metabolism and accumulation of lactic acid. There are three main types of shock: hypovolaemic shock, distributive shock and cardiogenic shock.

Hypovolaemia may be haemorrhagic or due to other causes, such as prolonged diarrhoea or vomiting. The volume of blood loss can be estimated based on the clinical findings. In healthy adults hypotension is not usually seen until 30% of the circulating blood volume is lost. In elderly patients or those taking β-blockers, tachycardia is not always seen.

Distributive shock refers to the clinical picture seen with sepsis, anaphylaxis and neurogenic shock. In sepsis, the release of bacterial exotoxins and endotoxins leads to an acute-phase response. Endogenous cytokines lead to peripheral vasodilatation and capillary leak. In anaphylaxis massive peripheral vasodilatation is mediated via histamine release from mast cells. Tachycardia will be seen early but hypoxia due to airway swelling and bronchoconstriction can lead to bradycardia. This is a sign of imminent cardiac arrest. In neurogenic shock the significance of the loss of the sympathetic chain varies depending on the level of the injury. High thoracic or cervical injuries can lead to life-threatening hypotension and bradycardia. This is due to the loss of sympathetically mediated vasoconstriction and compensatory tachycardia. Priapism will often be present in males, and this is a worrying sign in trauma victims as it signifies spinal cord injury.

Cardiogenic shock refers to a state of pump failure. This can be due to ischaemia, valvular problems or myocardial injury such as contusion or myocarditis. Blood pressure and heart rate can be either high or low, depending on the aetiology, but the fundamental problem remains one of failure of perfusion to the periphery.

Vincent JL, Ince C, Bakker J. Clinical review. Circulatory shock – an update: a tribute to Professor Max Harry Weil. *Crit Care* 2012; 16: 239.

Question A18: Pulse oximetry

The following are sources of inaccuracy in pulse oximetry monitoring of oxygen saturations:

A. Arterial oxygen saturations below 70%
B. Movement
C. Cyanide poisoning
D. Methaemoglobinaemia
E. Carbon monoxide poisoning

Answer: TTFTT

Short explanation

Pulse oximeters are calibrated between values of 70% and 100%, with potentially inaccurate derived values below 70%. Movement can lead to falsely low or absent readings. Cyanide poisoning has no effect on saturation monitoring. Methaemoglobinaemia leads to readings that tend toward 85% as levels rise. Carboxyhaemoglobin leads to falsely high readings.

Long explanation

The pulse oximeter is a critically important monitor in the intensive care unit, which gives rapid measurement of pulse rate, oxygen saturations and peripheral perfusion. Despite its simplicity and near-ubiquity, there are many potential sources of error that practitioners should be aware of.

The pulse oximeter consists of two light-emitting diodes (LEDs) on one side and a photocell on the other. One LED emits light at 660 nm (red), the other at 940 nm (infrared). These are shone through the patient's finger (or other body part) alternately, with a period of time when neither LED is on (to help eliminate the signal from ambient light). The amount of light transmitted through the finger onto the photocell results in an electrical signal relating to the amount of light absorbed by tissues at each wavelength. Oxygenated blood absorbs more infrared and less red light than deoxygenated blood. The amount of each wavelength transmitted is characteristic of a level of oxygen saturation, which is calibrated using healthy volunteers. For this reason, any readings below 70% are extrapolated, and hence potentially inaccurate.

There are two components to the signal: constant and pulsatile. The constant signal is due to ambient light and absorbance of LED light by tissue and venous blood. This signal is removed by the monitor. The pulsatile component of the signal relates to arterial blood light absorbance, and is the component displayed on the monitor. Excessive movement may interfere with this process and lead to falsely low readings or loss of signal altogether.

Changes to the light absorbance properties of the blood or tissues can lead to error. Nail varnish may reflect the light before it is allowed to reach the sensor, although in practice the signal is attenuated rather than abolished. Methaemoglobin has a different absorption spectrum to haemoglobin, and readings will tend towards 85% as methaemoglobin levels rise. Carboxyhaemoglobin (in carbon monoxide poisoning) has a similar absorption spectrum to oxyhaemoglobiin, and so readings are falsely high. Cyanide poisoning has no effect on haemoglobin or oxygen saturation measurement, although oxygen levels may be high due to reduced oxygen consumption by tissues.

Davis PD, Kenny GNC. *Basic Physics and Measurement in Anaesthesia*, 5th edn. London: Elsevier, 2005.

Question A19: Acute seizures

Concerning the causes of acute seizures:

A. Multiple sclerosis causes acute seizures in 2% of patients with the disease
B. Hypernatraemia can cause seizures
C. Patients must have two or more seizures to be diagnosed with epilepsy
D. Non-epileptic seizures usually involve incontinence
E. Febrile convulsions lead to epilepsy in most patients

Answer: TTTFF

Short explanation

Epilepsy is defined as recurrent (two or more) unprovoked epileptic seizures with no identifiable cause. Non-epileptic seizures are not usually associated with incontinence or tongue biting. Febrile convulsions are common in children and rarely lead to epilepsy.

Long explanation

Seizures are often seen in acutely unwell patients and therefore do not necessarily indicate an underlying diagnosis of epilepsy. However, epilepsy is a common condition, with a 2011 report from the Joint Epilepsy Council suggesting that approximately 1 in 103 people in the UK have epilepsy – a prevalence of 9.7 per 1000.

Trauma can cause seizures, particularly in those patients with depressed skull fracture or intracranial haemorrhage. Early seizures following trauma are predictive of long-term epilepsy.

Stroke and vascular accidents, either recent or in the past medical history, can be a cause of seizures in the elderly. The scarred brain tissue acts as a focus for epileptiform activity. Recurrent seizures are common in this group. In the elderly it is important to be aware of the fact that other electrolyte abnormalities and pathologies can lower the seizure threshold of an already aged and scarred brain. Deranged (both low and high) sodium, magnesium and calcium levels can all lead to seizures. Patients taking diuretics are at risk of slowly developing electrolyte abnormalities.

In sepsis, fever may also lower the seizure threshold. Intracranial infection must always be excluded in the patient presenting with acute seizures, particularly if there are other signs of sepsis or meningism. Encephalitis, meningitis or brain abscess can all present in this way. Adult patients presenting with a first seizure and no obvious cause should undergo imaging to look for an intracranial mass lesion. Brain tumours may require contrast-enhanced CT or MRI in order to be identified.

The management of acute seizures follows the algorithm used for status epilepticus, and an ABC approach should be employed. This includes benzodiazepines, antiepileptic drugs (such as phenytoin and levetiracetam) and general anaesthetic agents if required.

Brophy GM, Bell R, Claassen J, *et al*. Guidelines for the evaluation and management of status epilepticus. *Neurocrit Care* 2012; 17: 3–23.

Question A20: Disinfection and sterilisation

With respect to the cleaning of medical equipment:

A. Hydrogen peroxide treatment will sterilise an object
B. Pasteurisation is the removal of all viable microorganisms and infectious agents from an object
C. Sterilisation will effectively remove prions

D. Autoclaving an object will sterilise it
E. 2% glutaraldehyde will disinfect an object

Answer: FFFTT

Short explanation

Hydrogen peroxide treatment will disinfect an object. Sterilisation is the removal of all viable microorganisms and infectious agents from an object. This may not include prions.

Long explanation

Decontamination is the process of removing matter such that it is unable to reach a site in sufficient quantities to initiate infection or inflammation. It starts with cleaning and is followed by disinfection or sterilisation, as appropriate to the equipment.

Cleaning is the physical removal of foreign material from an object, reducing bioburden but not necessarily destroying all infectious agents. It may include the use of detergents, enzyme solutions and automated washers.

Disinfection is the reduction of all pathogenic material on an object but not complete removal of material such as spores. Disinfection includes chemical and thermal methods. Thermal methods with moist heat to 70–100 °C are reliable but will damage some equipment. Chemical methods include 2% glutaraldehyde for 20 minutes and 6–7.5% hydrogen peroxide for 30 minutes. Pasteurisation is a form of heat disinfection where an object is heated to 60–100 °C for up to 30 minutes.

Sterilisation is the removal of all viable microorganisms and infectious agents from an object. However, this may not include prions. Methods include pressurised steam (autoclaving), dry heat and ethylene oxide gas.

Al-Shaikh B, Stacey S. *Essentials of Anaesthetic Equipment*, 3rd edn. London: Elsevier Churchill Livingstone, 2007; pp. 237–8.

Question A21: The anterior triangle of the neck

Regarding the anterior triangle of the neck:

A. The common carotid artery divides at the level of the cricoid cartilage
B. The internal jugular vein travels in the carotid sheath lateral to the carotid artery
C. The vagus nerve travels posterior to the carotid sheath
D. The internal jugular vein is valveless
E. The carotid body contains baroreceptors and is found above the carotid bifurcation

Answer: FTFFF

Short explanation

The carotid sheath contains the common, internal and external carotid arteries (medial), the internal jugular vein (lateral), the vagus nerve (posterior), and the ansa cervicalis. The carotid bifurcation is at the level of the superior border of the thyroid cartilage. The carotid body contains chemoreceptors. The internal jugular vein has a valve just before its junction with the subclavian vein in the root of the neck.

Long explanation

The paired anterior triangles of the neck are bounded by the inferior border of the mandible, the anterior border of the sternocleidomastoid and the midline. Each contain suprahyoid and infrahyoid muscles, vessels, nerves, lymphatics and the thyroid and parathyroid glands. It is of particular relevance to intensive care as the site for central venous access and percutaneous tracheostomies.

The carotid sheath runs from the base of the anterior triangle to the base of the skull. It contains the common carotid artery, the internal jugular vein, the vagus nerve and the ansa cervicalis. The common carotid artery bifurcates within the sheath at the level of the superior border of the thyroid cartilage. Just above the bifurcation lies the carotid body, which contains chemoreceptors sensitive for PaO_2 and $PaCO_2$. The carotid sinus is a swelling in the internal carotid artery that contains baroreceptors and is involved in blood pressure control. The internal carotid artery ascends to enter the base of the skull to supply intracranial structures; the external carotid artery ascends and passes between the mandible and the ear, giving off multiple branches to supply extracranial structures of the face and head.

The internal jugular vein originates at the jugular foramen of the posterior fossa, draining blood from the brain as the continuation of the sagittal sinuses. It runs within the carotid sheath, lateral to the internal and common carotids, to the medial end of the clavicle, where it joins with the subclavian vein to form the brachiocephalic trunk. It contains a bicuspid valve just before this junction. The carotid sheath also contains the vagus nerve, which runs posterior to the vessels, and the ansa cervicalis.

Moore KL, Dalley AF, Agur AMR. *Clinically Oriented Anatomy*, 7th edn. Philadelphia, PA: Lippincott, Williams & Wilkins, 2013.

Question A22: Intubation and ventilation

The following are absolute indications for tracheal intubation and ventilatory support:

A. $PaO_2 < 8$ kPa (60 mmHg)
B. $PaCO_2 > 8$ kPa (60 mmHg)
C. GCS < 8
D. Septic shock with a severe metabolic acidosis
E. Ventilatory insufficiency from fractured ribs

Answer: FFFFF

Short explanation

There are no absolute indications for intubation and ventilation. Each patient must be assessed individually regarding acute condition, chronic comorbidities, alternatives to invasive ventilation and the likely benefit from ventilation.

Long explanation

One common reason for ventilation on the intensive care unit is respiratory failure, where it is used to improve gas exchange and correct hypoxia. Ventilation is also used to reduce the work of breathing in cases of respiratory and non-respiratory pathology, e.g. cardiac failure, metabolic acidosis. A severe metabolic acidosis that is unlikely to resolve quickly (e.g. diabetic ketoacidosis) may quickly result in the patient tiring from the increased work of breathing. Hypotension and reduced conscious level will contribute to this and provide further impetus for intubation and ventilation.

Ventilation also protects the airway if the patient's conscious level drops. Traditional teaching is that a patient's airway is at risk when the GCS is 8 or below, but this is simplistic and may not be applicable to all situations. For example, a patient with a severe head injury and a GCS of 8 should be intubated and ventilated to allow recovery and prevent complications from hypercapnia, hypoxia and aspiration. However, a patient with epilepsy may have a GCS of 8 in the post-ictal period, and provided appropriate care is taken with the airway and there are no adverse features or ongoing seizures that patient may be allowed to safely recover without intubation.

Respiratory failure may be defined as:

- type 1 (hypoxic): $PaO_2 < 8$ kPa (60 mmHg) when the patient is breathing room air
- type 2 (hypercapnic): $PaCO_2 > 6.7$ kPa (50 mmHg)

As respiratory failure may be acute, acute on chronic, or chronic, the need for ventilation should be determined on the basis of the history and examination findings of each patient. In general, hypoxia on maximal oxygen therapy or non-invasive ventilation should prompt consideration for ventilation. Equally, hypercapnia sufficient to cause a drop in pH (implying that it is above the usual level for the patient even if he or she normally retains CO_2) should prompt the institution of non-invasive or invasive ventilation.

Ventilatory insufficiency from fractured ribs is usually secondary to pain, and ventilation may be avoided with a good analgesic regimen. This is usually a thoracic epidural with or without further analgesia for other injuries.

Waldmann C, Soni N, Rhodes A. *Oxford Desk Reference: Critical Care*. Oxford: Oxford University Press, 2008; pp. 6–7.

Question A23: Venous blood gases

With respect to the measurement of venous blood gases:

A. Mixed venous oxygen saturation is normally 70%
B. Central venous saturations are generally 5% lower than mixed venous oxygen saturations
C. Mixed venous oxygen saturation is decreased by shunt in septic shock
D. Venous bicarbonate is usually 3–4 mmol/l higher in venous blood than in arterial
E. Venous pH is usually 0.03–0.05 pH units lower than arterial pH

Answer: TFFFT

Short explanation

Central venous saturations are generally 5% higher than mixed venous oxygen saturations. Mixed venous oxygen saturation is increased by shunt in septic shock. There is no difference in serum bicarbonate between venous and arterial samples.

Long explanation

The mixed venous oxygen saturation (SvO_2) is the oxygen saturation of the blood returning to the right side of the heart. It is a reflection of the oxygen extraction of the tissues.

A true mixed venous oxygen saturation (SvO_2) is obtained from the distal lumen of a pulmonary artery (PA) catheter. A PA catheter is associated with significant side effects, and many patients do not require one, so central venous oxygen saturations ($ScvO_2$) are often used instead. Normal SvO_2 is 60–80%. Normal $ScvO_2$ (from an internal jugular or subclavian vein) is > 70%.

Oxygen delivery to the tissues is shown by the following equation:

$$\text{Oxygen delivery } (DO_2) = \text{cardiac output (heart rate} \times \text{stroke volume)} \times \text{oxygen content (haemoglobin} \times SaO_2)$$

In critically ill patients, cardiac output may not be adequate to meet the tissue oxygen demand, assuming that the haemoglobin and oxygen saturations have been optimised. In this setting the tissues may extract more oxygen from the blood, thereby decreasing the SvO_2 or $ScvO_2$. If the values are normal it suggests that oxygen delivery is adequate. If low, fluid resuscitation, inotropes and vasopressors may be used to try to optimise the patient's cardiovascular status. The trend in SvO_2 or $ScvO_2$ is therefore useful to guide therapy.

If the SvO_2 or $ScvO_2$ is high, it implies that the oxygen delivery is surplus to need, that there is shunting away from the peripheries (e.g. septic shock) or that the tissues are unable to extract the oxygen (e.g. cyanide poisoning). Measurement of SvO_2 or $ScvO_2$ forms part of the Surviving Sepsis Campaign guidelines for goal-directed therapy.

It is also possible to monitor other variables with a central or mixed venous blood sample. Central and mixed venous pH is 0.03–0.05 pH units lower than arterial pH and the PCO_2 is 4–5 mmHg higher, with little or no difference in serum bicarbonate. However, the differences between arterial and venous measurements may be affected by the cardiovascular stability of the patient, and comparison and regular calibration with arterial blood gases is advised.

Dellinger RP, Levy MM, Rhodes A, *et al.* Surviving Sepsis Campaign. International guidelines for management of severe sepsis and septic shock: 2012. *Crit Care Med* 2013; 41: 580–637.

Ladakis C, Myrianthefs P, Karabinis A, *et al.* Central venous and mixed venous oxygen saturation in critically ill patients. *Respiration* 2001; 68: 279–85.

Theodore AC. Venous blood gases and other alternatives to arterial blood gases. *UpToDate* 2012. http://www.uptodate.com (accessed June 2014).

Question A24: Chest compressions in CPR

Chest compressions during cardiopulmonary resuscitation:

A. Should be at a rate of 100–120/minute
B. Increase the likelihood of VF being successfully defibrillated
C. Provide a circulation to the brain and heart that is at best 25% of normal
D. Should be continuous if a supraglottic airway has been inserted
E. Should be continued while the defibrillator is charging

Answer: TTTTT

Short explanation

This should be a straightforward question if you know the algorithm, as the five options presented here describe the perfect technique for chest compressions.

Long explanation

Chest compressions with minimal interruptions and of good quality are one of the few interventions in cardiopulmonary resuscitation that have been shown to improve outcome. Compressions should be started without delay if there are no signs of life (for bystanders) or after confirmation of cardiorespiratory arrest for no longer than 10 seconds (for trained healthcare personnel). The compressions should not be interrupted except briefly for defibrillation, pulse checks and, if absolutely necessary, for intubation/supraglottic airway placement (again, for no longer than 10 seconds). The compressions should be continued after the rhythm analysis during the period when the defibrillator is charging if staff have been trained appropriately. Obviously, however, defibrillator safety is of paramount importance, and the person in charge of the defibrillator has prime responsibility for ensuring that rescuers are clear.

Chest compressions work by direct compression of the heart generating forward blood flow. Even the highest-quality compressions only achieve up to 25% of normal brain and myocardial blood flow. Compressions will increase the amplitude and frequency of the VF waveform and therefore the likelihood of successful defibrillation. The cerebral perfusion pressure generated during CPR has also been correlated with the restoration of spontaneous circulation.

Chest compressions should be performed at a ratio of 30:2 breaths at a rate of 100–120/minute, compressing the chest by approximately 5–6 cm. Compressions should be continuous if an endotracheal tube or supraglottic airway is in situ, providing that ventilation is possible. If there is a significant leak with a supraglottic airway then a ratio of 30:2 may be required again.

Resuscitation Council (UK). Advanced life support algorithm. In *Advanced Life Support*, 6th edn. London: Resuscitation Council, 2011; Chapter 6.

Waldmann C, Soni N, Rhodes A. *Oxford Desk Reference: Critical Care*. Oxford: Oxford University Press, 2008; pp. 240–1.

Question A25: Intraosseous drug administration

Regarding the intraosseous (IO) route of drug administration, which of the following are correct?

A. It is a good alternative to central venous access for children requiring long-term antibiotic therapy
B. It should always be considered in the paediatric resuscitation scenario, where obtaining intravenous access is likely to be challenging
C. The iliac crest is the preferred location for access, because of its proximity to the skin
D. The incidence of serious complications such as skin necrosis or osteomyelitis is around 5%
E. The speed of drug onset following administration is likely to be slower than following intravenous administration

Answer: FTFFF

Short explanation

The speed of drug onset is comparable to that following intravenous administration. IO access is a short-term alternative to intravenous access only. The proximal tibia is the preferred location for access, because of its ease of identification. The incidence of serious complications is less than 1%.

Long explanation

Intraosseous (IO) cannulation is a reliable alternative to vascular access in children and is increasingly used in adults. Manual techniques include the use of standard wide-bore hypodermic or spinal needles (16–20 gauge), although this can prove technically difficult if the bone is particularly hard. Manual IO needles (14, 16 and 18 gauge) have been used routinely for many years, and a 'drilling motion' technique is used to penetrate the bone.

More recently battery-operated IO drill-like needles have been introduced. These automatic needles are efficient and easy to use even in adult bone. They have been used in the military for many years to obtain sternal IO access in soldiers with multiple injuries. During medical emergencies in children, for example polytrauma or cardiac arrest, the IO route should be considered early if intravenous access proves difficult. Some recommendations state that a maximum of three IV attempts should be made before the IO route is employed.

The marrow cavity is in continuity with the venous system, and therefore blood can be taken for routine tests as well as for cross-matching. The IO route should be employed for short periods only (a few hours) until IV access is obtained. Complications include fracture, compartment syndrome, osteomyelitis and skin necrosis. If strict aseptic technique is used for insertion, then osteomyelitis occurs in less than 1% of cases. There are no long-term effects on bone growth.

Day MW. Intraosseous devices for intravascular access in adult trauma patients. *Crit Care Nurse* 2011; 31: 76–89.

Question A26: Transfusion-related acute lung injury

Transfusion-related acute lung injury (TRALI):

A. Is more common if blood is donated by a multiparous woman
B. Is most common after red cell transfusion
C. Is a complication of intravenous immunoglobulin therapy
D. Is usually seen between 12 and 24 hours after transfusion
E. Is associated with high pulmonary artery wedge pressures

Answer: TFTFF

Short explanation

TRALI is seen in the first 6 hours after transfusion. It is most common with products containing high proportions of plasma, such as fresh frozen plasma (FFP), platelets and whole blood. Cardiac pressures are normal in TRALI.

Long explanation

Transfusion-related acute lung injury (TRALI) is defined by the SHOT (Serious Hazards of Transfusion) working group as 'acute dyspnoea with hypoxia and bilateral pulmonary infiltrates occurring during or within 6 hours of transfusion not due to circulatory overload or other likely cause'. Intracardiac pressures are normal, as TRALI is a cause of non-cardiogenic pulmonary oedema. Clinical features include hypoxia, tachypnoea, fever, tachycardia and hypotension.

Two pathogenic mechanisms have been proposed for the development of TRALI: immune and non-immune. Immune TRALI develops as a result of leukocyte antibodies in the plasma of donor blood directed against human leucocyte antigens (HLA) and human neutrophil alloantigens (HNA) in the recipient. Rarely, it is the recipient who has the antibodies. Forty per cent of patients have non-immune TRALI, with no identifiable antibodies in the donor or recipient. Lipid products released from the donor cell membranes may trigger the reaction in these cases. Non-immune TRALI is more common in critically ill patients.

In both types of TRALI, the end result is neutrophil activation and migration to the lungs. The neutrophils are trapped in the pulmonary vasculature and cause an inflammatory response due to release of oxygen free radicals and proteolytic enzymes. This results in acute lung injury, and 70% of patients will require ventilation. The mortality in TRALI is 6–9%.

Immune TRALI occurs in about 1 in 5000 units transfused and non-immune TRALI in 1 in 1100. TRALI is commonest with transfusions containing relatively more plasma, e.g. platelets and FFP. It can also be seen with red cell or immunoglobulin transfusion, however. TRALI is unpredictable, but its incidence has been significantly reduced by reducing transfusions, using male donors or nulliparous women only for plasma-containing products, and leucodepletion of blood.

Treatment of TRALI is supportive. Patients should be followed up by the transfusion service and the donor blood screened for antibodies.

Maxwell MJ, Wilson MJA. Complications of blood transfusion. *Contin Educ Anaesth Crit Care Pain* 2006; 6: 225–9.

Thachil J, Erinjeri JF, Mahambrey TD. Transfusion-related acute lung injury: a review. *J Intensive Care Med* 2009; 10: 207–11.

Question A27: Weaning from mechanical ventilation

Ventilatory modes useful in weaning a patient from mechanical ventilation include:

A. Synchronised intermittent mandatory ventilation (SIMV) with pressure support
B. Bilevel ventilation (BIPAP) with pressure support
C. Non-invasive ventilation (NIV)
D. Airway pressure-release ventilation (APRV)
E. Pressure-support ventilation without automatic tube compensation

Answer: FTTFT

Short explanation

SIMV is volume-controlled ventilation with or without pressure support for spontaneous breaths. It is not a suitable weaning mode when compared to others. APRV is generally used in patients with acute lung injury and acute respiratory distress syndrome (ARDS), where a high mean airway pressure improves alveolar recruitment and oxygenation with carbon dioxide clearance during the transient fall in airway pressure.

Long explanation

Weaning from mechanical ventilation describes the transition between full ventilatory support and spontaneous breathing, and the removal of any artificial airway. Prolonged ventilation is problematic both for the patient (increased morbidity and mortality) and for the organisation (increased length and cost of stay).

SIMV is volume-controlled ventilation with or without pressure support for spontaneous breaths. It is not a suitable weaning mode when compared to others because of the mandatory breaths. APRV is a ventilation mode that can be useful in patients with ARDS, where a high mean airway pressure improves alveolar recruitment and oxygenation with carbon dioxide clearance during the transient fall in airway pressure. It is not suitable for weaning, because of the unnatural respiratory pattern.

The most common mode of ventilation for weaning is pressure-support ventilation. Weaning may start with the patient on BIPAP, with reduction in ventilatory pressures, cardiovascular support and sedation as the patient's condition improves. This facilitates a switch to spontaneous ventilation with gradually reducing pressure support as the patient takes over the work of breathing. T-piece trials may then also be used, although there is little evidence that they are superior to simply reducing the pressure support the patient is receiving. Continuous positive airway pressure (CPAP) is the natural end-point of PSV weaning and may be the last step prior to extubation.

Automatic tube compensation aims to compensate for the non-linear pressure drop across the endotracheal tube during spontaneous breathing. The ventilator delivers a higher inspiratory pressure during inspiration and a reduced pressure during expiration to offset the increased work of breathing due to the tube. It can be used during spontaneous breathing trials, although it is probably most useful in patients with a narrow endotracheal tube in situ.

Non-invasive ventilation is generally used in patients with chronic obstructive pulmonary disease (COPD), where it may bridge the gap between ventilation and spontaneous breathing in patients with poor respiratory reserve. It is not currently recommended as a weaning tool in all patients, as it may lead to delayed reintubation and a poorer outcome should the patient fail the trial of extubation.

Boles JM, Bion J, Connors A, *et al*. Weaning from mechanical ventilation. Statement of the Sixth International Consensus Conference on Intensive Care Medicine. *Eur Respir J* 2007; 29: 1033–56.

Intensive Care Society. Weaning guidelines. http://www.ics.ac.uk/ics-homepage/guidelines-standards (accessed June 2014).

Waldmann C, Soni N, Rhodes A. *Oxford Desk Reference: Critical Care*. Oxford: Oxford University Press, 2008; pp. 16–17.

Question A28: Glasgow Coma Scale

Regarding the Glasgow Coma Scale (GCS):

A. It is a three-part scoring system giving a score of 0–15
B. The motor score is the most useful discriminator
C. It should only be applied to patients with head injuries
D. A score of ≤ 8 defines severe head injury and mandates intubation
E. It can be modified for use in children

Answer: FTFFT

Short explanation

The GCS was originally intended for use after head injury, but is commonly used in all patients with disturbances of consciousness. Modified versions exist for use in children. Scores range from 3 to 15, for eye opening (1–4), verbalisation (1–5), motor response (1–6). The last of these is the best discriminator of severity of brain injury. Patients with GCS < 9 are likely to have impairment of airway reflexes and often require intubation.

Long explanation

The Glasgow Coma Scale (GCS) was introduced in 1974 as a neurological scoring tool, to assess level of consciousness after head injury. Its role has since expanded and it is widely used in the prehospital environment, emergency departments, critical care and general wards. While GCS as a tool has the greatest validity in head-injury patients, its application to wider patient groups is also appropriate. It forms part of many critical illness severity scoring systems (e.g. APACHE, SAPS, SOFA) and can be used to stratify risk following insults such as brain injury and subarachnoid haemorrhage.

The most widely used version of the GCS has a 15-point scale, but the originally described version had only 14 points. The Modified GCS, which added an extra motor category, is now almost universal. The standard GCS cannot be used in young children, but several versions exist that are adapted to specific age groups.

GCS is the total of three scores, for eye opening, verbalisation and motor response. The best response in each category should be recorded. Each category has a minimum score of 1, and so the lowest possible GCS is 3/15. Scoring is as follows:

Eye response	Spontaneous opening	4
	Open in response to voice	3
	Open in response to pain	2
	Do not open	1
Verbal response	Oriented, coherent speech	5
	Confused speech	4
	Inappropriate words	3
	Unintelligible sounds	2
	No response	1
Motor response	Obeys commands	6
	Withdraws from painful stimulus	5
	Localises to painful stimulus	4
	Abnormal flexion to pain	3
	Abnormal extension to pain	2
	No response to pain	1

Painful stimuli should be peripheral (upper limb) to allow withdrawal, but central stimuli may also be used for clarification. The motor category is the best discriminator of the severity of brain injury.

Palazzo M. Severity of illness and likely outcome from critical illness. In Bersten AD, Soni N. *Oh's Intensive Care Manual*, 6th edn. Edinburgh: Butterworth-Heinemann, 2009, pp. 17–30.

Teasdale G, Murray G, Parker L, Jennett B. Adding up the Glasgow Coma Score. *Acta Neurochir Suppl (Wien)* 1979; 28: 13–16.

Question A29: Drowning

In the treatment of drowning victims:

A. Chest compressions should be started immediately in the presence of cardiac arrest
B. Cervical spine injury is common in drowning victims
C. Salt-water drowning causes more severe acute respiratory distress syndrome (ARDS) than fresh-water drowning
D. Antibiotics should be started after open-water drowning
E. Non-fatal fresh-water drowning is characterised by a dilutional hyponatraemia

Answer: FFFFF

Short explanation

Rescue breaths should be used prior to chest compressions. The severity of ARDS is not related to the type of water aspirated. Non-fatal drowning rarely results in electrolyte abnormalities. Antibiotics should only be started when there is evidence of infection. Cervical spine injury is uncommon (< 0.5%).

Long explanation

Drowning is defined as primary respiratory compromise as a result of submersion or immersion in a liquid, and it may be fatal or non-fatal. There has traditionally been a distinction between salt- and fresh-water drowning. Hypertonic salt water was thought to draw fluid into the lungs, increasing pulmonary oedema and causing hypertonic plasma. Fresh-water drowning was described as the opposite, with hypotonic fluid passing though the lungs to cause plasma dilution and volume overload. However, most non-fatal drowning casualties only aspirate between 3 and 4 ml/kg; blood volume changes require volumes of > 11 ml/kg, and electrolyte changes > 22 ml/kg.

Non-fatal drowning results in respiratory compromise due to reduced lung surfactant producing acute respiratory distress syndrome (ARDS). About 20% of non-fatal drowning victims will suffer a hypoxic brain injury. Arrhythmias are common after drowning, secondary to hypoxia or associated with hypothermia. An arrhythmia may also be the cause of the drowning episode. Patients may have a metabolic or respiratory acidosis, depending on the level of respiratory or cardiovascular compromise. Significant electrolyte imbalances are rare, although renal failure may occur due to hypoxia, shock or rhabdomyolysis. Haemolysis and coagulopathy are rare complications of non-fatal drowning.

Cardiopulmonary resuscitation is modified in drowning victims to take account of hypoxia as the primary cause in many cases and victims often being hypothermic. Resuscitation should commence with five rescue breaths before standard 30:2 compressions:ventilation. If the victim's core temperature is < 30 °C, defibrillation should only be attempted three times, and drugs should be given at twice the normal intervals until core temperature is > 30 °C.

Steroids and routine antibiotics are not recommended after non-fatal drowning unless otherwise indicated.

Survival after non-fatal drowning is difficult to predict, but cold water (< 10 °C) certainly appears protective. A long period of submersion or time to basic life support (> 10 minutes), a long resuscitation period (> 25 minutes) with persistent coma (GCS < 5) and severe acidosis (pH < 7.1 on admission) are poor prognostic signs.

Chandy D, Weinhouse GL. Drowning (submersion injuries). *UpToDate* 2013. http://www.uptodate.com (accessed June 2014).

Resuscitation Council (UK). *Advanced Life Support*, 6th edn. London: Resuscitation Council, 2011; pp. 127–9.

Question A30: Skin disinfection

Regarding skin disinfection:

A. 0.5% chlorhexidine has a concentration below the minimal inhibitory concentration (MIC) for most nosocomial bacteria
B. 2% chlorhexidine in 70% alcohol is recommended for skin disinfection prior to insertion of a central venous catheter
C. Aqueous 0.5% chlorhexidine is recommended for skin disinfection prior to insertion of an epidural catheter
D. 10% povidone–iodine has a similar efficacy to 2% chlorhexidine in preventing catheter-related bloodstream infections (CRBSI)
E. The use of acetone to remove skin lipids prior to insertion of a central venous catheter reduces CRBSI

Answer: FTTFF

Short explanation

Both 2% and 0.5% chlorhexidine have a concentration above the MIC for most nosocomial bacteria. Chlorhexidine is superior to 10% povidone–iodine solutions, and the use of acetone does not reduce CRBSI.

Long explanation

Microorganisms present on the skin around any invasive device are generally responsible for subsequent infection in that device. The higher the density of microorganisms, the greater the likelihood of infection, highlighting the need for rigorous decontamination of the skin prior to insertion of any invasive device.

Catheter-related bloodstream infection (CRBSI) is the presence of a bacteraemia caused by an intravenous catheter. The incidence is up to 16% of catheterisations. CRBSI is rare from peripheral or arterial cannulae, highest in dialysis catheters, and roughly equal in central venous catheters and pulmonary artery catheters. The site of placement also impacts on the likelihood of infection: femoral placement carries the highest risk, followed by internal jugular then subclavian vein cannulation. A central venous catheter care bundle incorporating all aspects from insertion to aftercare and removal has been shown to reduce CRBSI and should be employed in all patients with central venous access devices.

epic3 guidelines (2014) suggest the use of 2% chlorhexidine in 70% alcohol as being superior to povidone–iodine solutions. Both 0.5% and 2% chlorhexidine provide a concentration of chlorhexidine that is greater than the minimal inhibitory concentration (MIC) for most nosocomial bacteria and yeasts, although 2% chlorhexidine is thought to be more effective in preventing CRBSI. There have been reports of adhesive arachnoiditis with the use of chlorhexidine for central neuraxial procedures, so a number of bodies – including the Association of Anaesthetists of Great Britain and Ireland and the NAP 3 investigators on behalf of the Royal College of Anaesthetists – recommend the use of 0.5% chlorhexidine in 70% alcohol solutions rather than the 2% equivalent. The evidence for this, however, is by no means conclusive.

The application of organic solvents, such as acetone, to remove skin lipids before central venous catheter insertion is not recommended, as there is no evidence that the use of these agents reduces CRBSI and their use could increase local inflammation.

Cook TM, Counsell D, Wildsmith JAW. Major complications of central neuraxial block: report on the 3rd National Audit Project of the Royal College of Anaesthetists. On behalf of the Royal College of Anaesthetists Third National Audit Project. *Br J Anaesth* 2009; 102: 179–90.

Loveday HP, Wilson JA, Pratt RJ, *et al.* epic3: national evidence based guidelines for preventing healthcare-associated infections in NHS hospitals in England. *J Hosp Infect* 2014; 86 (Suppl 1): S1–70.

Question A31: Ventilator-associated pneumonia

Concerning ventilator-associated pneumonia (VAP):

A. VAP is associated with increased mortality and length of stay
B. VAP is defined as a pneumonia occurring after 48 hours of ventilation
C. Lung-protective ventilation (6 ml/kg IBW) reduces rates of VAP
D. Gastric ulcer prophylaxis with proton-pump inhibitors increases VAP rates
E. Selective decontamination of the digestive tract (SDD) reduces VAP rates

Answer: TFFTT

Short explanation

VAP is defined as a pneumonia occurring 48 hours or more after intubation. It is associated with increased ventilator days and length of stay, and it has an estimated attributable mortality of 9%. Effective prevention is key. Oral decontamination, SDD, head-up positioning, subglottic suctioning and reducing the duration of ventilation reduce VAP rates. Lung-protective ventilation reduces iatrogenic lung injury but not VAP.

Long explanation

Ventilator-associated pneumonia (VAP) is defined as a pneumonia occurring 48 hours or more after tracheal intubation. VAP may be diagnosed in patients intubated and ventilated for less than 48 hours if the pneumonia occurs after that period. It is the commonest nosocomial infection in ventilated patients. It is estimated to occur in 10–25% of ventilated patients and has been found to increase ventilator days and ICU and hospital length of stay. VAP has an estimated attributable mortality rate of 9%.

Diagnosis can be difficult, as there is no consensus on diagnostic criteria and critically ill patients often have multiple co-existent pathologies. The HELICS (Hospitals in Europe Link for Infection Control through Surveillance) criteria are complex but include: CXR changes; fever or leucocytosis with no other cause; change in lung condition (cough, sputum, dyspnoea, abnormal signs or worsening gas exchange); and positive microbiological culture.

Causative organisms in VAP are commonly colonising species of the oropharynx or gastrointestinal tract. The commonest organisms are *Pseudomonas aeruginosa, Staphylococcus aureus*, Enterobacteriaceae, *Haemophilus* and *Streptococcus* species. Bacterial drug resistance is widespread, and treatment can therefore be difficult.

Prevention is crucially important. Many simple interventions have been shown to reduce VAP rates, particularly if combined in a care bundle for use in all ventilated patients. Common components of ventilator care bundles include:

- Nursing in head-up position (> 30°)
- Oral decontamination (e.g. with chlorhexidine)
- Daily sedation holds (to reduce duration of ventilation)
- Hand washing
- DVT prophylaxis (no effect on VAP)
- Gastric ulcer prophylaxis (despite being associated with increased VAP rates)

Of these interventions, head-up positioning and oral decontamination are those recommended by the National Institute for Health and Care Excellence (NICE).

Other interventions shown to reduce rates of VAP are selective decontamination of the digestive tract (SDD: an intervention rarely used in the UK despite good evidence of reduced mortality), subglottic suctioning and the use of silver-coated endotracheal tubes. Lung-protective ventilation with tidal volumes of < 6 ml/kg reduces lung trauma and mortality in ARDS but not in VAP.

Hunter JD. Ventilator associated pneumonia. *BMJ* 2012; 344: e3325.

Valencia M, Torres A. Ventilator-associated pneumonia. *Curr Opin Crit Care* 2009; 15: 30–5.

Question A32: Measurement of drug plasma levels

Which of the following drug assays are routinely available to measure plasma levels?

A. Phenytoin
B. Tacrolimus
C. Flecainide
D. Digoxin
E. Sodium valproate

Answer: TTTTT

Short explanation

All of the above can be measured, allowing clinicians to assess whether drug levels are therapeutic. This is important when the therapeutic index is narrow, such as in the case of digoxin. It is also important for patients receiving immunosuppression following organ transplantation, for those with poorly controlled epilepsy, and for those with difficult-to-treat arrhythmias.

Long explanation

Plasma levels of most therapeutic drugs can be measured using laboratory assays, but many of these are used only for research purposes during drug development and are not routinely available for clinical use. For some agents, however, given the nature of their pharmacokinetics or pharmacodynamics, it is important that drug assays are routinely available. These drugs fall into a number of categories.

Firstly, drugs with a narrow therapeutic range and the potential for toxicity require monitoring. A narrow therapeutic range means that the therapeutic and toxic doses are close together. Hence, if distribution, metabolism and/or elimination is altered in any way then plasma levels may easily become subtherapeutic or toxic. Examples of such drugs include phenytoin, digoxin and lithium.

Another category includes drugs where the therapeutic plasma level is very important to achieve. This is the case for immunosuppressant medication such as tacrolimus, where inadequate dosing can have catastrophic consequences in transplant patients. Epilepsy medication, particularly for patients on multi-drug therapy and those with poorly controlled seizures, is another example where dosing can be altered depending on plasma levels. Monitoring can also be performed in these patients to check compliance. Dosing is often guided by plasma levels in drugs such as aminoglycosides, to avoid toxic effects such as renal failure and ototoxicity.

Ghiculescu R. Therapeutic drug monitoring: which drugs, why, when and how to do it. *Aust Prescr* 2008; 31: 42–4.

Question A33: Pulmonary function tests

Which of these statements about pulmonary function tests are correct?

A. FEV_1 is normal or increased in restrictive lung disease
B. Gas transfer of CO measures V/Q matching
C. PEFR monitoring can be used to predict exacerbations of asthma
D. Spirometry gives values for FEV_1, FVC, FRC and tidal volume
E. FEV_1/FVC ratio of $< 70\%$ is consistent with an obstructive lung disease

Answer: FTTFT

Short explanation

Spirometry gives values for all dynamic lung volumes (V_T, FVC, IRV etc.) but cannot measure residual volume (and hence FRC). FEV_1/FVC ratio is $< 70\%$ in COPD and normal or raised in restrictive lung disease (FEV_1 and FVC are both reduced). Daily PEFR measurements can give an early warning of asthma exacerbation and allow pre-emptive treatment. Gas transfer in normal lungs is a measure of diffusing capacity, but becomes a measure of V/Q mismatch in lung pathology.

Long explanation

Pulmonary function tests cover a variety of measures of ventilation, volume, diffusion and function, from simple bedside tests to complex or invasive investigations.

Ventilatory function

Peak expiratory flow rate (PEFR) can be assessed by a simple bedside test. A forced expiration from total lung capacity into a variable-orifice flowmeter gives a reproducible reading related to airflow limitation. It is used in asthma as daily monitoring to pre-empt exacerbations, or as part of risk stratification in asthma exacerbations.

Spirometry involves a forced expiration from total lung capacity to residual volume into a spirometer containing bellows. Important spirometry values are the forced vital capacity (FVC), the total volume of gas exhaled, and the forced expiratory volume (FEV_1: the volume expired in the first second). The ratio (FEV_1/FVC) is also used in diagnosis. Obstructive lung diseases (asthma, COPD) have low FEV_1 and low FEV_1/FVC ratios (< 70% for diagnosis of COPD). FVC may be increased (asthma), normal or reduced (COPD). Restrictive lung diseases (pulmonary fibrosis) have reduced FVC and FEV_1, in similar proportions, giving normal or high FEV_1/FVC ratios.

Volumes

Spirometry can give values for tidal volume (V_T), FVC and inspiratory and expiratory reserve volumes (IRV, ERV), but not for residual volume (RV), functional residual capacity (FRC) or total lung capacity (TLC). For these, helium dilution tests or body plethysmography are required.

Diffusion

Gas transfer is a measure or diffusion capacity of the lung. A small concentration of carbon monoxide (CO) is inhaled from residual volume to total lung capacity, held, and then expired into an analyser. The difference in CO concentrations and the PaCO can be used to calculate the diffusion capacity (DL_{CO}). The transfer coefficient (K_{CO}) also controls for lung volume. Any V/Q mismatch will affect these measures as much as alveolar disease.

Functional tests

Arterial blood gas testing, oxygen saturations, exercise tests and cardiopulmonary exercise tests (CPEX) are also tests of respiratory function, with important results, but they are not classed as pulmonary function tests

Kumar P, Clark ML. *Clinical Medicine*, 8th edn. Edinburgh: Saunders Elsevier, 2012.

Question A34: Smoke inhalation

With regards to smoke inhalation, which of the following are correct?

A. Early bronchoscopy and washout can be helpful
B. Upper airway swelling occurs rapidly, and intubation should be performed pre-hospital
C. Cut endotracheal tubes are preferred
D. Hoarseness is a common sign and does not signify airway compromise
E. Burns to the face, lips and eyebrows are a worrying sign

Answer: TFFFT

Short explanation

Upper airway swelling occurs over a few hours following the burn. Intubation may be required, but usually there is time to assess the patient and prepare a full anaesthetic team. Uncut endotracheal tubes are recommended, to account for subsequent facial swelling. Hoarseness is a worrying sign.

Long explanation

The management of the airway in patients with airway burns or inhalational injury is very important. The clinical history can identify those patients at risk of airway compromise. Patients involved in house fires or other fires in enclosed spaces are at particularly high risk of having inhaled hot, toxic gases. Inhalational injuries are rare in patients who have sustained flash burns. Upper airway thermal injury (above the larynx) can lead to extensive epiglottic and pharyngeal swelling. By the time the heat has reached the larynx it has usually cooled enough to prevent direct injury to the larynx. Stridor, change in voice and a swollen uvula are worrying signs.

Airway injury below the larynx is usually due to sloughing of the epithelium caused by inhalation of products of combustion. Patients may be breathless, have a cough or be wheezing. Bronchial lavage with 1.4% bicarbonate will often reveal carbonaceous deposits and can help neutralise acids and remove soot. It is important to remember the risk of carbon monoxide and cyanide poisoning in patients with inhalational injury. Standard pulse oximetry will not detect carboxyhaemoglobin, and co-oximetry should be performed to check levels. 100% oxygen should be administered to all patients with inhalational injury to reduce carboxyhaemoglobin levels.

Intubation should be considered but does not usually need to be performed immediately following the injury. Swelling occurs over many hours and so there is usually time for full assessment and preparation unless the patient is in extremis or presents late. An experienced anaesthetist or intensive care physician should be present, and alternative methods for securing the airway should be considered in case of failure to place an endotracheal tube. Equipment for front-of-neck access should be readily available, and staff must be familiar with it before embarking on intubation. Suxamethonium is safe to use in the first 24 hours following the burn. Thereafter life-threatening hyperkalaemia can occur and alternative agents should be used.

Bishop S, Maguire S. Anaesthesia and intensive care for major burns. *Contin Educ Anaesth Crit Care Pain* 2012; 12: 118–22.

Question A35: Cardiac output monitoring

Regarding the monitoring of cardiac output (CO):

A. Thermodilution with a pulmonary artery (PA) catheter is the gold standard
B. Pulse contour analysis (PCA) requires calibration with indicator studies
C. CO monitors use the Fick principle to calculate CO
D. The ability to accurately measure CO is more important than tracking changes
E. Fluid responsiveness is reflected by an observed increase in stroke volume (SV) after a fluid bolus

Answer: TFFFT

Short explanation

PA catheter thermodilution is the gold standard for assessing performance of other CO monitors. Some PCA systems are uncalibrated or use demographic and physical data. Most CO monitors do not use the Fick principle. Tracking changes, especially increases in SV after fluid boluses (fluid responsiveness), is more clinically useful than measurement of absolute values.

Long explanation

The measurement of cardiac output (CO) is becoming increasingly important in critical care with the focus on goal-directed therapy and demonstrations that inappropriate fluid therapy adversely affects outcomes. Identification of patients who increase their stroke volume in response to a fluid challenge (fluid responsiveness) has become a goal, and many CO monitors are now in existence to enable this. The absolute values of CO or stroke volume (SV) are less important than the change in these values over time and with fluid challenges.

The first method of estimating CO was described by Adolph Fick in 1870. The Fick principle states that the total amount of a substance produced or taken up by the body is equal to CO multiplied by the arteriovenous concentration difference. If the amount of substance and the arterial and venous concentrations are known, then CO can be calculated. Using pulmonary artery and peripheral arterial oxygen measurements, and assuming a value of oxygen consumption of 125 ml/min/m^2 body surface area (BSA), CO may be estimated. The Fick principle is also used by the non-invasive cardiac output (NICO) monitor, which compares CO_2 measured during normal ventilation and during periods of partial CO_2 rebreathing.

Indicator dilution methods are used by many CO monitors: cold saline (thermodilution) by PA catheters and pulse contour cardiac output (PiCCO) monitors, and lithium ions by lithium dilution cardiac output (LiDCO) monitors. CO is calculated by dividing the total amount of indicator by the integral of the concentration of indicator at a point downstream over time. Thermodilution by PA catheter is used as the gold standard in studies comparing methods of CO measurement.

Pulse contour analysis monitors analyse the arterial pressure waveform and calculate a value for SV (and hence CO) using measured, derived or calculated values for blood pressure, arterial compliance and systemic vascular resistance (SVR). Some monitors are calibrated with indicator dilution methods (PiCCO, LiDCO), others use demographic and physical data to estimate arterial compliance and SVR (FloTrac), and a third group uses the waveform alone (PRAM).

Other methods of CO estimation use oesophageal Doppler, transthoracic ultrasound, thoracic bioimpedance and bioreactance technology.

Marik PE. Noninvasive cardiac output monitors: a state-of-the-art review. *J Cardiothorac Vasc Anaesth* 2013; 27: 121–34.

Question A36: Mast-cell tryptase in anaphylaxis

With respect to mast-cell tryptase sampling after anaphylaxis:

A. A-tryptase is measured to ascertain if a reaction is anaphylaxis
B. The volume of intravenous resuscitation fluid should be taken into account
C. The assay has a high sensitivity
D. Samples taken more than 12 hours post mortem are unreliable
E. Tryptase levels are likely to be raised by myocardial infarction

Answer: FTFFT

Short explanation

B-tryptase is released in anaphylaxis. The assay measures both A- and B-tryptase and has a relatively low sensitivity. Post-mortem samples are reliable, as tryptase is no longer broken down after death.

Long explanation

Anaphylaxis is a severe, life-threatening, generalised or systemic hypersensitivity reaction. It may be classified into allergic anaphylaxis and non-allergic anaphylaxis – previously called 'anaphylactoid'. Allergic anaphylaxis occurs when exposure to a foreign antigen stimulates production of IgE antibodies that bind to mast cells and basophils. After further exposure to the antigen IgE cross-linking results in mast-cell degranulation and release of histamine, slow-reacting substance A, leukotrienes, tryptase and prostaglandins. The clinical features may be identical in allergic and non-allergic anaphylaxis, but in the latter IgE is not part of the pathological process.

Tryptase is a protease enzyme that has two subtypes: A and B. B-tryptase is stored in granules in mast cells and is released during anaphylaxis. A-tryptase is secreted by mast cells continuously in healthy people. A rise in serum tryptase indicates mast-cell degranulation but does not discriminate between allergic and non-allergic anaphylaxis. It is thought that the rise may be less marked in non-allergic anaphylaxis. During anaphylaxis, tryptase peaks at approximately 1 hour, and its half-life in the circulation is about 2 hours. Anaphylaxis caused by basophil or complement activation will not cause a rise in mast-cell tryptase. Samples should be taken as soon as treatment priorities allow, 1–2 hours post-reaction and at 24 hours for a baseline.

The assay for tryptase measures the sum of A- and B-tryptase and has a high specificity but low sensitivity, resulting in a relatively high number of falsely negative results. Because there is a wide variation in the baseline plasma concentration of tryptase, the change in concentration is more useful than the absolute concentration. Intravenous fluid replacement dilutes the blood and therefore the tryptase concentration. This should be taken into account.

After death, tryptase is no longer removed from the circulation so post-mortem samples are valid, although they have a lower predictive value than a sample taken during life. B-tryptase may be raised in trauma or myocardial infarction.

Association of Anaesthetists of Great Britian and Ireland. *AAGBI Safety Guideline: Suspected Anaphylactic Reactions Associated with Anaesthesia*. London: AAGBI, 2009.

Ryder SA, Waldmann C. Anaphylaxis. *Contin Educ Anaesth Crit Care Pain* 2004; 4: 111–13.

Sim K, Webster N. Anaphylaxis. In Waldmann C, Soni N, Rhodes A. *Oxford Desk Reference: Critical Care*. Oxford: Oxford University Press, 2008; pp. 456–7.

Question A37: Lumbar puncture

Regarding lumbar puncture (LP):

A. Blood-stained CSF is not diagnostic of subarachnoid haemorrhage (SAH)
B. Post-dural puncture headache (PDPH) is prevented by the use of a 25G pencil-point needle
C. Absolute contraindications include coagulopathy, patient refusal and local infection
D. LP should not be performed in patients with raised intracranial pressure
E. LP can be performed at any lumbar level

Answer: TFFFF

Short explanation

Blood in the CSF may be from local bleeding. Xanthochromia is highly suggestive of SAH. LP should be performed as low as possible (L4/5 or L5/S1), below the end of the spinal cord. Refusal and local infection are absolute contraindications; coagulopathy and raised ICP are relative contraindications, but extreme caution should be exercised in both circumstances. LP may be used to drain CSF in some cases of raised intracranial pressure. The size and shape of the needle has no effect on the incidence of PDPH.

Long explanation

Lumbar puncture is a procedure for removing cerebrospinal fluid (CSF) for therapeutic or diagnostic purposes. Indications for LP include:

- Diagnosis of meningitis and encephalitis
- Diagnosis of subarachnoid haemorrhage (xanthochromia)
- Diagnosis of multiple sclerosis, sarcoidosis, Guillain–Barré syndrome and other conditions
- Measurement of CSF pressure
- Therapeutic drainage of CSF (e.g. benign intracranial hypertension)
- Intrathecal injection (spinal anaesthesia, cytotoxic drugs, contrast)

Absolute contraindications are limited to patient refusal and local infection. Relative contraindications include raised intracranial pressure (ICP), sepsis, coagulopathy and congenital abnormalities (e.g. meningocoel). Extreme caution should be exercised for LP in the presence of raised ICP. Release of CSF pressure in the spine can lead to herniation of posterior fossa structures through the foramen magnum ('coning'), which leads to brainstem compression and death. However, raised ICP is a relative contraindication, as therapeutic drainage of CSF is performed in many cases (e.g. benign intracranial hypertension). Expert assistance should be sought. It is now routine to wait for results of CT brain before performing LP, in order to exclude raised ICP, but this should not lead to unacceptable delays in treatment for bacterial meningitis.

The procedure is performed under strict aseptic conditions. Patients are commonly placed in the lateral decubitus position with maximal head, neck, hip and knee flexion to reduce lumbar lordosis, but LP may be performed on the sitting patient (although CSF pressure measurement will be impaired). The needle should pass along the midline from the skin, between spinous processes of the lower lumbar vertebrae, through the ligamentum flavum, dura mater and arachnoid to enter the subarachnoid space. A paramedian approach is preferred by some clinicians and may be of benefit if midline LP is not possible for anatomical or other reasons. The level chosen for LP should be below the end of the spinal cord. This is usually around L2 in adults, but is lower in children and in the presence of spinal cord tethering. The L4/5 interspace is commonly chosen for this reason.

Complications include haemorrhage (including spinal or epidural haematoma), infection (cellulitis, meningitis, epidural or spinal abscess), post-dural puncture headache (PDPH), neurological damage (temporary and permanent) and cerebral herniation. PDPH can occur with any size or shape of needle.

Johnson KS, Sexton DJ. Lumbar puncture: technique, indications, contraindications, and complications in adults. *UpToDate* 2013. http://www.uptodate.com (accessed June 2014).

Kumar P, Clark ML. *Clinical Medicine*, 8th edn. Edinburgh: Saunders Elsevier, 2012.

Question A38: Antibiotic resistance

Regarding antibiotic resistance:

A. Free bacterial DNA is commonly found in the blood of intensive care patients
B. Genetic mutation is the most common mechanism of acquisition of resistance

C. Plasmids move independently of bacteria to spread resistance
D. Intrinsic resistance occurs as a result of genetic mutation
E. Transposons may insert DNA into either the bacterial chromosome or a plasmid to confer resistance

Answer: TFFFT

Short explanation

Intrinsic resistance refers to the inherent lack of activity of an antibiotic beyond its spectrum of activity. Intercell transfer of genetic material is the most common mechanism of acquisition of resistance. Plasmids cannot move independently of bacteria

Long explanation

Antibiotic resistance is when an organism will not be inhibited or killed by an antibacterial agent at concentrations of the drug achievable in the body after a normal dose. Antibiotic resistance may be intrinsic (natural) or acquired. Intrinsic resistance refers to the inherent lack of activity of an antibiotic beyond its spectrum of activity. Acquired resistance is when organisms previously sensitive to an antibiotic become resistant.

There are two mechanisms that allow a bacterium to become resistant: mutation and intercell transfer. Mutation occasionally confers resistance but in general has negative consequences for the bacterium. Intercell transfer is more important in the process of spreading resistance. Intercell transfer of genetic material may occur in four ways:

- Naked or free DNA released from bacteria killed by antibiotics may be taken up from the bloodstream and incorporated into the genetic makeup of another bacterium.
- Bacteriophage transduction: a viral vector transports the genetic material into the bacterium, where it is incorporated.
- Plasmid conjugation: plasmids are self-replicating circles of DNA that cannot move independently of the bacterium but may be transferred from one bacterium to another. They are the most common route of transmission of genetic information in bacteria seen in critical care.
- Transposons: small segments of DNA may move between plasmids or within the main chromosome of the bacterium.

Varley AJ, Williams H, Fletcher S. Antibiotic resistance in the intensive care unit. *Contin Educ Anaesth Crit Care Pain* 2009; 9: 114–18.

Waldmann C, Soni N, Rhodes A. *Oxford Desk Reference: Critical Care.* Oxford: Oxford University Press, 2008; pp. 228–9.

Question A39: Stress hyperglycaemia

The following physiological changes contribute to stress hyperglycaemia:

A. Increased cortisol levels
B. Reduced corticotrophin-releasing hormone (CRH) levels
C. Insulin resistance

D. Increased glycogenesis
E. Increased norepinephrine levels

Answer: TFTFT

Short explanation

Physiological stress activates the HPA axis and sympathetic nervous system. Increased CRH, ACTH and cortisol are seen, along with greatly increased levels of circulating catecholamines. These act to increase glycogenolysis, gluconeogenesis and insulin resistance, leading to increased glucose levels. This is an adaptive mechanism known as stress hyperglycaemia.

Long explanation

Stress hyperglycaemia is a term used to describe hyperglycaemia and insulin resistance in critical illness, including surgical insults and trauma. The degree of hyperglycaemia is related to the severity of insult to the body and is correlated with severity of illness or injury scores and type of surgery. Perhaps unsurprisingly, the degree of stress hyperglycaemia is also related to outcomes such as mortality, morbidity and length of stay.

Critical illness and stressors such as shock, sepsis, trauma and surgery lead to activation of the hypothalamus–pituitary–adrenal (HPA) axis and the sympathetic adrenal system. Increased corticotrophin-releasing hormone (CRH) release from the hypothalamus leads to increased adrenocorticotrophic hormone (ACTH) from the anterior pituitary and activation of the immune system. ACTH then stimulates cortisol release from the adrenal cortex. Activation of the locus coeruleus leads to increased epinephrine release from the adrenal medulla and norepinephrine release from sympathetic nerves.

Cortisol, epinephrine and norepinephrine activate gluconeogenesis, glycogenolysis and insulin resistance, which leads to hyperglycaemia. Stress hyperglycaemia is thought to be an adaptive response, freeing up fuel for the fight-or-flight response. In critical illness, mild stress hyperglycaemia may be protective, but excessive or prolonged stress responses become maladaptive and harmful. This may be reflected in the fact that tight glycaemic control (e.g. between 4 and 7 mmol/l) has been found to increase mortality (e.g. the NICE-SUGAR trial), while looser glycaemic control is widely recommended (e.g. in sepsis, stroke, myocardial infarction, trauma, head injury etc.).

Marik PE, Bellomo R. Stress hyperglycemia: an essential survival response! *Crit Care Med* 2013; 41: e93–94.

Question A40: Prognosis after out-of-hospital cardiac arrest

Following return of spontaneous circulation (ROSC) from out-of-hospital cardiac arrest (OHCA), the following are useful indicators of neurological outcome:

A. Fixed dilated pupils on admission
B. Isoelectric EEG
C. Post-arrest myoclonic status epilepticus
D. Absent somatosensory evoked potentials (SSEPs)
E. Loss of grey–white distinction on CT brain

Answer: FTTTF

Short explanation
Prognostication based on clinical condition at presentation or imaging after OHCA has too high a false-negative rate to be of use. Electrophysiological studies are diagnostic but require time, skill and expert interpretation. Myoclonus is a good marker, but easily mistaken for intentional myoclonus, which indicates preserved consciousness.

Long explanation
Prognostication for the OHCA victim could be of value to reduce unnecessary ICU admission with less distress for relatives, invasive procedures and expense. Any such test or scoring system should have as low a false-positive rate as possible. The circumstances of the OHCA and findings at admission (e.g. fixed dilated pupils, GCS of 3, prolonged no-flow time) have a poor predictive value, and scoring systems based on such findings and premorbid history (PAR score, OHCA score) should not be used to inform admission or treatment decisions.

Post-arrest myoclonic status is a reliable marker of hopeless neurological prognosis, but is difficult to accurately diagnose, as it is easily mistaken for Lance–Adams syndrome (intentional myoclonus, indicating preserved consciousness), which carries a good neurological prognosis.

Tests with a 0% false-positive rate include an isoelectic EEG in the first week after cardiac arrest and absent somatosensory evoked potentials (SSEPs). Both tests require expertise to perform and interpret and therefore may be of limited use. CT brain findings are not reliably associated with neurological prognosis

Temple A, Porter R. Predicting neurological outcome and survival after cardiac arrest. *Contin Educ Anaesth Crit Care Pain* 2012; 6: 283–7.

Question A41: Acute pulmonary oedema

Appropriate immediate management of acute cardiogenic pulmonary oedema includes:

A. Intravenous opiates
B. Norepinephrine
C. Haemofiltration
D. ACE inhibitors
E. Intra-aortic balloon pump (IABP)

Answer: TTTFT

Short explanation
Diamorphine and morphine cause venodilatation and relieve distress. Norepinephrine may be appropriate in cardiogenic shock once inotropes have been started. Haemofiltration can rapidly remove excess fluid. ACE inhibitors are important in treating heart failure, but should only be started once the patient is stable. IABPs may be used as a bridge to recovery or surgical therapy in reversible acute heart failure.

Long explanation
Acute pulmonary oedema is a life-threatening emergency. Pulmonary oedema may be cardiogenic or non-cardiogenic. Distinguishing between the two may be difficult, and relies on history, examination, investigations and monitoring the response to treatments. The commonest causes of acute cardiogenic pulmonary oedema include myocardial infarction, arrhythmias, cardiac structural lesions and

myocarditis. Assessment and initial management should be simultaneous, with particular focus on oxygenation, arrhythmias, shock, ischaemia and acute structural lesions. Invasive monitoring, including arterial blood pressure, central venous pressure and cardiac output monitoring should be considered.

The first line of treatment should be an intravenous bolus of a loop diuretic such as furosemide, at a dose of 50 mg or 2.5 times the patient's regular oral dose. A venodilator effect causes relief of symptoms prior to the diuretic effect. Hypoxic patients should be given oxygen therapy titrated to saturation levels. Patients with significant distress or anxiety may be treated with morphine or diamorphine, which not only reduce distress but are thought to cause venodilatation.

Shocked patients or those with systolic BP < 85 mmHg should be started on an inotropic drug, such as dobutamine. In patients taking β-blockers, levosimendan or phosphodiesterase inhibitors may be appropriate. Hypertensive patients may be started on a vasodilator such as glyceryl trinitrate.

Persistent hypoxia may be treated initially with non-invasive ventilation or continuous positive airway pressure (CPAP), although intubation and ventilation is often required. Inadequate diuresis (< 100 ml) may be treated with increased doses of loop diuretic, addition of a secondary diuretic (aldosterone antagonists, thiazides), haemodialysis or haemofiltration.

Persistent shock or hypotension despite inotropes may require the addition of a vasoconstrictor (e.g. norepinephrine) or mechanical circulatory support (IABP or left ventricular assist device (LVAD)). Mechanical devices should be restricted to reversible causes of cardiogenic shock, including structural lesions, myocarditis and ischaemic disease around the time of revascularisation.

An underlying cause to the development of acute pulmonary oedema should be sought and treated as a matter of urgency. This may include cardiac catheterisation, valvular surgery, antibiotics, pacing or cardioversion.

McMurray JJV, Adamopoulos S, Anker SD, *et al.* ESC guidelines for the diagnosis and treatment of acute and chronic heart failure 2012. The Task Force for the Diagnosis and Treatment of Acute and Chronic Heart Failure 2012 of the European Society of Cardiology. *Eur Heart J* 2012; 33: 1787–847.

Question A42: Hypokalaemia

The following ECG changes are characteristic of hypokalaemia:

A. Bradycardia more commonly than tachycardia
B. Delta waves
C. T-wave inversion
D. ST depression
E. U waves

Answer: FFTTT

Short explanation

Delta waves are a slurred upstroke in the QRS complex seen in patients with Wolff–Parkinson–White syndrome. Bradycardia is sometimes seen in hypokalaemia, but tachycardia is more characteristic.

Long explanation

Hypokalaemia is defined as a serum potassium of < 3.5 mmol/l, and it may be caused by inadequate intake, excessive loss, or intracellular shift of potassium. Clinical features are rare until the potassium is very low, and are non-specific with generalised weakness, nausea and vomiting, and constipation. Cardiac arrhythmias may be fatal and unpredictable. Patients are more at risk from adverse sequelae of hypokalaemia if they have underlying heart disease or are taking digoxin.

ECG changes include a predisposition to tachycardia (although bradycardia may also occur), U waves, ST depression and T-wave inversion. U waves occur after the T wave and are often seen in the precordial leads V4–6. The QT interval may also be prolonged.

Treatment of hypokalaemia includes management of the underlying cause and potassium replacement. This may be by enteral or parenteral routes, with intravenous replacement preferred in the emergency setting. The rate of replacement should not generally exceed 20 mmol/hour, because of the risk of precipitating ventricular fibrillation. Hypomagnesaemia should be treated, as it may cause refractory hypokalaemia. Chronic hypokalaemia may be managed with potassium-sparing diuretics.

O'Neil P, Webster N. Electrolyte disorders. In Waldmann C, Soni N, Rhodes A. *Oxford Desk Reference: Critical Care*. Oxford: Oxford University Press, 2008; pp. 410–11.

Question A43: Antifungal agents

With respect to antifungal agents used in critical care:

A. Echinocandins have the best side-effect profile of the antifungal agents
B. Fluconazole should be first line for invasive aspergillosis
C. Amphotericin B is fungistatic
D. Oral fluconazole is 100% bioavailable
E. Amphotericin B exhibits dose-limiting nephrotoxicity

Answer: TFFTT

Short explanation

Fluconazole is not effective against *Aspergillus*, and amphotericin B is fungicidal.

Long explanation

There are three main groups of systemic antifungal treatment used in intensive care:

1. Polyenes, e.g. amphotericin B

Polyenes bind ergosterol in the fungal cell wall, resulting in cell death. They have a broad spectrum of activity against most fungi. Amphotericin B exhibits dose-limiting nephrotoxicity, which is usually reversible and should be monitored with blood tests. Infusions may cause fever, chills and rigors ameliorated by the use of antihistamines and paracetamol.

2. Azoles, e.g. fluconazole, itraconazole and voriconazole

Azoles act by inhibiting ergosterol synthesis and therefore disrupting the fungal cell wall. Fluconazole is active against most *Candida* species but is not effective against *Aspergillus*. Oral fluconazole is 100% bioavailable. Itraconazole has a broader spectrum of activity against yeasts and is active against *Aspergillus*. Voriconazole is active against all *Candida* species and is the first-line treatment for invasive aspergillosis.

3. Echinocandins, e.g. caspofungin, anidulafungin
Echinocandins inhibit fungal cell-wall synthesis. They are fungicidal against *Candida* and fungistatic against *Aspergillus*. They may be used synergistically with polyenes and azoles. They are only available in intravenous formulations, because of low oral bioavailability, but they exhibit good side-effect tolerability and few drug interactions.

Bellman R. Clinical pharmacokinetics of systemically administered antimycotics. *Curr Clin Pharmacol* 2007; 2: 37–58.
Iyer S. Antifungals. In Waldmann C, Soni N, Rhodes A. *Oxford Desk Reference: Critical Care*. Oxford: Oxford University Press, 2008; pp. 230–1.

Question A44: Core temperature measurement

The following sites allow accurate measures of core temperature:

A. Tympanic membrane
B. Nasopharynx
C. Bladder
D. Groin
E. Forehead

Answer: TTTFT

Short explanation

Core temperature monitoring is key to the safe practice of therapeutic hypothermia. The gold-standard measure of core temperature is of blood by a pulmonary artery (PA) catheter. Good correlation with the gold standard is seen with measures from the oesophagus, bladder, rectum, nasopharynx and infrared measures of forehead and tympanic membrane. Peripheral monitoring has poor correlation with core temperature.

Long explanation

Therapeutic hypothermia is in widespread use for the management of patients following cardiac arrest and is advocated in other conditions such as traumatic brain injury, stroke and hepatic failure. Safe practice of therapeutic hypothermia relies on the accurate measurement of core temperature. The gold standard for core temperature measurement is blood by a pulmonary artery (PA) catheter.

Thermistor-based temperature probes may be used to estimate core temperature. Common sites that have been found to correlate well with the gold standard of temperature measurement are the rectum, urinary bladder and nasopharynx, although the latter may be cooled by inspiratory gases if not placed accurately.

Infrared thermometers are also well correlated with core temperature. Common sites of use of infrared thermometers are the tympanic membrane and forehead, sites which are thought to be more indicative of brain temperature.

Peripheral sites do not accurately correlate with core temperature and should not be used to guide therapeutic hypothermia.

Polderman KH, Herold I. Therapeutic hypothermia and controlled normothermia in the intensive care unit: practical considerations, side effects, and cooling methods. *Crit Care Med* 2009; 37: 1101–20.

Question A45: Chronic obstructive pulmonary disease

Chronic obstructive pulmonary disease (COPD):

A. Is classified for severity on the basis of forced expiratory volume in 1 second (FEV_1) measurements
B. Requiring ICU admission confers a 50% 1-year mortality
C. Is responsible for approximately 40% of patients admitted in type 2 respiratory failure
D. Treated with long-term oxygen therapy has improved mortality
E. Should be treated with non-invasive ventilation as a first-line therapy for $PaCO_2 > 6$ kPa

Answer: TTFTF

Short explanation

COPD is responsible for approximately 10% of patients admitted in type 2 respiratory failure. The indications for non-invasive ventilation for an acute exacerbation are $PaCO_2 > 6$ kPa and pH < 7.35.

Long explanation

Chronic obstructive pulmonary disease (COPD) is characterised by progressive, minimally reversible and chronic airflow obstruction. It is predominantly caused by smoking. Severity is defined on the basis of forced expiratory volume in 1 second (FEV_1) measurements, and divided into mild, moderate and severe.

Concern is often raised over patients receiving high-flow, uncontrolled oxygen, because of the risk of type 2 respiratory failure from a loss of hypoxic ventilatory drive. COPD is responsible for only 10% of patients admitted with type 2 respiratory failure, but it is good practice to ensure that all patients receive appropriate oxygen therapy to avoid hyperoxia.

Management of an acute exacerbation of COPD centres on:

- treatment of the underlying cause (e.g. antibiotics for a bacterial infection)
- reducing bronchospasm and inflammation (bronchodilators and steroids)
- reducing the work of breathing (non-invasive ventilation (NIV))
- supportive care (controlled oxygen, nutrition)

Not all patients with COPD will be appropriate for admission to ICU. However, NIV has been shown to reduce mortality, reduce the need for intubation and speed up recovery in patients admitted with acute hypercapnic respiratory failure. The indications for NIV for an acute exacerbation are $PaCO_2 > 6$ kPa *and* pH < 7.35 when medical management has failed. For patients admitted to hospital requiring NIV or ICU admission, the 1-year mortality is approximately 50%.

Long-term oxygen therapy is indicated for patients with a resting PaO_2 of < 7.3 kPa when they do not have an acute exacerbation. If used for > 15 hours a day it has been shown to reduce mortality.

Lumb AL, Biercamp C. Chronic obstructive pulmonary disease and anaesthesia. *Contin Educ Anaesth Crit Care Pain* 2014; 14: 1–5.

National Clinical Guideline Centre. *Chronic Obstructive Pulmonary Disease: Management of Chronic Obstructive Pulmonary Disease in Adults in Primary and Secondary Care*. London: National Clinical Guideline Centre, 2010. http://guidance.nice.org.uk/CG101/Guidance/pdf/English (accessed June 2014).

Waldmann C, Soni N, Rhodes A. *Oxford Desk Reference: Critical Care*. Oxford: Oxford University Press, 2008; pp. 254–5.

Question A46: Burns

Regarding the differences between partial- and full-thickness burns, which of the following are correct?

A. Partial-thickness burns are usually painless
B. Full-thickness burns are usually more extensive than partial-thickness burns
C. Full-thickness burns can include loss of hair follicles and nerve endings
D. A white and rubbery appearance indicates a full-thickness burn
E. Partial-thickness burns often require escharotomy

Answer: FFTTF

Short explanation

Partial-thickness burns are often very painful due to preservation of nerve fibres and endings. The extent of the burn area is not usually related to whether it is partial- or full-thickness. In large burns there is often a mixture of partial- and full-thickness burn. Partial-thickness burns occasionally require escharotomy.

Long explanation

Burns can be classified into superficial, partial- and full-thickness. First-degree or superficial burns often present as an area of painful erythema. There are no blisters and the burn consists of damage to the epithelium only. It is similar to sunburn. This type of burn would be expected to heal within a week and does not usually require surgical intervention. If the burnt area is large, fluid resuscitation will be required.

Second-degree burns are also classed as partial-thickness. These involve damage to the entire epidermal layer and part of the underlying dermis. Blisters will be present in addition to painful areas of erythema. There is often extensive swelling. Healing takes between 10 and 21 days, and surgical intervention may be required. Infection is a risk in these burns. In less deep partial-thickness burns there is severe pain. In deeper partial-thickness burns sensation can be impaired to a variable degree.

Third-degree or full-thickness burns lead to destruction of all epidermal and dermal elements. The burn extends into subcutaneous fat or deeper and can involve muscle and bone. The skin can appear white and leathery. These burns are generally not painful, although areas surrounding the deep burn are often partial-thickness and hence very painful.

An escharotomy involves surgical excision of the eschar (the burn) and superficial fascia in order to permit the cut edges to separate and restore blood flow to unburned tissue distal to the eschar. This is sometimes performed in circumferential burns to permit ventilation, or in compartment syndrome to permit perfusion.

Alharbi Z, Piatkowski A, Dembinski R, *et al.* Treatment of burns in the first 24 hours: simple and practical guide by answering 10 questions in a step-by-step form. *World J Emerg Surg* 2012; 7: 13.

Question A47: Extracorporeal membrane oxygenation

When planning extracorporeal membrane oxygenation (ECMO) treatment:

A. Patients with cardiorespiratory failure are suitable for venovenous ECMO
B. Patients should have a reversible cause or be on a transplant list

C. Venoarterial ECMO can be used as a bridging device prior to insertion of a ventricular assist device
D. Arteriovenous ECMO is useful to increase blood oxygenation
E. Carbon dioxide clearance is more efficient than oxygenation

Answer: FTTFT

Short explanation

Venoarterial ECMO is used for cardiorespiratory support, venovenous ECMO for respiratory support, and arteriovenous ECMO for carbon dioxide clearance.

Long explanation

Extracorporeal membrane oxygenation (ECMO) is becoming increasingly recognised for the treatment of patients with cardiorespiratory failure. ECMO allows gas exchange outside the body and originated with technology used in cardiopulmonary bypass machines. Its use in neonates and children with reversible respiratory failure is well documented, but its use in adults has been limited until recently.

ECMO circuits can be set up in three ways:

(1) Venoarterial ECMO (VA-ECMO): cannula in inferior vena cava or right atrium leads to oxygenator and pump; blood is returned to the aorta or femoral artery. As the heart and lungs can be completely bypassed, this is generally used in patients who require both cardiac and respiratory support, and can be used directly after cardiopulmonary bypass as the cannula positions are similar.
(2) Venovenous ECMO (VV-ECMO): cannula from femoral vein to oxygenator and pump, blood returned to internal jugular or femoral vein. This can be used for any potentially reversible cause of acute respiratory failure but does not reduce myocardial workload or oxygen consumption.
(3) Arteriovenous ECMO (AV-ECMO): uses the patient's own cardiac output to drive circuit, with no pump. This is used solely for carbon dioxide removal.

ECMO is most efficient for carbon dioxide removal, because of the increased solubility and better diffusion properties of carbon dioxide compared to oxygen.

Any patient considered for ECMO should have a reversible cause for his or her condition; established multi-organ failure is a contraindication. With cardiac conditions it may be used as a bridging tool until a ventricular assist device or cardiac transplantation can take place. The greatest success has been seen in young patients with H1N1 viral pneumonia, as they have few comorbidities and a reversible cause for respiratory failure.

Hung M, Vuylsteke A, Valchanov K. Extracorporeal membrane oxygenation: coming to an ICU near you. *J Intensive Care Soc* 2012; 13: 31–7.

Martinez G, Vuylsteke A. Extracorporeal membrane oxygenation in adults. *Contin Educ Anaesth Crit Care Pain* 2012; 12: 57–61.

Peek GJ, Mugford M, Tiruvoipati R, *et al*. Efficacy and economic assessment of conventional ventilator support versus extracorporeal membrane oxygenation for severe adult respiratory failure (CESAR): a multicentre randomised controlled trial. *Lancet* 2009; 374: 1351–63.

Question A48: Delayed cerebral ischaemia

Regarding delayed cerebral ischaemia (DCI) following subarachnoid haemorrhage (SAH):

A. DCI may be effectively prevented with oral nimodipine

B. Digital subtraction angiography (DSA) is the best investigation for vasospasm
C. Maintenance of euvolaemia is as effective as hypervolaemia in treating DCI
D. Haemodilution is only effective in patients with high haematocrits
E. DCI in patients with unsecured aneurysms can still be treated with hypertension

Answer: TTTTT

Short explanation

Nimodipine has strong evidence of benefit in prevention of DCI and should be used in all SAH patients for 21 days. DSA is the gold-standard investigation for vasospasm. Euvolaemia should be the aim rather than hypervolaemia. Haemodilution should not be used except in cases of erythrocytosis. Hypertension with vasopressors and inotropes is effective at reducing DCI and may be used with caution even in patients with unsecured aneurysms.

Long explanation

Delayed cerebral ischaemia (DCI) is a cause of delayed neurological deterioration following subarachnoid haemorrhage (SAH). It overlaps and often co-occurs with vasospasm and is now the major cause of morbidity and mortality following SAH. Breakdown products of haemoglobin are thought to be the causative agent in the development of vasospasm and DCI. All patients should be closely monitored for signs and symptoms of clinical deterioration while receiving preventive agents. Nimodipine reduces the likelihood of DCI and has strong evidence of benefit following SAH. It should be administered for 21 days following SAH.

Investigation of neurological deterioration may start with routine tests and CT imaging of the brain. The gold-standard investigation for vasospasm is digital subtraction angiography, although CT angiography is almost as sensitive. Transcranial Doppler ultrasound is commonly used to assess the extent of vasospasm.

Traditional treatment of DCI is known as 'triple H' therapy: hypervolaemia, hypertension and haemodilution. Of these, the only intervention with evidence of benefit is hypertension. Vasopressors, inotropes or a combination may be used to increase the cerebral perfusion pressure. Stepwise increments with neurological assessment should be employed, to avoid excessive hypertension. In patients with unsecured aneurysms, hypertensive therapy should be attempted with caution following risk–benefit analysis. Haemodilution has not been shown to be effective in isolation and is only recommended in patients with high erythrocyte counts. Likewise, hypervolaemia alone has not been shown to improve outcomes, and so the focus should be on maintaining euvolaemia.

Triple H therapy is not without risks, and not always effective. Other strategies include endovascular approaches, such as balloon angioplasty and intra-arterial vasodilators. The latter is recommended for cases of DCI refractory to standard therapy; the former has little evidence of benefit and is risky, so should be undertaken with caution.

Diringer MN, Bleck TP, Claude Hemphill J, *et al*. Critical care management of patients following aneurysmal subarachnoid hemorrhage: recommendations from the Neurocritical Care Society's Multidisciplinary Consensus Conference. *Neurocrit Care* 2011; 15: 211–40.

Steiner T, Juvela S, Unterberg A, *et al*. European Stroke Organization guidelines for the management of intracranial aneurysms and subarachnoid haemorrhage. *Cerebrovasc Dis* 2013; 35: 93–112.

Question A49: Meropenem

Meropenem:

A. Does not require dose reduction in acute kidney injury
B. Is a β-lactam antibiotic
C. Is contraindicated in patients with a penicillin allergy
D. Is effective against methicillin-resistant *Staphylococcus aureus* (MRSA) infections
E. Is ineffective against extended-spectrum β-lactamase (ESBL) Enterobacteriaceae

Answer: FTFFT

Short explanation

Meropenem requires dose adjustment according the glomerular filtration rate. It should be used with caution in patients with a penicillin allergy. It has good anaerobic cover but is not useful in MRSA infection.

Long explanation

Meropenem is a carbapenem antibacterial agent. It has one of the broadest spectrums of activity of all antibacterials, covering Gram-positive, Gram-negative and anaerobic organisms. It is ineffective against extended-spectrum β-lactamase (ESBL) Enterobacteriaceae because of very high β-lactamase resistance. It is not effective against MRSA or *Enterococcus faecium*, and some strains of *Pseudomonas* are meropenem resistant.

Meropenem is a β-lactam antibiotic, and therefore patients with a penicillin allergy may exhibit cross-sensitivity. This is most likely in patients with immediate hypersensitivity reactions such as anaphylaxis. A patient with a vague history of rash after penicillin should not be excluded from treatment with meropenem where indicated. Meropenem requires dose reduction according to the glomerular filtration rate. The dose should also be reduced in renal replacement therapy, as clearance is reduced.

Peck TE, Hill SA, Williams M. Antimicrobials. In *Pharmacology for Anaesthesia and Intensive Care*, 2nd edn. Cambridge: Cambridge Press, 2006; pp. 311–35.

Thirunavakkarasu S, Lynch G. Antibiotics in critical care: an introduction. *Anaesthesia Tutorial of the Week* 2010; 168. http://www.aagbi.org/sites/default/files/168-Antibiotics-in-Critical-Care-an-introduction.pdf (accessed June 2014).

Question A50: ECG changes

Specific ECG changes are characteristically associated with certain conditions. Which of the following associations are correct?

A. COPD – P mitrale
B. Paracetamol overdose – prolonged QT interval
C. Hypothermia – U waves
D. Hyperchloraemia – widened QRS complex
E. High digoxin levels – concave ST elevation in chest leads

Answer: FFFFF

Short explanation

COPD is associated with P pulmonale, due to cor pulmonale and right ventricular hypertrophy; P mitrale is associated with mitral regurgitation. Paracetamol (acetaminophen) overdose and hyperchloraemia have no characteristic ECG changes.

U waves are found in hypokalaemia; hypothermia is associated with J waves. Digitalis effect is down-sloping ST segments; concave ST elevation in chest leads is associated with pericarditis.

Long explanation

Many conditions have characteristic ECG changes, which may aid diagnosis, indicate disease severity or guide treatment.

The P wave may be small or absent in hyperkalaemia, enlarged in cor pulmonale from chronic lung disease (P pulmonale) and bifid or biphasic in mitral regurgitation (P mitrale). The PR interval is lengthened in first-degree heart block, hyperkalaemia and use of drugs such as β-blockers and digoxin. Short PR intervals are seen in Wolff–Parkinson–White syndrome.

Widened QRS complexes are seen in conduction deficits, ventricular hypertrophy, hyperkalaemia, Wolff–Parkinson–White syndrome and overdose of any drug which blocks sodium channels. Common drugs include tricyclic antidepressants, local anaesthetics, type 1a and 1c antiarrhythmics, antimalarials and antiepileptics.

ST changes are seen in many conditions, including ischaemic heart disease, digoxin toxicity ('reverse tick' ST depression), pericarditis (saddle-shaped ST elevation), conduction deficits and hypokalaemia (ST depression).

Causes of prolonged QT include congenital causes, electrolyte imbalance (hypokalaemia, hypomagnesaemia, hypocalcaemia), drugs (antiarrhythmics including amiodarone, macrolides, antihistamines, tricyclic antidepressants etc.), myocardial infarction and other cardiac disease.

Prominent U waves are seen in bradycardia and severe hypothermia. J waves are seen in hypercalcaemia and hypothermia.

Chan TC, Brady WJ, Harrigan RA, Ornato JP, Rosen P. *ECG in Emergency Medicine and Acute Care*. Philadephia, PA: Elsevier Mosby, 2005.

Surawicz B, Knilans T. *Chou's Electrocardiography in Clinical Practice*, 6th edn. Philadephia, PA: Saunders, 2008.

Question A51: Delirium

With regards to the assessment of delirium, which of the following are correct?

A. The CAM-ICU assessment tool can be performed on patients who are intubated
B. The DSM-IV criteria can only be used by psychiatrists in the identification of delirium
C. The Intensive Care Delirium Screening Checklist (ICDSC) requires a qualified doctor to carry out the assessment
D. The CAM-ICU assessment tool cannot be used if a patient is sedated
E. The CAM-ICU assessment and ICDSC have been shown to have high sensitivity in identifying patients with delirium

Answer: TFFFT

Short explanation

The CAM-ICU assessment tool can be used on patients who are intubated and sedated but cannot always be completed, depending on the patient's level of consciousness. The DSM-IV criteria are usually used by psychiatrists but can be applied by any health professional with the required knowledge. All these tests can be used by nursing and medical staff.

Long explanation

Delirium is common on the ICU, and there are many assessment tools available to identify delerious patients. The formal psychiatric assessment involves use of the DSM-IV criteria. This is very extensive and can take up to 40 minutes to complete. A prior knowledge and understanding is not vital, but it is unlikely that an intensive care practitioner would routinely be able to use this tool in clinical practice.

Delirium is probably underdiagnosed, and so newer more simple tools have been developed to allow the multidisciplinary team to assess patients accurately and in a sensible time frame during clinical practice. The CAM (Confusion Assessment Method) has recently been adapted for ICU (CAM-ICU). The CAM-ICU is a point-in-time, objective, non-verbal assessment and has been validated in a number of studies for intubated patients. The Intensive Care Delirium Screening Checklist (ICDSC) has also been well validated. Both these tests are relatively quick to perform and require little specific training of intensive care staff members.

The ICDSC is more subjective than the CAM-ICU and requires the nurse to assess the patient over the course of the nursing shift. Both tests have been shown to have high sensitivity (> 97%), but the CAM-ICU has a better specificity than the ICDSC. The CAM-ICU has been shown to be better at predicting outcome than the ICDSC.

There are other tools available, but they are less widely used in clinical practice. They include the CAM, the Delirium Rating Scale (DRS-R98), the Memorial Delirium assessment Scale (MDAS) and the Nursing Delirium Screening Scale (NuDESC).

Alce T, Page V, Vizcaychipi M. Delirium uncovered. *J Intensive Care Soc* 2013; 14: 53–9.

Girard T, Jackson J, Pandharipande P, *et al*. Delirium as a predictor of long-term cognitive impairment in survivors of critical illness. *Crit Care Med* 2010; 38: 1513–20.

Ouimet S, Kavanagh B, Gottfried S, Skrobik Y. Incidence, risk factors and consequences of ICU delirium. *Intensive Care Med* 2007; 33: 66–73.

Van Rompaey B, Elseviers M, Schuurmans M, *et al*. Risk factors for delirium in intensive care patients: a prospective cohort study. *Crit Care* 2009; 13: R77.

Question A52: Bacterial meningitis

Causes of bacterial meningitis include:

A. *Haemophilus influenzae*
B. *Staphylococcus aureus*
C. *Listeria monocytogenes*
D. *Streptococcus pneumoniae*
E. *Staphylococcus epidermidis*

Answer: TTTTT

Short explanation

All of the above organisms can be responsible for bacterial meningitis. *Staphylococcus epidermidis* and *S. aureus* should be considered particularly after neurosurgery.

Long explanation

Meningitis is infection or inflammation of the meninges and subarachnoid space. Infection may be caused by viruses, bacteria, fungi or protozoa.

Bacterial meningitis is a serious, life-threatening disease that can occur at any age. The most likely bacterial pathogen alters with age group. In neonates it is commonly caused by group B streptococci, *Escherichia coli* or *Listeria monocytogenes*. In infants and children, *Neisseria meningitidis*, *Haemophilus influenzae* and *Streptococcus pneumoniae* have all been implicated and are the subject of vaccination programmes. Adult cases are most commonly due to *S. pneumoniae, N. menigitidis* or *L. monocytogenes*. After neurosurgery, normal skin flora may be responsible, including *Staphylococcus aureus* and *S. epidermidis*. Empirical antibiotic cover should be broad spectrum, usually third-generation cephalosporins, with the addition of amoxicillin if *Listeria* is suspected. Co-administration of antiviral agents is common until viral meningo-encephalitis is excluded.

Aseptic meningitis is a generic term for cases where bacteria cannot be isolated from the cerebrospinal fluid. The differential diagnosis for aseptic meningitis includes viral meningitis, partially treated bacterial meningitis, tuberculous meningitis, fungal meningitis, subarachnoid haemorrhage, lymphoma or sarcoidosis. The most common causes of aseptic meningitis are viral infections, most commonly enterovirus or Coxsackie. Rarely, it is possible to have meningeal micrometastases from disseminated carcinoma.

Gillian P. Meninigitis. In Waldmann C, Soni N, Rhodes A. *Oxford Desk Reference: Critical Care*. Oxford: Oxford University Press, 2008; pp. 364–5.

Kennedy AM. Meningitis and encephalomyelitis. In Bersten AD, Soni N. *Oh's Intensive Care Manual*, 6th edn. Edinburgh: Butterworth-Heinemann, 2009; pp. 583–92.

Question A53: Pulmonary embolism risk

Risk factors for pulmonary embolus include:

A. Renal replacement therapy on ICU
B. Lightning strike
C. Factor V Leiden mutation
D. Rheumatoid arthritis
E. Cardiac failure

Answer: TTTTT

Short explanation

All of these represent a potential risk factor for pulmonary embolism and should be taken into consideration when risk-stratifying patients for anticoagulation.

Long explanation

Hospitalised patients, and particularly those admitted to critical care, are at increased risk of developing venous thromboembolism (VTE), which contributes significantly to their morbidity and mortality. Post-mortem studies have shown that the incidence of pulmonary embolism (PE) is as high as 27% and the incidence of image-proven deep venous thrombosis (DVT) in critically ill patients is much higher, depending upon the screening methods and diagnostic criteria used.

Most critically ill patients have multiple risk factors for VTE, and many are present prior to admission such as surgery, trauma, burns, sepsis, malignancy, immobilisation, increased age, heart or respiratory failure and previous VTE. Any chronic inflammation such as rheumatoid arthritis or inflammatory bowel disease may predispose to VTE.

Underlying thrombophilia such as that conferred by protein C or S deficiency, antiphospholipid syndrome or factor V Leiden mutation will contribute significantly to the patient's overall risk of developing VTE. Factor V Leiden mutation is a hypercoagulability state caused by a mutation in the gene that codes for factor V, rendering it immune to inactivation by activated protein C.

Additional risk factors acquired on ICU are immobilisation, chemical paralysis, central venous catheterisation, sepsis, vasopressors and haemodialysis.

Davies AR, Pilcher DR. Pulmonary embolism. In Bersten AD, Soni N. *Oh's Intensive Care Manual*, 6th edn. Edinburgh: Butterworth-Heinemann, 2009; pp. 387–98.

Hunt B, Retter A. *Venous Thromboprophylaxis in Critical Care: Standards and Guidelines*. Intensive Care Society, 2008. http://www.ics.ac.uk/professional/standard_safety_quality/standards_and_guidelines/guielines_for_venous_thromboprophylaxis_in_critical_care_2008 (accessed June 2013).

National Institute for Health and Care Excellence. *CG144: Venous Thromboembolic Diseases: the Management of Venous Thromboembolic Diseases and the Role of Thrombophilia Testing*. London: NICE, 2012. http://www.nice.org.uk/cg144 (accessed June 2014).

Question A54: Renal replacement therapy discontinuation

The following are evidence-based criteria for discontinuation of renal replacement therapy (RRT):

A. pH > 7.30
B. Serum urea < 10 mmol/l
C. Serum potassium < 5 mmol/l
D. Urine output > 450 ml/day
E. Serum creatinine < 200 μmol/l

Answer: FFFTF

Short explanation

A urine output > 450 ml/day is the only criterion for which there is any evidence. The other parameters may be desirable physiologically and biochemically before RRT is discontinued.

Long explanation

There are no established criteria that absolutely define the point at which renal replacement therapy (RRT) can be terminated, other than futility and the decision to withdraw life-supporting treatment. The available evidence indicates that urine output is probably the best predictor of renal recovery, and a low urine output is predictive for recommencing RRT. The Beginning and Ending Supportive Therapy for the Kidney (BEST Kidney) study defined a threshold urinary output of 450 ml/day as predictive for not requiring further RRT. Postoperatively, the risk of early re-dialysis after weaning from RRT occurs with a urinary output < 100 ml/8 hours.

In practice, it is common to establish biochemical normality or near normality – to have seen an improvement in the underlying condition requiring RRT and to have achieved a reduction in cardiovascular and respiratory support supplied to the patient. Without these preconditions, the likelihood of normal renal function being re-established is small.

Uchino S, Bellomo R, Morimatsu H, *et al*. Discontinuation of continuous renal replacement therapy: A post hoc analysis of a prospective multi-center observational study. *Crit Care Med* 2009; 37: 2576–82.

Wu VC, Ko WJ, Chang HW, *et al*. Risk factors of early redialysis after weaning from postoperative acute renal replacement therapy. *Intensive Care Med* 2008; 34: 101–8.

Question A55: Brain death

Following diagnosis of brain death:

A. Myocardial damage often occurs
B. There is commonly hypotension followed by hypertension
C. Patients are at greater risk of hypothermia
D. Diabetes insipidus is a common feature
E. Patients commonly develop an active inflammatory response and/or disseminated intravascular coagulation (DIC)

Answer: TFTTT

Short explanation

Brain death causes a surge in catecholamines, leading to vasoconstriction, hypertension, tachycardia and myocardial damage. This is usually followed by loss of sympathetic tone, with vasodilatation and hypotension. Intracerebral damage leads to loss of pituitary function, with diabetes insipidus a prominent feature. The release of inflammatory mediators by the dying brain leads to systemic inflammation and coagulopathy and/or DIC.

Long explanation

There are many physiological changes associated with brainstem death, which can make the management of these patients in ICU and the operating theatre problematic, with consequences for the condition of the organs to be retrieved. Awareness of the issues and pre-emptive action are required to optimise the chances of successful organ donation and transplantation.

There is usually a period of raised intracranial pressure (ICP) prior to brain death, which may be prolonged and/or extreme. The cardiovascular response to this raised ICP (Cushing's response) includes vasoconstriction, hypertension and bradycardia. This is associated with a huge increase in circulating catecholamine levels ('catecholamine storm'), with further vasoconstriction and tachycardia. This can lead to visceral ischaemia, greatly increased myocardial work and ischaemic damage in up to 25% of donation-after-brain-death (DBD) donors. Pulmonary oedema occurs in up to 18% of DBD donors, due to a combination of neurogenic and cardiogenic causes. Following the catecholamine storm, there is loss of sympathetic tone, leading to vasodilatation and hypotension.

Damage to the pituitary and hypothalamus leads to homeostatic disruption, particularly diabetes insipidus, hypothyroidism and insulin resistance. Hypothermia is common, owing to a combination of hypothalamic dysfunction, reduced metabolism and vasodilatation. Systemic inflammation is also relatively common; in addition to pre-existing inflammation, the dying brain releases an array of inflammatory mediators leading to a SIRS response and coagulopathy or DIC in up to one-third of DBD donors.

Gordon JK, McKinley J. Physiological changes after brain stem death and management of the heart-beating donor. *Contin Educ Anaesth Crit Care Pain* 2012; 12: 225–9.

Question A56: Ethanol intoxication

With regards to patients who are intoxicated with ethanol, which of the following are correct?

A. Outcome following traumatic brain injury is worse if the patient is intoxicated at time of injury compared with a similar injury in a sober patient
B. A metabolic alkalosis is the commonest acid–base derangement seen
C. Insulin and dextrose infusion is recommended in patients with alcoholic ketoacidosis
D. Outcome following major burns is worse in intoxicated than in non-intoxicated patients
E. Alcoholic ketoacidosis is most commonly seen in patients with chronic alcohol dependence

Answer: FFFTT

Short explanation

Traumatic brain injuries are more common in patients who are intoxicated with ethanol, but outcome in patients who are intoxicated at the time of injury has not been found to be any worse than in non-intoxicated patients. A metabolic acidosis is the commonest acid–base derangement seen; this may represent alcoholic ketoacidosis, which should be treated with intravenous dextrose and saline to avoid hypoglycaemia.

Long explanation

The number of alcohol-related acute care hospital admissions is increasing. Many of these are for minor complaints and injuries which do not require critical care involvement. Patients admitted to critical care due to trauma-related injuries such as brain injuries and major burns are often found to be intoxicated with ethanol, which may contribute to the aetiology of the accident itself. Intoxicated trauma patients with head injuries have not been clearly shown to have worse outcomes than those who are not intoxicated at time of injury, once adjustments for injury severity are made. The biggest difference shown is that they are more likely to have unsuspected injuries. In contrast, burn patients who are intoxicated at time of injury have a sixfold increase in mortality compared with non-intoxicated patients with similar injury.

It is important to be aware of the impact of ethanol intoxication upon biochemical and physiological parameters. Alcoholic ketoacidosis is usually seen in chronic alcohol abusers who partake in a period of binge drinking. It is seen in fewer than 10% of cases of acute alcohol intoxication. Patients have usually had a period of reduced food intake and vomiting. This stimulates lipolysis and generation of free fatty acids due to low insulin levels, resulting in ketone body formation. This leads to a metabolic acidosis similar to that seen in diabetic ketoacidosis (DKA). The metabolic picture can be mixed with a respiratory alkalosis. Vomiting can also cause a metabolic alkalosis. The metabolic acidosis is usually a high anion gap acidosis, but hyperchloraemic acidosis (seen in DKA) is rare. The depletion of glycogen stores in these patients means that hypoglycaemia is common, and treatment involves the administration of dextrose and saline. Insulin is not usually required. The acid–base derangement usually corrects very quickly, and administration of sodium bicarbonate is only rarely necessary.

Corrigan JD. Substance abuse as a mediating factor in outcome from traumatic brain injury. *Arch Phys Med Rehabil* 1995; 76: 302–9.

De Wit M, Jones D, Sessler C, Zilberberg M, Weaver M. Alcohol-use disorders in the critically ill patient. *Chest* 2010; 138: 994–1003.

Kraut J, Kurtz I. Toxic alcohol ingestions: clinical features, diagnosis and management. *Clin J Am Soc Nephrol* 2008; 3: 208–25.

Question A57: Stress ulcer prophylaxis

Stress ulcer prophylaxis in ICU:

A. Should be given to all ventilated patients
B. Increases the risk of *Clostridium difficile* infection
C. Reduces ICU mortality
D. Leads to the side effect of interstitial nephritis more commonly with proton-pump inhibitors (PPIs) than with histamine H_2 receptor antagonists (H_2RAs)
E. Is associated with lower rates of ventilator-associated pneumonia (VAP) when PPIs are used, compared with H_2RAs

Answer: FTFTF

Short explanation

PPIs should be given to patients with a risk factor for gastrointestinal bleeding. Stress ulcer prophylaxis may be associated with increased *Clostridium difficile* infection. No mortality benefit has been demonstrated. Stress ulcer prophylaxis with both PPIs and H_2RAs has been shown to reduce clinically significant bleeding, but increase the risk of VAP. Interstitial nephritis is associated with PPI use.

Long explanation

The prevention of gastric stress ulceration in critically ill patients is commonplace but not without controversy. Critically ill patients are at increased risk of developing stress ulcers owing to an imbalance in acid production and protective mucus and bicarbonate secretion. Increased acid secretion is seen at times of stress and in conditions such as head injury. Reduced mucus and bicarbonate secretion is seen in patients treated with steroids and NSAIDs and those with reduced visceral perfusion (including vasopressor usage). Finally, reflux of bile salts leads to reduced gastric mucus.

H_2 receptor antagonists (H_2RAs) such as ranitidine are competitive antagonists at histaminergic receptors on the acid-secreting enterochromaffin cells in the stomach. Proton-pump inhibitors (PPIs) are irreversible inhibitors of the H^+/K^+ pump responsible for secreting acid into the gastric lumen. H_2RAs are known to have a shorter half-life than PPIs and to exhibit tachyphylaxis. PPIs have been shown to be more effective than H_2RAs at reducing upper gastrointestinal bleeding. No mortality benefit has been demonstrated with prophylaxis with either class of drug.

Stress ulcer prophylaxis is not without risks, however. Ventilator-associated pneumonia (VAP) rates are higher in patients treated with H_2RAs or PPIs. There is no difference in VAP rate between the two classes of drugs. Other concerns include an increased risk of *Clostridium difficile* infection in patients on stress ulcer prophylaxis. Interstitial nephritis is associated with PPI use.

Therefore, only patients at increased risk of stress ulceration should receive prophylaxis. This includes patients ventilated for > 48 hours, patients on certain medications (corticosteroids, NSAIDs etc.), patients with previous GI bleeding and those with coagulopathy. The presence of stress ulcer prophylaxis on ventilator care bundles and as a quality marker for ICU may mean that patients at low risk are being treated unnecessarily, with increased risk of VAP as a result.

Alhazzani W, Alenezi F, Jaeschke RZ, Moayyedi P, Cook DJ. Proton pump inhibitors versus histamine 2 receptor antagonists for stress ulcer prophylaxis in critically ill patients: a systematic review and meta-analysis. *Crit Care Med* 2013; 41: 693–705.

Marik PE, Vasu T, Hirani A, Pachinburavan M. Stress ulcer prophylaxis in the new millennium: a systematic review and meta-analysis. *Crit Care Med* 2010; 38: 2222–8.

Question A58: Intra-aortic balloon pump

With regards to the intra-aortic balloon pump (IABP) which of the following are correct?

A. The balloon inflates during systole to improve cardiac output
B. Cardiac output is improved by up to 20%
C. Post-acute MI ventricular septal defect is an indication for use
D. Aortic stenosis is a contraindication to its use
E. The balloon should be left in situ for 6 hours once it has been weaned off in case of deterioration

Answer: FTTFF

Short explanation

The balloon inflates during diastole to increase diastolic aortic root pressure and therefore improves coronary artery perfusion, which is usually passive. Aortic regurgitation is a contraindication to its use. It may be used in decompensated aortic stenosis. The balloon should not be left in situ once it is turned off, because of a high risk of thrombus formation.

Long explanation

Intra-aortic balloon pump (IABP) therapy is often reserved for use in specialist centres and in patients with acute cardiogenic shock. Common indications include acute myocardial infarction, acute mitral regurgitation, acute ventricular septal defect, weaning from cardiopulmonary bypass following cardiac surgery, acute cardiogenic shock and refractory left ventricular failure. It is important to appreciate that IABP use is only a temporary measure and should be reserved for reversible conditions or for patients awaiting definitive surgery or percutaneous procedures.

The basic principle underlying the function of the IABP is counterpulsation. Balloon inflation in the descending aorta during diastole results in an increased aortic root diastolic pressure and therefore improved flow to the coronary arteries. This leads to improved myocardial oxygen delivery and cardiac output. The balloon deflates during systole, which reduces the left ventricular afterload. Renal blood flow also improves due to the increased cardiac output.

The balloon pump is usually inserted into the femoral artery by a cardiologist or cardiac surgeon experienced in the technique. The balloon is inflated with helium, as it is inert in case of rupture. The tip of the balloon should lie just distal to the origin of the left subclavian artery in the descending aorta. Fluoroscopy is usually used to confirm placement. The balloon is connected to an electronic console that times inflation and deflation based on either the ECG or the aortic blood pressure, which is also monitored by the balloon. The arterial pressure waveform will show a second 'peak', which is the diastolic pressure augmentation achieved by the balloon inflation. The patient should be weaned from the balloon when inotropic support has reduced or definitive treatment has been performed. This is done by reducing the ratio of the balloon inflation to the patient's own heart rate. Once the balloon has stopped it should be removed, because there is a high risk of thrombus formation and distal embolisation.

Krishna M, Zacharowski K. Principles of intra-aortic balloon counterpulsation. *Contin Educ Anaesth Crit Care Pain* 2009; 9: 24–8.

Question A59: Rhabdomyolysis

The following are recognised causes of rhabdomyolysis:

A. Statins
B. Diabetic ketoacidosis (DKA)
C. Epilepsy
D. Isoflurane
E. Gentle exercise

Answer: TTTTF

Short explanation

Rhabdomyolysis is the pathological breakdown of striated muscle. It can lead to renal failure and death. It may be caused by crush injuries, hypoperfusion of muscles, extreme muscle activity (seizures or vigorous exercise), hyperthermia, malignant hyperthermia (caused by anaesthetic agents), drugs (statins, cocaine, alcohol) and metabolic disturbance (hypokalaemia, hypocalcaemia, DKA).

Long explanation

Rhabdomyolysis is the pathological breakdown of striated muscle. Necrosis allows intracellular contents to enter the circulation, particularly myoglobin, potassium, phosphate and creatine kinase (CK). Hyperkalaemia and hypocalcaemia (due to calcium sequestration) can lead to dysrhythmias. Other complications include compartment syndrome from muscle oedema (which can lead to further rhabdomyolysis), hypovolaemia, disseminated intravascular coagulation (DIC) and acute kidney injury (AKI), owing to the nephrotoxic nature of myoglobin.

Causes of rhabdomyolysis include:

- trauma – crush injuries, burns and electrical injury
- limb ischaemia – vascular disease or postural hypoperfusion
- hyperthermia – malignant hyperthermia (MH), heat stroke, neuroleptic malignant syndrome (NMS)
- exertion – vigorous exercise, status epilepticus
- drugs – statins, cocaine, alcohol, antipsychotics, anaesthetics (MH)
- infections – *Streptococcus*, *Clostridium*, viral myositis, HIV, Epstein–Barr virus (EBV), malaria
- metabolic – hypokalaemia, hypocalcaemia, DKA, hyperosmolar non-ketotic acidosis (HONK)
- genetic – metabolic enzyme deficiencies

Management of rhabdomyolysis is mainly supportive, with treatment of the underlying cause. Large volumes of fluid are commonly required, and invasive monitoring is usually necessary. Urinary alkalinisation with sodium bicarbonate is commonplace. Renal replacement therapy may be required for hyperkalaemia and renal failure. Fasciotomies may be required to treat ongoing compartment syndrome and prevent further rhabdomyolysis.

Bosch X, Poch E, Grau J. Rhabdomyolysis and acute kidney injury. *N Engl J Med* 2009; 361: 62–72.

Question A60: Diabetic ketoacidosis

With regards to the assessment and management of a patient with diabetic ketoacidosis (DKA), which of the following are correct?

A. DKA most commonly occurs in patients without a previous diagnosis of diabetes mellitus
B. Hyperglycaemia commonly causes a falsely elevated measured plasma sodium concentration
C. The cause of DKA is often not found
D. An elevated anion gap metabolic acidosis is a key feature of DKA
E. An elevated white cell count is often seen in DKA even in the absence of infection

Answer: FFTTT

Short explanation

While an episode of DKA may be the first presenting feature of diabetes mellitus in some patients, the majority of episodes of DKA occur in patients in whom the diagnosis of diabetes mellitus has already been established. Hyperglycaemia can cause a falsely low sodium concentration. DKA can occur due to intercurrent infection, vomiting or omission of insulin.

Long explanation

Diabetic ketoacidosis (DKA) is a medical emergency and is common among patients with type 1 diabetes mellitus. More recently some people have recognised DKA as a feature of type 2 diabetes mellitus, although this is uncommon. The diagnosis requires that the patient has a blood sugar > 14 mmol/l, the presence of urinary or plasma ketones, a pH < 7.3 and a serum bicarbonate < 18 mmol/l. There are other biochemical markers that may be abnormal in DKA. The amylase can be raised even in the absence of pancreatitis. Often the serum potassium level is high at presentation but there is usually a total body deficit of potassium. The serum potassium will drop as glucose and acidosis is corrected, and levels must therefore be checked regularly throughout treatment. Hyperglycaemia causes a dilutional hyponatraemia; the actual serum sodium can be calculated from the following formula:

$$\text{Corrected Na}^+ = \text{measured Na}^+ + (((\text{serum glucose} - 100) / 100) \times 1.6)$$

A key feature of DKA is an elevated anion gap metabolic acidosis. The anion gap can be calculated as follows:

$$\text{Anion gap} = (\text{serum Na}^+ + \text{K}^+) - (\text{serum HCO}_3^- + \text{Cl}^-)$$

The commonest cause for DKA is infection such as a urinary tract infection. Other common causes include non-compliance with insulin therapy, undiagnosed type 1 diabetes and other stresses such as alcohol, myocardial infraction and pancreatitis. In 40% of cases the cause is never identified.

Hardern R, Quinn N. Emergency management of diabetic ketoacidosis in adults. *Emerg Med J* 2003; 20: 210–13.

Question A61: Sepsis

In the case of a general surgical patient with severe sepsis:

A. The patient should be operated on within 6 hours unless resuscitation is required
B. The mortality rate is < 10%
C. A predicted mortality score of ≥ 5% indicates a high-risk patient

D. In septic shock, a delay to surgery of > 12 hours increases mortality rates to 60%
E. All patients with predicted mortality ≥ 10% should receive postoperative care on HDU or ICU

Answer: FFTTT

Short explanation

Patients with surgical disease and severe sepsis should be operated on within 6 hours, with resuscitation beforehand. Hospital mortality rate for these patients is > 25%, and 30-day mortality for emergency laparotomy is around 15%. A 12-hour delay for shocked patients is estimated to increase mortality to > 60%. The high-risk patient is defined as one with predicted mortality of ≥ 5%. If the score is ≥ 10%, patients should receive postoperative care in HDU or ICU.

Long explanation

Emergency general surgical patients have among the highest mortality, morbidity and complication rates of any patient group. Cases are commonly complex and high risk, but often performed by junior members of staff out of hours without critical care input. Since 2010, several reports and studies have been published highlighting the substandard care that this patient group sometimes receives, and outlining standards of care and good practice. Foremost among these is the RCS(Eng) report from 2011, *The Higher Risk General Surgical Patient.*

Patients with sepsis of any origin should have early resuscitative measures as described in the Surviving Sepsis Campaign guidelines. Within the first hour, patients should receive intravenous fluids, have their lactate measured, have bacterial cultures sent and receive broad-spectrum antibiotics appropriate for the suspected site of infection. If a source of sepsis can be identified that is amenable to surgical or radiological therapy, then this should occur within a timescale appropriate to the condition of the patient:

- septic shock: immediately
- severe sepsis: as soon as possible; within 6 hours
- sepsis: as soon as possible (not between 10 pm and 7 am); within 18 hours
- no SIRS: as soon as possible within working hours.

Overall hospital mortality is > 25%. 30-day mortality following laparotomy is around 15%. A 12-hour delay in source control in septic shock is estimated to increase mortality to 60% or higher.

Risk assessment should occur, using a tool such as the P-POSSUM score. A predicted mortality score of ≥ 5% defines the high-risk surgical patient. Any patient with predicted mortality ≥ 10% should have consultant surgical and anaesthetic care, and should receive postoperative care in HDU or ICU.

Royal College of Surgeons of England, Department of Health. *The Higher Risk General Surgical Patient: Towards Improved Care for a Forgotten Group.* London: RCS England, 2011.

Saunders DI, Murray D, Pichel AC, Varley S, Peden CJ. Variations in mortality after emergency laparotomy: the first report of the UK Emergency Laparotomy Network. *Br J Anaesth* 2012; 109: 368–75.

Question A62: Eclampsia

With regards to severe eclampsia, which of the following are correct?

A. It is the commonest reason for maternal admission to the intensive care unit
B. High-resistance uterine spiral arteries persist due to deficient placental implantation
C. Seizures are due to ischaemia caused by cerebral vasoconstriction
D. Because of volume depletion, aggressive fluid resuscitation should be commenced without delay
E. Phenytoin loading should be started after two seizures

Answer: TTTFF

Short explanation

Despite the fact that most patients are volume depleted, fluid resuscitation must be carefully titrated. Even small fluid boluses can lead to pulmonary oedema, because of reduced left ventricular compliance. Seizures should initially be managed with a magnesium infusion, and the airway should be protected. Anticonvulsants are very rarely indicated, as seizures are usually short-lived and self-terminating.

Long explanation

Despite the dramatic reduction in maternal mortality in the developed world over the last few decades, severe eclampsia still remains a major cause of maternal morbidity and mortality. The pathophysiology is not fully understood but probably relates to abnormal placental implantation in the first trimester. In normal pregnancies the fetal cytotrophoblast cells invade the uterine spiral arteries, which become low-resistance vessels as the pregnancy progresses. If this process is abnormal, the arteries remain high-resistance vessels, leading to the release of mediators into the systemic circulation which bring about widespread vasoconstriction and vasospasm. There is thought to be an immunological basis for the disordered placentation, and certain risk factors have been identified. These include primigravidas, multigravidas with a new partner and patients with autoimmune diseases.

Systemic hypertension developing after 20 weeks gestation and proteinuria are the diagnostic features of pre-eclampsia. Severe pre-eclampsia exists if the blood pressure is > 170/110 mmHg, with proteinuria > 300 g/day, hepatic epigastric pain, elevated liver enzymes or bilirubin, headaches, visual disturbance, clonus, hyperreflexia, thrombocytopenia, DIC, haemolysis or pulmonary oedema. The disease is renamed eclampsia if the patient suffers a seizure.

Seizures are usually short-lived and self-terminate. Benzodiazepines are not usually required and should in fact be avoided. A magnesium loading dose followed by an infusion should be commenced immediately to prevent further seizures. This has an added benefit of treating hypertension, although blood pressure should be carefully monitored, as abrupt reduction can be problematic. Renal failure may require renal replacement therapy but usually recovers following delivery and resolution of the condition. Delivery of the fetus and placenta remains the definitive treatment, and for this reason most intensive care admissions are post-partum. Pulmonary oedema can develop quickly and after seemingly small volumes of intravenous fluid. For this reason, fluid restriction is usually instigated, and invasive monitoring should be considered in patients with haemodynamic instability. Coagulopathy is not uncommon, and patients may require blood product transfusion to prevent or treat post-partum haemorrhage. Central venous pressure monitoring should be considered in these patients to guide fluid balance. Diuretics should be considered for those with oliguria, although this usually improves following delivery.

Ciantar E, Walker J. Pre-eclampsia, severe pre-eclampsia and hemolysis, elevated liver enzymes and low platelets syndrome: what is new? *Womens Health* 2011; 7: 555–69.

Question A63: Systolic heart failure

The following treatments have been shown to reduce mortality in systolic heart failure (heart failure with left ventricular ejection fraction < 40%)

A. Loop diuretics
B. Mineralocorticoid receptor antagonists (MRAs)
C. β-adrenergic receptor antagonists
D. Statins
E. Non-dihydropyridine calcium-channel blockers

Answer: FTTFF

Short explanation

All patients with systolic heart failure (LVEF < 40%) should be treated with an ACE inhibitor and a β-blocker, as tolerated. Those with persisting symptoms should also receive an MRA. Statins have not been shown to be of benefit in systolic heart failure, although they are beneficial in many other related conditions. Most calcium-channel blockers (except amlodipine and felodipine) are negatively inotropic and can worsen heart failure. Loop diuretics may be used for symptom control, but there is no evidence that they reduce mortality.

Long explanation

Heart failure is the failure of the heart to deliver the required amount of oxygen to respiring tissues despite adequate filling. Systolic heart failure describes a condition in which the left ventricular ejection fraction is reduced to below 35–40%. Patients with diastolic dysfunction require a different treatment strategy.

In critical care, patients with systolic heart failure may be encountered following admission for conditions unrelated to their heart disease. As they recover, heart failure therapy should be reinstituted and the opportunity taken to optimise therapy in a controlled environment.

ACE inhibitors have been shown to be beneficial in systolic heart failure in a number of trials and meta-analyses (e.g. CONSENSUS, SOLVD, SAVE, AIRE, TRACE). Patients intolerant of ACE inhibitors may be equally well treated with angiotensin II receptor antagonists.

β-Blockers have equally strong evidence of benefit in terms of reduced mortality and hospitalisation due to heart failure (e.g. COPERNICUS, MERIT-HF, SENIORS, BEST, COMET). Many patients in the trials supporting ACE inhibitor and β-blocker use were on both agents, and so the recommendation is for patients to be started on dual therapy, as tolerated.

Mineralocorticoid receptor antagonists have good evidence of reduced mortality and hospitalisation and should be started in patients who remain in systolic failure (LVEF < 35% or NYHA class III–IV) after treatment with an ACE inhibitor and β-blocker. Examples of trials include RALES, EMPHASIS-HF and EPHESUS.

There are other recommended therapies in systolic heart failure with less strong evidence of benefit. These include digoxin, ivabradine and a combination of hydralazine and isosorbide dinitrate.

Loop diuretics are commonly used for symptom control in systolic heart failure but have not been shown to improve mortality or morbidity, reduce length of stay or prevent hospitalisation. Many patients with systolic heart failure are treated with statins for another indication, but there is no evidence of benefit in systolic heart failure. Most early studies of the efficacy of statins excluded patients with systolic heart failure but recent trials of statins in heart failure have shown no benefit. Calcium-channel blockers, except amlodipine and felodipine, should be avoided in systolic cardiac failure as they are negatively inotropic and exacerbate heart failure.

McMurray JJV, Adamopoulos S, Anker SD, *et al*. ESC guidelines for the diagnosis and treatment of acute and chronic heart failure 2012. The Task Force for the Diagnosis and Treatment of Acute and Chronic Heart Failure 2012 of the European Society of Cardiology. *Eur Heart J* 2012; 33: 1787–847.

Question A64: Myasthenia gravis

Regarding myasthenia gravis (MG):

A. MG affects central more than peripheral muscles
B. The Tensilon (edrophonium) test is the most sensitive and specific diagnostic test for MG
C. Almost all patients have autoantibodies to postsynaptic acetylcholine receptors
D. Vital capacity (VC) < 15 ml/kg is an indication for intubation
E. Plasma exchange is the most effective treatment for myasthenic crisis

Answer: TFTTT

Short explanation

MG is an autoimmune disease affecting the neuromuscular junction. Up to 90% of people have detectable autoantibodies. The Tensilon test is of low sensitivity and specificity. Oculomotor, bulbar and proximal muscles are primarily affected. Myasthenic crisis is a medical emergency. VC < 15 ml/kg, bulbar palsy and respiratory failure are indications for intubation.

Long explanation

Myasthenia gravis (MG) is an autoimmune disease that affects the neuromuscular junction, often associated with thymus gland disease. Up to 90% of cases have identifiable IgG antibodies to the postsynaptic nicotinic acetylcholine receptor. Around 70% of the rest have autoantibodies to a muscle-specific receptor kinase. Autoantibody tests are highly specific but costly. The Tensilon (edrophonium) test is used for diagnosis in urgent cases but has low sensitivity and specificity. An increase in strength within 45 seconds of 2–10 mg edrophonium is a positive result.

Clinical features are of a fatiguable weakness of skeletal muscles, primarily of the oculomotor, bulbar and proximal limb muscles. Ptosis is a common presenting feature, with weakness progressing caudally as the disease progresses. Myasthenic crisis occurs in up to 20% of patients, especially in those with thymic disease. Respiratory muscle weakness can develop and should be monitored with vital capacity (VC) measurements. Indications for intubation include a VC < 15 ml/kg, bulbar palsy or respiratory failure.

MG is treated with anticholinesterase medications and immunosuppression (e.g. corticosteroids). Thymectomy is effective in those patients with thymic dysfunction. Myasthenic crisis is most effectively treated with plasma exchange. Intravenous immunoglobulin may be as effective, but trial data are currently equivocal. Long-term steroids are usually required after treatment of myasthenic crisis.

Gajdos P, Chevret S, Toyka K. Intravenous immunoglobulin for myasthenia gravis. *Cochrane Database Syst Rev* 2008; (1): CD002277.
Green DM. Weakness in the ICU. *Neurologist* 2005; 11: 338–47.

Question A65: Diagnosis of death

Diagnosis of death:

A. Is made by a doctor
B. Can be determined by somatic, cardiorespiratory or neurological criteria
C. Requires demonstration of the loss of consciousness and loss of cardiac output
D. Takes 5 minutes using cardiorespiratory criteria in the UK
E. Is impossible to determine neurologically in massive craniofacial injuries

Answer: FTFTF

Short explanation

Death is the simultaneous, irreversible loss of the capacities for consciousness and breathing. Determination of death can use somatic, cardiorespiratory or neurological criteria. Somatic criteria include decapitation and putrefaction and do not require a doctor for diagnosis. Cardiorespiratory death is defined as continuous apnoeic asystole for 5 minutes (UK) and loss of consciousness. Neurological death can be diagnosed by brainstem testing or ancillary tests of cerebral perfusion or function.

Long explanation

Death has been defined as the irreversible loss of the capacity for consciousness combined with irreversible loss of the capacity to breathe. The diagnosis of death can be made by one of three criteria.

Somatic determination of death is the oldest method and requires only simple inspection of the body to demonstrate the loss of capacity for respiration and consciousness. Conditions unequivocally associated with death include decapitation, rigor mortis, incineration and decomposition. Diagnosis of death in these cases does not need to be made by a doctor; for instance, ambulance crews have 'recognition of life extinct' criteria.

Diagnosis of death by cardiorespiratory criteria requires examination of the patient to determine loss of capacity for respiration and consciousness. It requires observation of continuous apnoeic asystole for a period of 5 minutes in the UK (times differ internationally), followed by testing for capacity for consciousness (pupillary response to light, corneal reflex, central painful stimulus). Clinical examination or arterial and ECG monitoring may be used for observation of apnoeic asystole.

Diagnosis of death by neurological criteria (brainstem death) must be made by two doctors with five years' registration, one of whom must be a consultant. Patients must be in a state of apnoeic coma with a diagnosis of irreversible brain damage of known aetiology. There should be no exclusion criteria present (e.g. sedative drugs, hypothermia, hypoglycaemia) and the patient should be haemodynamically stable. Six tests of brainstem reflexes are performed, followed by apnoea testing. The tests must be performed twice for a diagnosis of death. In cases where testing is not possible, ancillary tests of cerebral function (e.g. cerebral angiography, EEG) must be performed for diagnosis of death by neurological criteria.

Oram J, Murphy P. Diagnosis of death. *Contin Educ Anaesth Crit Care Pain* 2011; 11: 77–81.

Question A66: Acute liver failure

Regarding acute liver failure:

A. Coagulopathy, jaundice and encephalopathy must be present to make the diagnosis
B. It may be diagnosed if encephalopathy follows jaundice within 6 months
C. The commonest cause worldwide is paracetamol toxicity
D. Clinical examination commonly reveals signs of chronic liver disease
E. It is often caused by hepatitis B and C viruses

Answer: TTFFF

Short explanation

Acute liver failure has a diagnostic triad of coagulopathy, jaundice and encephalopathy, occurring within 6 months (hyperacute 0–1 week; acute 1–4 weeks; subacute 4–26 weeks) in the absence of signs of chronic liver disease. The commonest cause worldwide is viral hepatitis (A, B, E). Acute liver failure caused by hepatitis C is extremely rare.

Long explanation

Acute liver failure (ALF) is uncommon, with around 400 cases occurring in the UK each year. However, mortality rates exceed 50% without transplantation. The diagnosis of ALF is based on the triad of jaundice, loss of synthetic function (coagulopathy) and encephalopathy, in the absence of signs of chronic liver disease. The rate of progression from the onset of jaundice to the development of encephalopathy is used to categorise liver failure into hyperacute (0–1 week), acute (1–4 weeks) and subacute (4–26 weeks). ALF in patients with chronic liver disease is termed a decompensation, or acute on chronic liver failure, and has different causes, management and prognosis to ALF.

Causes of ALF vary according to geography. In many developed countries the commonest cause is paracetamol (acetaminophen) toxicity (over half of all UK cases), although this is comparatively uncommon in other Western nations (e.g. Spain, Germany) and very rare in the developing world. The commonest cause worldwide is viral hepatitis caused by hepatitis A, B and E. Acute hepatic failure caused by hepatitis C is extremely rare. Other causes are:

- toxins (drugs, environmental)
- autoimmune disease (autoimmune hepatitis, primary biliary cirrhosis (PBC), primary sclerosing cholangitis (PSC))
- hepatic ischaemia
- pregnancy-related (fatty liver, HELLP)
- inherited disease (Wilson's, Budd–Chiari syndrome)

Bernal W, Auzinger G, Dhawan A, Wendon J. Acute liver failure. *Lancet*, 2010; 376: 190–201.

Question A67: Lumbar puncture

The following structures will be traversed during a midline lumbar puncture (LP):

A. Interspinous ligament
B. Pia mater
C. Supraspinous ligament
D. Arachnoid mater

E. Ligamentum flavum

Answer: TFTTT

Short explanation

During midline LP, the needle passes through skin, subcutaneous tissues and fat, supraspinous ligament, interspinous ligament, ligamentum flavum, dura mater, arachnoid mater.

Long explanation

Lumbar puncture (LP) is a common diagnostic procedure in intensive care, particularly in cases of suspected meningitis, encephalitis, subarachnoid haemorrhage or patients with unexplained neurological symptoms. LP should not be performed in patients with evidence of raised intracranial pressure. Information available from LP includes CSF pressure, biochemical make-up and the presence of immunological and microbiological abnormalities.

The procedure should be performed in strictly aseptic conditions. Patients may be sitting, although pressure measurements are only reliable in the lateral recumbent position. LP should not occur at a vertebral level above the level at which the spinal cord ends: L1–2 in adults, but lower in children or patients with spinal cord tethering. Commonly, the L3–4 or L4–5 interspace is chosen. This can be identified by use of the intercristal line (a horizontal line connecting the iliac crests), which usually passes through the L4 vertebra.

If a midline approach is chosen, then the structures through which the needle passes prior to accessing the CSF in the subarachnoid space are:

- skin
- subcutaneous tissues and fat
- supraspinous ligament (runs along the tips of the spinous processes)
- interspinous ligament (connects adjacent spinous processes in the midline)
- ligamentum flavum (connects laminae)
- dura mater
- arachnoid mater

The pia mater, which has a mesh-like consistency, is the innermost layer of the meninges and is therefore attached directly to the brain and spinal cord.

Moore KL, Dalley AF, Agur AMR. *Clinically Oriented Anatomy*, 7th edn. Philadelphia, PA: Lippincott, Williams & Wilkins, 2013.

Question A68: Neutropenic sepsis

In a case of neutropenic sepsis:

A. It is defined as fever (> 38 °C) in a patient with neutrophil count < 1.0×10^9/l
B. Broad-spectrum antibiotics should be started within 8 hours
C. Antibiotics should not be delayed for taking of blood and other samples for culture
D. Empirical therapy should include antibacterial and antifungal agents
E. Tunnelled lines may be safely left in situ in neutropenic patients with bacteraemia

Answer: FFTFT

Short explanation

Neutropenic sepsis, defined as a fever (T > 38 °C) or evidence of infection in a patient with a neutrophil count < 0.5×10^9/l, is a medical emergency. Empirical antibiotics should be started within 1 hour of presentation and not delayed by sampling for cultures. First-line treatment is antibacterial unless there is known or suspected fungal or viral infection. Tunnelled lines should not be removed routinely from febrile neutropenic patients, but cultured through and vigilantly observed.

Long explanation

Neutropenic sepsis is a medical emergency. It is defined as a fever (T > 38 °C) or other signs or symptoms of clinically important sepsis in a patient with a neutrophil count < 0.5×10^9/l. It should be suspected in any patient undergoing anticancer treatment who becomes unwell. Immediate assessment should focus on identifying any requirement for organ support and identifying a source of infection. Samples should be sent for microbiological culture. These should include peripheral blood and blood from any indwelling lines, along with urine, swabs and other samples as clinically indicated.

Early empirical antibacterial therapy should be started as soon as possible. This should start within 1 hour of presentation and should not be delayed for taking samples for microbiological culture. Initial therapy should be antibacterial unless there is reason to suspect a fungal or viral infection (e.g. previous known invasive candidiasis). The first-line antibacterial agent recommended by NICE is piperacillin with tazobactam. There is currently no recommendation for the use of aminoglycosides, nor glycopeptides in patients with indwelling lines, unless there are particular indications or local policies for their use.

Other antimicrobial agents should be added if there are specific patient indications or local guidelines. These circumstances may include: intolerance of a particular agent, known colonisation or previous infection with a resistant organism, suspected fungal or viral infection, or microbiological advice. If no response is seen with 2–3 days, microbiological advice should be sought and alternative agents used, including antifungal or antiviral agents.

Patients with neutropenia commonly have tunnelled, indwelling intravenous catheters. These should have cultures taken from them at the time of presentation but should not be removed routinely as part of the acute management of neutropenic sepsis. This is because intravenous access will be required for treatment, and to reduce the risks associated with further attempts at short- and long-term venous access. In cases not responsive to initial therapy, with high suspicion of line infection, known line colonisation or tunnel infection, then indwelling lines should be removed.

Other management of patients with neutropenic sepsis includes general supportive measures (fluids, nutrition, DVT prophylaxis etc.), organ support as required, isolation to reduce the risk of further infection and granulocyte-colony stimulating factor. This is an agent which stimulates the production of white blood cells from the bone marrow, reducing the duration of neutropenia and enhancing the host immune response.

Dellinger RP, Levy MM, Rhodes A, *et al.* Surviving Sepsis Campaign. International guidelines for management of severe sepsis and septic shock: 2012. *Crit Care Med* 2013; 41: 580–637.

National Institute for Health and Care Excellence. *CG151: Neutropenic Sepsis: Prevention and Management of Neutropenic Sepsis in Cancer Patients*. London: NICE, 2012. http://www.nice.org.uk/cg151 (accessed June 2014).

Question A69: Short bowel syndrome

With regards to short bowel syndrome, which of the following are correct?

A. Intestinal remnant length is the primary determinant of outcome in patients with short bowel syndrome
B. Short bowel syndrome will develop in most patients once 50% of the small intestine is lost
C. Bile salt malabsorption is unusual in patients with large terminal ileum resections
D. Iron deficiency is common in patients who have had significant ileal resections
E. Cholelithiasis is a common problem and has a higher incidence in patients receiving total parenteral nutrition (TPN)

Answer: TFFFT

Short explanation

Short bowel syndrome becomes more common once two-thirds of the small intestinal length is lost. Bile salts are absorbed in the terminal ileum and so malabsorption occurs in patients who have undergone partial or whole ileal resection. Iron is absorbed in the duodenum and proximal jejunum, so deficiency is rare as these are usually intact even in patients who have undergone large resections.

Long explanation

Normal adults have between 275 and 850 cm of small bowel; women tend to have less than men. There are a number of conditions which can lead to the development of short bowel syndrome. Extensive intestinal resection may be performed to treat cancer, irradiation, mesenteric vascular disease, Crohn's disease and postoperative complications after other abdominal surgery. It is more useful to refer to the remaining length of small bowel when discussing short bowel syndrome. Once there is less than 200 cm remaining, nutritional and/or fluid supplements are likely to be required. Patients with less than 120 cm of small bowel, who do not have colon in continuity, are likely to require permanent total parenteral nutrition (TPN). If there is colonic continuity then patients may tolerate as little as 60 cm of small bowel without requiring permanent TPN.

Patients may be categorised according to the segment of bowel resected and the nature of any anastomoses or stomata. Patients with jejunal resection have a jejunal–ileal anastomosis; these are unlikely to develop significant nutritional deficiency. Others have a jejunoileal resection, colectomy and formation of stoma (jejunostomy); these usually have severe nutritional and fluid deficiencies immediately following surgery. Finally, patients with jejunoileal resection and resulting jejunocolic anastomosis tend to develop nutritional problems over a longer period of time.

The presence of nutritional deficiencies depends on the anatomical remnants following resection. The most common nutritional deficiencies are of those substances which are predominantly absorbed in the ileum. These are vitamin B_{12} deficiency, fat malabsorption and hypomagnesaemia. Bile salt malabsorption also occurs despite increased hepatic synthesis. Over time, the bowel of patients with a jejunocolic anastomosis does undergo some functional adaptation such as slowing of gastric emptying and small bowel transit time. This means that requirements for nutritional supplements may reduce. Those patients with a jejunostomy rarely display signs of intestinal adaptation, and so nutritional requirements remain the same.

Nightingale J, Woodward J. Guidelines for management of patients with a short bowel. *Gut* 2006; 55 (Suppl IV): iv1–12.

Seetharam P, Rodrigues G. Short bowel syndrome: a review of management options. *Saudi J Gastroenterol.* 2011; 17: 229–35.

Question A70: Necrotising fasciitis

Necrotising fasciitis:

A. Is most commonly polymicrobial
B. Is rarely caused by fungal infection
C. Spreads between the dermis and superficial fascia
D. Should not be treated with clindamycin as first-line unless the patient has a penicillin allergy
E. Is a cause of hypocalcaemia

Answer: TTFFT

Short explanation

Necrotising fasciitis occurs at the level of the subcutaneous fat and deep fascia. Clindamycin should be given to all patients, as it reduces toxin production.

Long explanation

Necrotising fasciitis is a severe soft tissue infection with a mortality of around 25%. It may be classified by the bacterial cause of the infection:

- Type I: polymicrobial, most commonly Gram-positive cocci, Gram-negative rods and anaerobes. It generally occurs on the trunk or perineum of diabetic or immunocompromised patients or those with peripheral vascular disease.
- Type II: group A *Streptococcus* infection, usually on limbs and associated with toxic shock syndrome. Includes methicillin-resistant *Staphylococcus aureus* (MRSA) infection.
- Type III: rare monomicrobial infection, usually caused by a bacterium in the *Vibrio* class. It carries a very high mortality.
- Type IV: fungal necrotising fasciitis with *Candida*, which is very rare.

Infection of the soft tissues occurs through a wound or by spread from an internal organ, such as a perforated viscus or the urogenital tract. Toxins and enzymes released by bacteria allow spread through fascial planes, interruption of the microcirculation, tissue ischaemia and cell death. Skin necrosis is a late sign, as the infection starts at the level of the subcutaneous fat and deep fascia. This is in contrast to cellulitis, where infection is at the junction between the dermis and superficial fascia. The key clinical finding to differentiate necrotising fasciitis is pain disproportionate to the clinical findings.

The diagnosis is usually clinical, although findings of fascial necrosis and myonecrosis at surgery are pathognomonic. Blood tests may show features associated with severe sepsis including leucocytosis, leucopenia, coagulopathy and thrombocytopenia. Abnormal renal and hepatic function, a metabolic acidosis and high serum lactate concentrations may also occur. Muscle damage leads to a rise in creatinine kinase, and hypocalcaemia occurs with fat necrosis and calcium deposition in necrotic tissue.

Antibiotic therapy should be broad-spectrum, including clindamycin, which reduces toxin production in streptococcal infection. Intravenous immunoglobulin may also be used in staphylococcal and streptococcal infections to reduce exotoxin production. Hyperbaric oxygen has been used in *Clostridium* infections.

Necrotising fasciitis can spread quickly and often requires extensive and multiple surgical debridements followed by reconstruction. As risk factors for necrotising fasciitis include immunosuppression and chronic disease, it follows that these patients are very high risk.

Davoudian P, Flint NJ. Necrotising fasciitis. *Contin Educ Anaesth Crit Care Pain* 2012; 12: 245–50.

Question A71: Acute adrenal insufficiency

Causes of adrenal insufficiency in critically ill patients include:

A. Heparin-induced thrombocytopenia (HIT)
B. Sepsis
C. HIV
D. Addison's disease
E. Asthma

Answer: TTTTT

Short explanation

HIT can lead to bilateral adrenal vein thromboses resulting in failure of the adrenal glands. Abnormal function of the hypothalamic–pituitary–adrenal (HPA) axis is common in sepsis. The adrenal gland is the most commonly affected endocrine gland in HIV by organisms such as cytomegalovirus (CMV). Addison's disease is a cause of primary adrenal failure. Patients taking long-term synthetic glucocorticoids, even inhaled steroids, have a suppressed HPA axis.

Long explanation

Acute adrenal insufficiency is a problem encountered in many critically ill patients. The ability to increase cortisol production during times of physiological stress is important for the body to survive critical illness. The commonest cause of acute adrenal insufficiency in intensive care patients is sepsis and the systemic inflammatory response syndrome (SIRS). There are, however, particular patient groups who have adrenal insufficiency due to other causes.

Primary adrenal failure is caused by autoimmune disease (Addison's), adrenal infiltration (for example tuberculosis) or HIV. Tuberculosis has been overtaken by HIV as the commonest cause of primary adrenal failure. Infections such as cytomegalovirus (CMV), *Cryptococcus neoformans, Toxoplasma gondii* and fungi can all infect the adrenal glands and cause failure.

Secondary adrenal failure occurs in patients who are taking exogenous steroids for illnesses such as rheumatoid arthritis, inflammatory bowel disease and chronic lung conditions. The degree of adrenal suppression depends on the dose, frequency and length of treatment. Recovery of the adrenal glands can be delayed for up to 1 year if corticosteroids are taken for more than 30 days. Inhaled corticosteroids can suppress the HPA axis to varying degrees.

Whatever the cause, it is important to remember that the adrenal insufficiency may not be apparent during health. However, during times of stress, the adrenal glands may be unable to mount the normal response.

Marik P, Zaloga G. Adrenal insufficiency in the critically ill: a new look at an old problem. *Chest* 2002; 122: 1784–96.

Question A72: Cerebral blood flow measurement

With regards to the measurement of cerebral blood flow, which of the following are correct?

A. There is good-quality evidence that measurement of cerebral oxygenation ($PbrO_2$) can guide treatment and improve outcome in traumatic brain injury
B. If cerebrovascular autoregulation is lost the CPP target value should be between 50 and 70 mmHg
C. Cerebral oxygenation ($PbrO_2$) measured using a miniaturised Clark electrode correlates well with regional cerebral blood flow
D. It is recommended that patients with a severe but potentially survivable traumatic brain injury and an abnormal CT scan have ICP monitoring
E. Microdialysis catheters allow measurement of non-ischaemic forms of brain tissue hypoxia

Answer: FFTTT

Short explanation

There are currently only a few small and medium-sized studies which have assessed the usefulness of $PbrO_2$ in patients with brain injury. There is a need for larger randomised trials to determine the usefulness of this tool. If cerebral autoregulation is lost then it may be necessary to target cerebral perfusion pressure (CPP) values > 70 mmHg to ensure adequate tissue perfusion.

Long explanation

Raised intracranial pressure (ICP) is recognised as being a problem in a number of acute brain pathologies in the critically ill adult. It is one of a number of 'secondary insults' which can occur following traumatic brain injury and is also a problem in patients with spontaneous intracranial haemorrhage, hypoxic brain injury and fulminant hepatic failure. Raised ICP can lead to reduced cerebral perfusion and subsequent tissue damage.

The evidence for outcome benefits from active treatment of raised ICP is not strong, but randomised controlled trials would in all likelihood be denied ethical approval. Unfortunately, despite the fact that measurement of ICP allows the cerebral perfusion pressure (CPP) to be determined, this does not always reflect perfusion to the brain, either globally or regionally. Global perfusion may be adequate, but in areas where the brain is already damaged, perfusion, and more importantly oxygenation, may not be adequate.

There are a number of cerebral oxygenation ($PbrO_2$) measurement technologies being developed to help guide clinicians. The miniaturised Clark electrode allows measurement of cerebral oxygenation and also measures brain temperature, which is also known to be relevant in traumatic brain injury. Regional measurement of $PbrO_2$ has been shown to be more sensitive to changes in regional oxygenation than global measures such as arteriojugular venous oxygen content difference.

Prospective randomised controlled trials are required to determine if this costly and delicate technology can improve outcome in patients with brain injury.

Andrews P, Citerio G, Longhi L, *et al.* NICEM Consensus on neurological monitoring in acute neurological disease. *Intensive Care Med* 2008; 34: 1362–70.

Question A73: Clearance of solutes in RRT

Clearance of solutes during renal replacement therapy depends on:

A. Haemofiltration flow rate
B. Dialysis flow rate
C. Vascular access device properties
D. Solute molecular size
E. Membrane sieving coefficient

Answer: TTTTT

Short explanation

Solute clearance is dependent on molecular size, the membrane sieving coefficient, the circuit flow rate (and vascular access device properties), and the flow rates used for haemofiltration and dialysis fluids.

Long explanation

Renal replacement therapy (RRT) works by using a semi-permeable membrane to filter water and solutes via diffusion and ultrafiltration (convection). During diffusion, movement of solutes across the membrane is from a high concentration to a low concentration. Diffusion is limited by the thickness, surface area and diffusion coefficient of the membrane. A dialysis fluid flowing in the opposite direction to the blood maintains the concentration gradient. With ultrafiltration, water is pushed across a semi-permeable membrane under pressure and solutes follow. This is limited by the pore size of the membrane.

It is clear that both the haemofiltration and dialysis flow rate are important in determining clearance. The circuit flow will also depend on the lumen of the vascular access device and associated tubing. Kinked tubing will reduce or stop flow.

The molecular size of the solute to be filtered is also important, as is its protein binding. The membrane sieving coefficient determines the amount of solute that passes through the pores of the membrane. In general a molecular size of < 12 kDa is required for solutes to be filtered. Generally speaking, only the free fraction of a protein-bound substance will be filtered.

Hall NA, Fox AJ. Renal replacement therapies in critical care. *Contin Educ Anaesth Crit Care Pain* 2006; 6: 197–202.

Waldmann C, Soni N, Rhodes A. *Oxford Desk Reference: Critical Care*. Oxford: Oxford University Press, 2008; pp. 68–9.

Question A74: Platelet transfusion

Regarding platelet transfusions:

A. Platelets should be stored at 37 °C
B. Platelet transfusions should be ABO-compatible
C. Nearly one-third of transfused platelets will be sequestered in the spleen
D. One unit of platelet concentrate increases the platelet count by 10×10^9/l per m^2 body surface area
E. The shelf-life of platelets is 5 days

Answer: FTTTT

Short explanation

Platelets should be stored at 20–26 °C with constant agitation.

Long explanation

Units of platelets may be derived from a single donor or a pool of 4–6 donors. The higher the number of donors the greater the risk of adverse events, including infection or immune reactions such as transfusion-related lung injury (TRALI). Platelet packs are made of specialised polyolefin plastic which allows aeration of the platelets and extends the shelf-life to 5 days. Platelets should be stored at 20–26 °C with constant agitation.

One unit of platelet concentrate increases the platelet count by 10×10^9/l per m^2 body surface area, but nearly one-third of transfused platelets will be sequestered in the spleen. Platelets express HLA class I antigens, so in theory ABO compatibility is not required. As they are derived from whole blood, however, contamination with red or white blood cells can trigger an incompatibility reaction, and therefore platelet transfusion are always ABO- and rhesus-compatible. HLA-matched platelets should be used in patients with HLA antibodies (e.g. haematology or transplant patients).

Power I, Kam P. Physiology of blood. In *Priniciples of Physiology for the Anaesthetist*, 2nd edn. London: Hodder Arnold; p. 291.

Question A75: Metabolic acidosis

Physiological effects of a metabolic acidosis include:

A. Increased myocardial contractility
B. Tachycardia
C. Increased serum ionised calcium concentration
D. Shift of the oxyhaemoglobin dissociation curve to the left
E. Renal vasoconstriction

Answer: FTTFT

Short explanation

Acidosis will shift the oxyhaemoglobin dissociation curve to the right, increasing oxygen delivery to the tissues, and is associated with a reduction in myocardial contractility.

Long explanation

A metabolic acidosis is defined as a serum pH < 7.35 due to excess hydrogen ions or bicarbonate loss. Acidosis alters homeostasis via direct biochemical effects on physiological functions and indirect effects through alteration of endocrine or autonomic nervous system function.

Acidosis has a direct negative inotropic effect by inhibition of the slow inward calcium current and diminished calcium release from the sarcoplasmic reticulum. Acute respiratory acidosis causes more myocardial depression than acute metabolic acidosis. The myocardial depressant effect is offset by catecholamine release but this compensation is lost below a pH of 7.2. Catecholamine release results in a tachycardia and may precipitate atrial and ventricular tachycardias. Acidosis causes vasodilatation in coronary arteries, muscles and uterus but systemic, renal and splanchnic vasoconstriction accompanied by a reduction in gastrointestinal motility.

A metabolic acidosis will elicit a compensatory response with hyperventilation, which occurs more slowly than with a respiratory acidosis as the blood–brain barrier is more permeable to carbon dioxide than to hydrogen ions. Acidosis shifts the oxyhaemoglobin dissociation curve to the right, increasing oxygen delivery to the tissues. Hydrogen ions bind to albumin and in excess will displace calcium, thereby increasing serum ionised calcium concentrations. Chronic acidosis may lead to calcium mobilisation from bones. Intracellular potassium is exchanged for hydrogen ions, leading to a rise in serum potassium concentrations. Severe acidosis may lead to confusion and a drop in conscious level.

Power I, Kam P. Acid–base physiology. In *Priniciples of Physiology for the Anaesthetist*, 2nd edn. London: Hodder Arnold; pp. 251–68.

Question A76: Paracetamol overdose

With regards to the management of patients with paracetamol (acetaminophen) overdose, which of the following are correct?

A. The toxic metabolite of paracetamol which causes liver damage is glutathione
B. The antidote *N*-acetyl-cysteine is a sulphydryl donor
C. *N*-acetyl-cysteine should not be administered to patients presenting with staggered overdose
D. Most patients should be considered to be on the low-risk line of the nomogram
E. Liver transplantation should be considered in patients with high lactate at admission

Answer: FTFFT

Short explanation

The toxic metabolite of paracetamol is *N*-acetyl-p-benzoquinoneimine (NAPQI), which is only produced in large quantities once the normal conjugation pathway for paracetamol metabolism becomes saturated. The treatment nomogram is not useful in staggered overdose, and clinicians should have a low threshold for commencing acetyl-cysteine. There are no longer 'high-risk' and 'low-risk' lines. All patients should be treated on the same nomogram.

Long explanation

Paracetamol (acetaminophen) overdose remains a major cause of morbidity and mortality in the UK. It is still one of the leading causes of acute liver failure requiring transplantation, although in recent years the incidence has fallen, due to tighter controls on over-the-counter paracetamol preparations. Accidental overdose remains a problem: many cold and flu remedies contain paracetamol, and patients can unknowingly ingest toxic quantities if they take regular paracetamol in addition. Therapeutic doses vary with age and weight, and recently there has been a move to reducing doses administered to small adults (under 50 kg).

Peak plasma levels following an overdose will occur at approximately 4 hours. However, if the overdose is accidental over a number of days or staggered then it is impossible to determine when the peak level will occur. Similarly in patients with delayed gastric emptying, such as with co-administration of codeine, peak plasma levels may be delayed.

When paracetamol is ingested in overdose, its normal metabolism via conjugation becomes saturated and it is instead metabolised to *N*-acetyl-p-benzoquinoneimine (NAPQI), which is toxic to hepatocytes. NAPQI is conjugated with glutathione sulphydryl groups to a non-toxic metabolite. Patients who are at a higher risk of toxicity are those who have depleted levels of glutathione and those who have induced enzymes which catalyse the rate of formation of NAPQI. Patients with depleted levels of glutathione include those who have anorexia, cystic fibrosis, failure to thrive, AIDS, alcoholism and cachexia. Patients taking antiepileptic medication and excess alcohol are at risk of having enzyme induction. In the past these patients were treated along a different nomogram to those deemed 'low risk'. As of 2012 all patients are to be treated along the same nomogram, as assessment of risk factors in the acute setting is neither straightforward nor accurate.

N-acetyl-cysteine (NAC) should be administered intravenously according to the nomogram available in the *British National Formulary* (BNF). The dose is calculated based on the patient's weight. Non-allergic anaphylactic ('anaphylactoid') reactions are not uncommon, and patients can become pyrexial, tachycardic and short of breath. Bronchospasm and hypotension are rare. Usually the symptoms settle with antihistamine and fluid resuscitation and slowing of the rate of the initial acetylcysteine bolus. Fatal adverse reactions are extremely rare and usually related to incorrect dose calculation.

Supportive treatment of the patient includes fluid administration, glucose control and renal support if necessary. Further treatment may require referral to a regional liver unit for consideration of transplantation. This should be considered early in large overdoses, and in patients with any of the following:

- arterial pH < 7.3
- hepatic encephalopathy grade 3 or 4, creatinine > 300 μmol/l and prothrombin time > 100 seconds
- arterial lactate > 3.5 mmol/l on admission or > 3 mmol/l 24 hours after paracetamol ingestion or after fluid resuscitation. Most deaths are due to late presentation or accidental staggered overdoses.

Ferner R, Dear J, Bateman N. Management of paracetamol poisoning. *BMJ* 2011; 342: d2218.

Thompson G, Fatima S, Shah N, Kitching G, Waring W. Impact of amending the acetylcysteine marketing authorisation on treatment of paracetamol overdose. *ISRN Toxicology* 2013; 2013: ID 494357.

Question A77: Weaning from tracheostomy

Weaning methods for a patient with a temporary tracheostomy include:

A. Cuff deflation
B. Use of a 'Swedish nose'
C. Removal of heat and moisture exchange (HME) filter from a T-piece to reduce work of breathing
D. Downsizing to a minitracheostomy
E. Reducing the tracheostomy tube size

Answer: TTFTT

Short explanation

T-pieces often do not include an HME filter. However the patient is ventilated or given supplementary oxygen with a tracheostomy, it should be humidified to reduce secretion drying and risk of tube obstruction.

Long explanation

Tracheostomy is a common procedure in intensive care. Once confined to patients with upper airway obstruction or malignancy, it now has numerous indications including prolonged mechanical ventilation, weaning from ventilation, failure of airway protective reflexes, secretion management and obstructive sleep apnoea.

Management of the patient with a tracheostomy includes meticulous hygiene measures for the tracheostomy, with the use of an inner cannula where possible, good oral hygiene, lung-protective ventilation and physiotherapy. Regardless of the means of delivery to the patient with a tracheostomy, gas-flow should be humidified to reduce secretion drying and risk of tube obstruction. The patient should be assessed regularly for the ability to wean from the ventilator, and assessments should be undertaken to assess swallow safety. Communication aids or the use of speaking valves where possible greatly contribute to patient wellbeing.

Weaning from a tracheostomy may be achieved in a number of ways. Common techniques include cuff deflation, use of a fenestrated tube, downsizing of the tube or use of a minitracheostomy. Tracheostomy tubes should generally be changed monthly after insertion to prevent the formation of granulation tissue around the tube. The tract forms around the tube within 7–10 days of insertion; tube changes before this may be fraught with difficulty.

Cook T, Woodall N, Frerk C. *Major Complications of Airway Management in the United Kingdom*. 4th National Audit Project of The Royal College of Anaesthetists and The Difficult Airway Society. London: Royal College of Anaesthetists, 2011.

Regan K, Hunt K. Tracheostomy management. *Contin Educ Anaesth Crit Care Pain* 2008; 8: 31–5.

Question A78: Refeeding syndrome

With regards to refeeding syndrome, which of the following are correct?

A. The hallmark biochemical feature is hyperphosphataemia
B. During starvation, plasma electrolytes are usually maintained in the normal range
C. Refeeding syndrome does not usually occur if starvation has been less than 14 days
D. Refeeding syndrome does not occur if patients receive total parenteral nutrition
E. Patients with anorexia nervosa and alcohol dependence are at high risk of refeeding syndrome

Answer: FTFFT

Short explanation

The hallmark biochemical feature is hypophosphataemia, in addition to hypokalaemia and hypomagnesaemia. Refeeding syndrome can occur following short periods of starvation (< 5 days) in high-risk patients. Refeeding syndrome occurs in patients receiving both enteral and parenteral nutrition.

Long explanation

Refeeding syndrome describes the dangerous shifts in fluid and electrolytes seen when malnourished patients receive artificial or oral feeding. In severe cases, patients can have respiratory and cardiac failure, which may lead to death. The hallmark biochemical feature is hypophosphataemia, usually accompanied by hypokalaemia and hypomagnesaemia. Intensive care patients are at a higher risk of refeeding syndrome than general hospital inpatients, because they are more likely to have periods of starvation and receive artificial nutrition.

Refeeding syndrome arises from the way in which the body adapts to starvation. The brain adapts to use ketone bodies as its main energy source and the liver decreases its rate of gluconeogenesis to preserve protein. Intracellular cations move to the extracellular space to maintain normal plasma concentrations of potassium, magnesium and phosphate. This results in shrinkage of the intracellular volume and reduced total body stores of these electrolytes. Upon refeeding, insulin levels increase, stimulating fat, glycogen and protein synthesis. These processes all require electrolytes such as phosphate and magnesium. Insulin also stimulates potassium transport into the cells. This results in a reduction in the plasma levels, which can be profound. In addition to these electrolytes, carbohydrate metabolism requires thiamine, which is often deficient in patients who are malnourished. Thiamine levels can therefore become extremely low in refeeding syndrome.

Mehanna HM, Moledina J, Travis J. Refeeding syndrome: what it is, and how to prevent and treat it. *BMJ* 2008; 336: 1495–8.

Rio A, Whelan K, Goff L, Reidlinger D, Smeeton N. Occurrence of refeeding syndrome in adults started on artificial nutrition support: prospective cohort study. *BMJ Open* 2013; 3 (1): 3e002173.

Question A79: Pleural effusions

Pleural effusions are usually transudates in the following conditions:

A. Hypoalbuminaemia
B. Pneumonia
C. Squamous cell lung cancer
D. Right ventricular failure
E. Pulmonary tuberculosis

Answer: TFFFF

Short explanation

Transudative pleural effusions are due to systemic imbalance of Starling forces. Common causes include left ventricular failure, hepatic cirrhosis, hypoalbuminaemia and nephrotic syndrome. Exudative effusions are due to local disease and inflammation. Common causes include pneumonia, malignancy, pulmonary embolism, tuberculosis and autoimmune disease.

Long explanation

The distinction between transudative and exudative pleural effusions is based on gross appearance and laboratory analysis of the fluid (Light's criteria). Transudates are usually clear and have low protein (< 0.5 the value of serum protein levels) and lactate dehydrogenase (LDH) (< 0.6 serum LDH) levels, whereas exudates are often cloudy with high protein and LDH levels.

Transudates are caused by systemic imbalance of Starling forces leading to an increased net flow of fluid from the pulmonary capillaries to the pleural space. Conditions which increase hydrostatic pressure (e.g. left ventricular failure) or reduce colloid oncotic pressure (e.g. hypoalbuminaemia) are associated with transudates. Common causes include left ventricular failure, hepatic cirrhosis, hypoalbuminaemia and nephrotic syndrome.

Exudates are caused by local disruption or inflammation of the pleura leading to abnormal pleural fluid formation. Common causes of exudative pleural effusions are pneumonia, malignancy (lung, breast, haematological), pulmonary embolus, pancreatitis, autoimmune disease and tuberculosis. Further laboratory analysis may help distinguish between different aetiologies: low glucose suggests infection or malignancy; pH < 7.2 suggests empyema; high amylase suggests pancreatitis or oesophageal rupture.

Sahn S. The differential diagnosis of pleural effusions. *Western J Med* 1982; 137: 99–108.

Question A80: Levosimendan

Levosimendan:

A. Is a synthetic catecholamine
B. Causes inotropy and vasodilatation
C. Antagonises intracellular calcium
D. Increases myocardial oxygen demand
E. Is not affected by concomitant β-blocker use

Answer: FTFFT

Short explanation

Levosimendan is an inodilator drug that acts directly on the mechanism of contraction, by increasing the sensitivity of troponin C to calcium in the myocyte. Contractility increases without increasing intracellular calcium levels or affecting diastolic relaxation. Secondary effects on peripheral potassium channels cause vasodilatation and hence reduced cardiac work.

Long explanation

Standard inotropes act to increase contractility by a common final pathway that leads to increased myocardial calcium levels by manipulating the sympathetic stimulatory pathway. This is achieved by stimulation of cell-surface receptors (e.g. dobutamine, β-adrenergic receptors) or by increasing levels of intracellular secondary messengers (e.g. enoximone, a phosphodiesterase inhibitor, preventing breakdown of cAMP). Secondary messenger production is dependent on the interaction between ligand and cell-surface receptor, which can be blocked by other medications (e.g. β-blockers) or reduced by down-regulation.

Levosimendan is an inodilator drug that has a mode of action distinct from other current treatments, bypassing these pathways and acting directly on the mechanism of contraction. Its primary action is to increase the sensitivity of troponin C to calcium in the myocyte, which increases contractility without increasing intracellular calcium levels or affecting diastolic relaxation. Secondary effects on peripheral potassium channels cause vasodilatation and hence reduced cardiac work. Cardiac output is increased without increasing myocardial oxygen demand.

Levosimendan has been shown to be more effective than dobutamine at improving cardiac output and reducing morbidity in decompensated heart failure, although no mortality benefit has been shown. It is also used in left ventricular failure secondary to myocardial infarction, in cardiogenic shock, and in acute heart failure in patients treated with β-blockers

Although no major trials have shown a significant improvement in mortality compared with other therapies, there is enough evidence of haemodynamic improvement to consider levosimendan as part of the treatment of acute heart failure and cardiogenic shock.

Mathieu S, Craig G. Levosimendan in the treatment of acute heart failure, cardiogenic and septic shock: a critical review. *J Intensive Care Soc* 2012; 12: 15–24.

Question A81: Oxygen therapy effects

Concerning the effects of oxygen therapy, which of the following are correct?

A. Acute tracheobronchitis is a late sign of oxygen toxicity
B. Central nervous system oxygen toxicity occurs with hyperbaric oxygen therapy
C. Acute tracheobronchitis is unusual in patients receiving normobaric oxygen therapy
D. Oxygen-induced diffuse alveolar damage is pathologically similar to ARDS
E. Acute tracheobronchitis and CNS oxygen toxicity are usually reversible complications

Answer: FTFTT

Short explanation

Acute tracheobronchitis is the earliest sign of pulmonary oxygen toxicity and is seen in patients receiving high levels (> 50%) of normobaric oxygen therapy. It can start to develop as early as 4 hours after commencing therapy with > 95% oxygen. It is also seen in patients receiving hyperbaric oxygen therapy, where it occurs as early as 3 hours into treatment.

Long explanation

The toxic effects of oxygen can be divided into those seen with normobaric oxygen therapy and those seen predominantly with hyperbaric oxygen therapy. For critical care physicians, it is more relevant to concentrate on the potential side effects seen when administering high levels of normobaric oxygen. There is also a lot of controversy surrounding this subject, particularly in specialised areas such as neonatal care. In resuscitation of the newborn, there is still little consensus over whether room air or supplementary oxygen should be used. The current evidence suggests that there is little benefit of hyperoxia in this group and there may be a higher incidence of severe hypoxic ischaemia encephalopathy if high levels of oxygen are administered. Whether air is actually superior to oxygen is as yet unclear.

When adult patients are given high levels of oxygen (> 50%) there is a latent period of up to 24 hours where no symptoms are present. After this time, symptoms of acute tracheobronchitis can develop. These include tickling sensations in the throat, substernal distress, inspiratory pain, cough and retrosternal burning sensations. Tracheal secretions will also be increased. The changes usually resolve within a few days after stopping oxygen therapy. Diffuse alveolar damage occurs when patients are exposed to high levels of oxygen for longer periods of time. Pathologically, the characteristics are similar to those seen in acute respiratory distress syndrome (ARDS), and the damage can result in chronic lung disease. It is, however, difficult to distinguish between the permanent oxygen-related lung damage, the effects of mechanical ventilation, and of the effects of the disease process itself, such as ARDS.

Hyperbaric oxygen therapy can lead to CNS and ophthalmic complications. CNS signs include dizziness, headache, tinnitus and twitching. The most dramatic effect is a generalised tonic–clonic seizure, which is usually self-limiting. Ophthalmic effects include a reversible myopia and cataract formation after multiple sessions of hyperbaric oxygen therapy. Hyperbaric oxygen therapy sessions are limited to short sessions, usually less than 2 hours, and at pressures below the threshold for CNS toxicity.

Bitterman H. Bench-to-bedside review: oxygen as a drug. *Crit Care* 2009; 13: 205.

Question A82: Arrhythmia management

With regards to the management of arrhythmias on the intensive care unit, which of the following are correct?

A. Excessive bradycardia can lead to torsades de pointes
B. Sotalol can precipitate life-threatening ventricular arrhythmias due to QT interval shortening
C. Magnesium should be administered for treatment of torsades de pointes only when the plasma level is low
D. Procainamide is useful for the treatment of all types of ventricular tachycardias
E. Atropine can be administered to prevent polymorphic ventricular tachycardia

Answer: TFFFT

Short explanation

Sotalol prolongs the QT interval and this can lead to the development of torsades de pointes. Magnesium has been used successfully in the treatment of resistant torsades de pointes even when the plasma level is normal. Procainamide is useful for the treatment of monomorphic ventricular tachycardia but can prolong the QT interval and lead to torsades de pointes so should be avoided in patients with either of these conditions.

Long explanation

Cardiac arrhythmias are common in patients on the intensive care unit. There are many possible precipitating factors. Myocardial ischaemia due to pre-existing coronary artery disease can become relevant in patients with sepsis or following major surgery. Other factors include electrolyte abnormalities, acid–base disturbance and administration of pro-arrhythmic agents. It is important to distinguish between the haemodynamically stable and unstable patient, as this will affect the choice of treatment and the urgency of administration.

Atrial fibrillation is by far the commonest arrhythmia encountered in hospital patients, and treatment options include electrical DC cardioversion, intravenous amiodarone, β-blockers and digoxin. Rate control is probably the key to treatment, although rhythm control may be more important in patients with poor ventricular function who rely on atrial systole for adequate cardiac output.

Ventricular tachycardias include polymorphic VT and torsades de pointes. These arrhythmias are likely to deteriorate into ventricular fibrillation, cardiac arrest and death if they are not treated promptly. Haemodynamically unstable patients should undergo immediate DC cardioversion, whereas stable patients may be managed pharmacologically. Monomorphic VT should be treated with amiodarone intravenously. Procainamide is an alternative. Polymorphic VT is often caused by electrolyte abnormalities, myocardial ischaemia, QT prolongation or some antiarrhythmic agents. These factors should be considered and reversed if present. Atropine or overdrive pacing (atrial or ventricular) can be administered to increase the heart rate and suppress the polymorphic VT. Intravenous amiodarone is also indicated in this situation. In patients with arrhythmias due to acute myocardial ischaemia, reperfusion therapy is indicated and pharmacological agents may not be necessary.

Torsades de pointes is polymorphic VT with prolonged QT interval. It can be precipitated by administration of drugs which prolong the QT interval in susceptible patients (those with already lengthened QT interval such as in Romano–Ward syndrome). It is often paroxysmal and preceded by a slow base rhythm. Treatment involves discontinuation of the offending agent, correction of electrolyte abnormalities and administration of magnesium. A 2 g bolus followed by another 2 g bolus can be administered, although this recommendation has not been derived from randomised controlled trials.

Trappe HJ. Treating critical supraventricular and ventricular arrhythmias. *J Emerg Trauma Shock* 2010; 3: 143–52.

Question A83: Syndrome of inappropriate antidiuretic hormone secretion

Regarding the diagnosis and management of the syndrome of inappropriate antidiuretic hormone secretion (SIADH), which of the following are correct?

A. Patients are usually hypovolaemic
B. Urine osmolality is inappropriately high
C. Demeclocycline can be administered
D. Urinary sodium is usually > 40 mmol/l
E. Plasma uric acid levels are usually high

Answer: FTTTF

Short explanation

The commonest cause of hyponatraemia in hospital patients is SIADH. Patients with SIADH are usually euvolaemic or slightly hypervolaemic, although this is not detectable clinically and does not cause oedema. Uric acid levels are usually low, probably due to plasma volume expansion.

Long explanation

Hyponatraemia is a common finding in hospital patients and can be a significant cause of morbidity and mortality, depending upon the underlying aetiology. Significant hyponatraemia (< 125 mmol/l) has been shown to be an independent risk factor for mortality irrespective of the underlying cause. Critical care patients are at an increased risk of hyponatraemia due to the high incidence of hepatic, renal and cardiac failure in these patients. In addition they may have head injuries, be receiving diuretics, have received intravenous fluid therapy or be relatively deficient in glucocorticoids and mineralocorticoids. All of these scenarios can contribute to disordered fluid and electrolyte balance leading to hyponatraemia.

The syndrome of inappropriate antidiuretic hormone secretion (SIADH) is almost certainly not a single condition, and there are variations in the biochemical and physiological findings depending on the aetiology. SIADH is classed as euvolaemic hyponatraemia, although the plasma volume is often slightly expanded due to suppression of plasma renin and elevation of plasma natriuretic peptides. Other causes of euvolaemic hyponatraemia include hypotonic fluid administration (including following bladder irrigation during urological procedures) and inappropriate fluid replacement following exercise. Adrenocorticotrophic hormone (ACTH) deficiency can also mimic SIADH and is thought to be quite common among patients with head injury, due to pituitary trauma. A short synacthen test or early-morning cortisol level should be performed in suspected cases.

The diagnostic criteria for SIADH have changed over the years but now include five criteria. First, hypo-osmolality must be present, with serum osmolality < 280 mosm/kg or plasma sodium concentration < 134 mmol/l. Second, there must be inappropriate urinary concentration for hyponatraemia (Uosm > 100 mosm/kg).

Third, the patient must be clinically euvolaemic. Fourth, there must be elevated urinary sodium (> 40 mosm/l) with normal dietary salt and water intake. Finally, hypothyroidism, diuretics and glucocorticoid deficiency need to be excluded as alternative causes, the latter particularly in neurosurgical conditions.

Water restriction remains the mainstay of treatment for SIADH. Fluid restriction to 800 ml per day is generally recommended – and this includes all fluid, including that found in food. Unfortunately patients will often feel inappropriately thirsty, which can lead to non-compliance. Hypertonic saline and loop diuretics may be used in the short term for correction of sodium but are unlikely to be useful in the longer term in patients with a cause of ongoing SIADH (e.g. lung carcinoma). Demeclocycline causes nephrogenic diabetes insipidus as a side effect and so can be used to treat SIADH. It can cause renal failure and takes 2–3 days to take effect but is a potential option for long-term treatment. Lithium has a similar effect but is not useful clinically due to the high risk of toxicity and the necessity for levels to be checked regularly.

Hannon MJ, Thompson CJ. The syndrome of inappropriate antidiuretic hormone: prevalence, causes and consequences. *Eur J Endocrinol* 2010; 162: S5–12.

Zietse R, van der Lubbe N, Hoorn EJ. Current and future treatment options in SIADH. *NDT Plus* 2009; 2 (Suppl 3): iii12–19.

Question A84: Open abdomen

With regards to leaving a patient with an open abdomen, which of the following are correct?

A. A Bogota bag allows active drainage of fluid out of the abdomen
B. Negative-pressure devices have been shown to be superior to a Bogota bag
C. Complications of leaving a patient with an open abdomen include the development of ventral hernias and intestinal fistulas
D. An open-abdomen technique is recommended in patients with acute pancreatitis and high intra-abdominal pressure
E. Abdominal compartment syndrome can recur in patients who have undergone decompressive laparotomy and have an open abdomen

Answer: FTTFT

Short explanation

A Bogota bag is a type of temporary abdominal closure system which has been used extensively in clinical practice. It is a plastic bag sutured into the borders of the laparotomy wound. It does not allow active drainage of fluid out of the abdomen. Decompressive laparotomy in patients with acute pancreatitis has a high mortality rate and should only be used as a last resort once medical management has failed.

Long explanation

Intra-abdominal hypertension and abdominal compartment syndrome have become well-recognised complications in critically ill surgical and trauma patients. Patients with severe acute pancreatitis and burns can also develop these complications. Increasing recognition of these conditions has led to improved monitoring of abdominal pressures and earlier intervention in suspected cases.

Many patients who undergo surgery are left with a laparostomy, or 'open abdomen', to try to prevent abdominal hypertensive complications. This is most common in patients undergoing emergency laparotomy for ruptured abdominal aortic aneurysm or ischaemic colitis.

In the past the open wound was covered with a sterile plastic bag or a 'Bogota' bag, which is sutured into the skin or fascia of the anterior abdominal wall. This does not routinely allow drainage of fluid from the abdomen unless an outlet is provided. More recently, evidence has shown that vacuum-assisted closure devices improve outcome in patients with an open abdomen. The devices allow active drainage of fluid and exudate out of the abdominal cavity, which can help reduce oedema and intra-abdominal pressure further.

The open-abdomen technique is not equally effective in all patients with abdominal compartment syndrome. Evidence has shown that the mortality rate is very high in patients with severe acute pancreatitis, and this method cannot be routinely recommended for these patients.

There are a number of complications that can occur in patients with an open abdomen. Early complications include recurrence of intra-abdominal hypertension, particularly when there are adhesions and also bacterial infection. Later complications include the development of enteric fistulae and anterior abdominal wall hernias as the abdominal wall closes.

Batacchi S, Matano S, Nella A, *et al*. Vacuum assisted closure device enhances recovery of critically ill patients following emergency surgical procedures. *Crit Care* 2009; 13: R194.

De Waele J, Hoste E, Blot S, Decruyenaere J, Colardyn F. Intra-abdominal hypertension in patients with severe acute pancreatitis. *Crit Care* 2005; 9: R452–7.

Mentula P, Leppäniemi A. Prophylactic open abdomen in patients with postoperative intra-abdominal hypertension. *Crit Care* 2010; 14: 111.

Question A85: Aspirin overdose

Which of the following statements about the management of aspirin overdose are correct?

A. Plasma levels should be measured 4 hours or more after ingestion
B. Plasma levels > 300 mg/l indicate severe toxicity and are likely to require haemodialysis
C. Tinnitus is a late sign of overdose and indicates severe toxicity
D. During urine alkalinisation plasma pH should not exceed 7.65
E. Urinary alkalinisation should be continued even if haemodialysis is commenced

Answer: TFFFT

Short explanation

Plasma levels of 300–500 mg/l indicate mild toxicity. Plasma levels of 500–700 mg/l indicate moderate toxicity. Plasma levels > 750 mg/l indicate severe toxicity. Tinnitus is an early sign of overdose and indicates mild toxicity. Plasma pH should not exceed 7.55 during urine alkalinisation.

Long explanation

Aspirin (salicylate or salicylic acid) overdose has reduced dramatically over the last few decades. This has mirrored the reduction in paracetemol overdose, brought about by tighter controls on over-the-counter purchase of analgesia tablets. However, it is still a potentially serious condition, particularly when large overdoses are taken. Aspirin toxicity can be graded as mild, moderate or severe, based on plasma levels measured after a minimum of 4 hours following ingestion.

Plasma levels of 300–500 mg/l indicate mild toxicity. Plasma levels of 500–700 mg/l indicate moderate toxicity. Plasma levels > 750 mg/l indicate severe toxicity. Staggered overdoses, where tablets are ingested over a longer period instead of all at once, and ingestion of enteric coated tablets renders these values unhelpful. Ingestion of enteric coated tablets can mean that peak plasma levels are not reached for up to 12 hours following ingestion. In this circumstance upper GI endoscopy can be useful to wash out and remove undigested tablets.

In mild and early overdose symptoms may include lethargy, nausea, tinnitus and dizziness. As toxicity progresses, tachypnoea, hyperthermia, sweating, dehydration, incoordination and restlessness develop. In severe toxicity, convulsions, cerebral oedema, oliguria, renal failure, cardiovascular failure and coma can develop. Aspirin is an acid and leads to metabolic acidosis in moderate and severe poisoning. Elimination is increased by alkalinisation of the urine; an increase in urine pH from 5 to 8 will increase elimination by 10–20 times. A urine pH of 7.5 or higher should be aimed for. Sodium bicarbonate should be administered to achieve these values.

In severe poisoning there may be oliguria, which results in slow elimination of salicylate despite adequate alkalinisation. Haemodialysis is the next step. It reduces morbidity and mortality and should be considered in all patients. In particular, children, the elderly, and those with metabolic acidosis, coma, seizures, acute kidney injury or pulmonary oedema should be considered early for haemodialysis.

Dargan P, Wallace C, Jones A. An evidence based flowchart to guide the management of acute salicylate (aspirin) overdose. *Emerg Med J* 2002; 19: 206–9.

Question A86: Heparin-induced thrombocytopenia

With regards to heparin-induced thrombocytopenia (HIT), which of the following are correct?

A. A reduction in the platelet count of > 25% after day 14 of heparin exposure strongly suggests HIT
B. Severe thrombocytopenia (platelet count < 15×10^9/l) is common in HIT
C. New arterial or venous thrombosis may occur before thrombocytopenia in patients with HIT
D. The presence of anti-PF4/heparin antibodies is diagnostic for HIT
E. The platelet count will generally recover within 2 weeks once heparin is discontinued

Answer: FFTFT

Short explanation

Typically patients with HIT develop thrombocytopenia between day 5 and 14 following heparin exposure. The platelet count is usually decreased by > 50% from baseline, although the severity of thrombocytopenia is not as severe as in other immune thrombocytopenic disorders. The presence of antibodies to heparin or PF4 on laboratory testing is not diagnostic, as not all antibodies are pathogenic.

Long explanation

Heparin-induced thrombocytopenia (HIT) is an immune-mediated condition which has potentially fatal consequences. Surgical and female patients are at a higher risk of developing the condition. The clinical syndrome is characterised by significant thrombocytopenia (platelet count < 50% of baseline) and spontaneous venous and arterial thromboses in 30–70% of patients. The platelet count does not usually fall as low as in other immunogenic thrombocytopenic conditions and rarely falls below 20×10^9/l. Thrombosis can occur in the absence of thrombocytopenia or before it develops. The risk of thrombosis appears to be related to the magnitude of the platelet fall and not to the absolute number. Bleeding is rare.

In the majority of cases, the condition is triggered by exposure to unfractionated and low-molecular-weight heparin within the preceding 5–14 days. HIT is much commoner with unfractionated heparin. As it is an antibody-mediated response, some patients will develop the clinical syndrome earlier than 5 days following exposure to heparin if they have previously been exposed in the preceding 100 days and produced antibodies. This means that the thrombocytopenia can occur abruptly and patients may feel unwell immediately following administration of heparin, with fever, shivering and skin lesions at the injection site.

Heparin interacts with a platelet-activating protein, platelet factor 4 (PF4). This creates the heparin-PF4 antigen, which can provoke an antibody response. The IgG antibodies to the heparin-PF4 antigen attach to the surface of platelets, leading to activation, aggregation and further acceleration of the process. This results in thrombocytopenia and thrombosis.

Diagnosis involves using the '4T' scoring system followed by locally available laboratory investigations. The 4T score was developed as a screening tool in the diagnosis of HIT; it calculates a score of between 0 ad 8, with the higher the score the more likely the diagnosis of HIT. In an analysis of the reliability of the 4T score, a low score had a negative predictive value of 0.998, making it an extremely useful negative screening tool. Laboratory investigations are generally good at excluding the diagnosis, but positive test results in isolation do not necessarily confirm the diagnosis.

Treatment of suspected or confirmed cases includes stopping all administration of heparin (including heparin flushes) and switching to prophylactic danaparoid in the case of suspected HIT. Thrombosis can occur following cessation of heparin. In patients with confirmed HIT, therapeutic doses of anticoagulant may be required, particularly if thrombosis is confirmed. All future administration of heparin must be avoided.

Sakr Y. Heparin-induced thrombocytopenia in the ICU: an overview. *Crit Care* 2011; 15: 211.

Selleng K, Warkentin T, Greinacher A. Heparin-induced thrombocytopenia in intensive care patients. *Crit Care Med* 2007; 35: 1165–76.

Question A87: Drug-induced nephrotoxicity

Mechanisms of drug-induced nephrotoxicity include:

A. Cyclosporin, constriction of efferent arteriole
B. Non-steroidal anti-inflammatory drugs (NSAIDs), crystal formation
C. Aminoglycosides, renal cell toxicity
D. Rifampicin, rhabdomyolysis
E. Radiocontrast dye, renal cell toxicity

Answer: TFTFT

Short explanation

NSAIDs are associated with altered intraglomerular haemodynamics or chronic interstitial nephritis. Rifampicin is associated with acute interstitial nephritis (an idiosyncratic allergic reaction, non-dose-dependent).

Long explanation

Drug-induced nephrotoxicity may be responsible for up to 20% of cases of acute kidney injury. Patient factors increasing the likelihood of drug-induced nephropathy include increasing age, underlying renal insufficiency, hypovolaemia, diabetes, heart failure and sepsis. The use of alternative non-nephrotoxic drugs, dose adjustment and monitoring of serum plasma levels help to decrease the incidence of nephrotoxicity. All patients should have their renal function monitored before, during and after treatment with nephrotoxic medications, and modifiable risk factors such as hypovolaemia should be corrected. The toxic effects of drugs are mediated in the following ways:

- Altered intraglomerular haemodynamics
  - non-steroidal anti-inflammatory drugs (NSAIDs)
  - ACE inhibitors and angiotensin receptor blockers
  - calcineurin inhibitors (e.g. cyclosporin, tacrolimus)
- Tubular cell toxicity
  - aminoglycoside antibiotics
  - amphotericin B
  - antiretrovirals
  - radiology contrast dye
- Inflammation
  - gold
  - hydralazine
  - lithium
  - allopurinol
  - antibiotics (β-lactams, rifampicin, sulfonamides; vancomycin; aciclover)
  - diuretics (loop and thiazide)
  - NSAIDs
  - phenytoin
  - proton-pump inhibitors
  - ranitidine
- Crystal nephropathy
  - ampicillin
  - ciprofloxacin
  - antivirals (e.g. aciclovir, foscarnet, ganciclovir)
  - methotrexate
- Rhabdomyolysis
  - statins
  - drugs of abuse (ketamine, heroin, cocaine and methamphetamine)
- Thrombotic microangiopathy
  - clopidogrel
  - ticlopidine
  - cyclosporin
  - quinine

Bellomo R. Acute renal failure. In Bersten AD, Soni N. *Oh's Intensive Care Manual*, 6th edn. Edinburgh: Butterworth-Heinemann, 2009; pp. 509–14.

Question A88: MDMA

Which of the following statements about MDMA are correct?

A. It is a Class A drug in the UK
B. Intake can lead to a clinical syndrome similar to malignant hyperthermia

C. Inhibition of ADH can result in water overload and hyponatraemia
D. Peak core body temperature > 39 °C usually results in development of rhabdomyolysis
E. Serotonin, norepinephrine and dopamine reuptake inhibition in the central nervous system results in euphoria

Answer: TTFFT

Short explanation

MDMA (3,4-methylenedioxymethamphetamine) or ecstasy stimulates increased antidiuretic hormone (ADH) secretion from the posterior pituitary, which can result in severe hyponatraemia. Other effects include a hyperthermic syndrome that can lead to rhabdomyolysis, disseminated intravascular coagulation (DIC) and multi-organ failure. Temperatures > 42 °C are highly likely to result in death.

Long explanation

MDMA, more commonly known as ecstasy, is a frequently ingested, Class A illegal recreational drug. Some statistics suggest that up to 2 million tablets are consumed weekly in the UK alone. Tablets are often sold containing other chemicals such as amphetamine, methamphetamine and ketamine.

MDMA causes increased release and reduced reuptake of serotonin (5-HT), dopamine and norepinephrine in the central nervous system. This causes improved mood and euphoria, but also affects the regulation of body temperature, appetite, thirst and the neuroendocrine system. Increased levels of prolactin, adrenocorticotrophic hormone (ACTH), cortisol and antidiuretic hormone (ADH) are seen following ingestion. Increased levels of ADH can result in water retention and hyponatraemia, which can lead to cerebral oedema and death. This is worsened when people drink large volumes of water and sweat excessively.

The syndrome of hyperthermia, rhabdomyolysis, DIC and multi-organ failure is well described. Risk factors include dancing and being in a hot and crowded environment. The syndrome probably has some overlap with malignant hyperthermia, neuroleptic malignant syndrome and severe heat stroke. Prognosis is poor if intensive care is not instituted early, and a peak core body temperature > 42 °C is strongly predictive of poor outcome. Cooling measures and rehydration are as important as organ support. Dantrolene has been used, although evidence is not strong.

Serotonin syndrome can also be provoked by ingestion of MDMA, again with overlap with the hyperthermic syndromes. Sudden adult death is also commoner in this population, probably related to cardiac arrhythmias. Liver failure can occur in isolation, although it is usually associated with the hyperthermic syndrome and multi-organ failure. A common cause of death in people ingesting ecstasy is trauma, particularly due to driving while under the influence of drugs.

Organ support should be commenced as early as possible, with consideration of early invasive monitoring and renal replacement therapy. The sympathomimetic effects of MDMA can be treated with labetolol due to its α- and β-blocking properties. Cooling should be active and aggressive. Alkalinisation of urine may protect the kidneys from myoglobinuria. Fluid restriction should be started in patients with hyponatraemia. Patients with serotonin syndrome should be paralysed, intubated and ventilated.

Hall A, Henry J. Acute toxic effects of 'ecstasy' (MDMA) and related compounds: overview of pathophysiology and clinical management. *Br J Anaesth* 2006; 96: 678–85.

Question A89: Subarachnoid haemorrhage investigations

Which of the following investigations can be used to diagnose or predict cerebral vasospasm following subarachnoid haemorrhage?

A. Digital subtraction angiography (DSA)
B. CT angiography (CTA)
C. CT perfusion imaging (CTP)
D. Transcranial Doppler ultrasonography (TCD)
E. Intracortical EEG

Answer: TTTTT

Short explanation

Neurological deterioration following subarachnoid haemorrhage has a number of underlying causes other than rebleeding. Vasospasm is a problematic complication but is a radiological diagnosis. DSA is the gold-standard investigation for detection of arterial narrowing. CTA is up to 95% specific and correlates well with DSA. The other modalities are inferior to DSA and CTA but are still of value.

Long explanation

Delayed neurological deterioration (DND) can occur following subarachnoid haemorrhage (SAH). It is a significant cause of morbidity and mortality that is not due to rebleeding. There are a number of causes of this, including delayed cerebral ischaemia (DCI), hypoxia, electrolyte disturbance, infection, fever, hydrocephalus, convulsive and non-convulsive seizures. These should be excluded in all patients with deteriorating neurological signs. Patients with higher-grade SAH are at higher risk of complications, which are less likely to be detected clinically because ongoing coma or sedatives can mask the clinical signs.

DCI is a clinical diagnosis, whereas vasospasm is a radiological diagnosis made when arterial narrowing is seen on imaging investigations. Both can be asymptomatic or can lead to cerebral infarction. DSA is the gold-standard investigation for vasospasm but CTA has been shown to correlate well with DSA in some studies. Neither of these modalities assess the adequacy of perfusion, and so CT perfusion imaging can be used to give some indication of this and can help predict the need for endovascular intervention. It does not image the posterior fossa particularly well, and clinical studies have so far been small. TCD has relatively good specificity but only moderate sensitivity compared to DSA. It has been used routinely in some centres for a long time, and as a non-invasive investigation it is quite safe. EEG findings of reduced alpha variability have been shown to be indicative of DCI, and intracortical EEG may be superior to surface EEG. Brain tissue oxygen monitoring and cerebral microdialysis have so far been used only in small studies.

Diringer MN, Bleck TP, Claude Hemphill J, *et al.* Critical care management of patients following aneurysmal subarachnoid hemorrhage: recommendations from the Neurocritical Care Society's Multidisciplinary Consensus Conference. *Neurocrit Care* 2011; 15: 211–40.

Question A90: Ionising radiation

With regards to ionising radiation:

A. 1 gray (Gy) is equivalent to 1 sievert (Sv) when comparing radiation dose from alpha particles

B. Haematopoietic dysfunction is the first manifestation of acute radiation syndrome
C. The risk of malignancy is dependent on the dose
D. Ultraviolet light is an example of non-ionising radiation
E. The dose rate for radiation decreases as the square of the distance from the source

Answer: FFFTT

Short explanation

1 Gy is equivalent to 20 Sv when comparing radiation dose from alpha particles. Gastrointestinal upset is the first sign of acute radiation syndrome, and the risk of malignancy with dose is a stochastic effect.

Long explanation

Radiation is energy in the form of particles or electromagnetic waves, and it is classified as non-ionising or ionising.

Non-ionising radiation includes light, ultraviolet and infrared radiation, and will generally only cause tissue damage by the transfer of thermal energy, as the energy is generally only sufficient to cause atomic vibration. Conversely, ionising radiation has a shorter wavelength and sufficient energy to displace electrons, forming ions and free radicals. Examples of ionising radiation are:

- alpha particles: do not penetrate skin but harmful if ingested, e.g. polonium-210
- beta particles: penetrate subcutaneous tissues, e.g. iodine-131
- x-rays/gamma rays: penetrate through tissue

Ionising radiation damages tissue directly (DNA damage, cell membrane disruption) and indirectly (free radical generation).

Radiation exposure may be deterministic (i.e. dose dependent – as seen in the reduction in blood counts) or stochastic (i.e. the probability of occurrence, but not the severity, is determined by the dose – as in the development of malignancy).

Radiosensitivity refers to the difference in tissue damage seen with a radiation dose to different organs. Rapidly dividing cells are the most sensitive to damage.

Radiation dose is described by two units:

- The gray (Gy): the absorption of 1 joule of ionising radiation by 1 kg of matter.
- The sievert (Sv): a derived unit of dose-equivalent radiation which also calculates the biological effect of the dose from the energy of the radiation type causing the exposure.

For gamma and x-rays 1 Gy = 1 Sv. For alpha particles 1 Gy = 20 Sv. The dose rate is also important: the higher the dose over the shorter the time, the more tissue damage occurs. The distance from the source is also important, as the dose rate decreases as the square of the distance from the source.

Acute radiation syndrome has four phases:

- Prodromal phase (minutes to a week post-exposure, depending on radiation dose): anorexia, apathy, nausea, vomiting, diarrhoea, fever, tachycardia, headache, fluid shifts and electrolyte imbalance.
- Latent phase (inversely related to dose): improvement in signs and symptoms.
- Manifest illness with central nervous system, gastrointestinal and cutaneous symptoms, accompanied by immunosuppression, the systemic inflammatory

response syndrome, disseminated intravascular coagulation and multi-organ failure.
- Recovery or death.

Dainiak N. Biology and clinical features of radiation injury in adults. *UpToDate* 2014. http://www.uptodate.com (accessed June 2014).

Taylor J, Chandramohan M, Simpson KH. Radiation safety for anaesthetists. *Contin Educ Anaesth Crit Care Pain* 2013; 13: 59–62.

Exam B: Questions

Question B1

Regarding the localisation of myocardial infarction (MI) and myocardial blood supply:

A. The left circumflex artery supplies the lateral and posterior walls of the left ventricle
B. The right coronary artery (RCA) usually supplies the sinoatrial node
C. ST elevation in leads I, II and aV_F usually indicates an inferior MI
D. ST elevation in V_6, I and aV_L suggests distal RCA occlusion
E. Proximal left anterior descending (LAD) artery occlusion causes extensive anterolateral infarction

Question B2

Regarding the mechanics of ventilators:

A. Pressure-controlled ventilators are flow-cycled
B. Volume-controlled ventilators are time-cycled
C. Flow triggering is more sensitive than pressure triggering
D. Flow is constant with volume-controlled ventilation
E. Flow is constant with pressure-controlled ventilation

Question B3

The following are features of acute cardiogenic pulmonary oedema on chest radiograph (CXR):

A. Enlarged upper-zone vessels
B. Cardiomegaly
C. Kerley B lines
D. Increased vascular pedicle width
E. Prominent horizontal fissure

Question B4

Regarding the venous drainage of the leg:

A. The great saphenous vein may be cannulated anterior to the medial malleolus
B. The short saphenous vein runs anterior to the lateral malleolus
C. The popliteal vein becomes the femoral vein at the inguinal ligament
D. The great saphenous vein runs from the arch of the foot to the femoral triangle
E. The short saphenous vein becomes the popliteal vein at the knee

Question B5

Estimates of the following may be derived from the arterial pressure waveform:

A. Stroke volume
B. Myocardial contractility
C. Systemic vascular resistance (SVR)
D. Intravascular filling
E. Arterial compliance

Question B6

Regarding electrical safety, which of the following are correct?

A. Moist skin surfaces reduce the risk of microshock
B. Microshock is defined as current flow of less than 1 amp
C. Pulmonary artery catheters would are classed as type BF electrical equipment
D. Floating circuits improve the safety of operating theatres
E. UK mains electricity is supplied at 50 Hz 240 V alternating current

Question B7

Septic shock:

A. Is defined as sepsis with hypotension
B. Has both pathogen and host aetiological factors
C. Invariably leads to an increase in cardiac output
D. Leads to multi-organ failure and death in up to 50% of cases
E. Is usually characterised by high levels of IL-1, IL-5 and TNF-γ

Question B8

With regards to the assessment of acute kidney injury using the RIFLE criteria:

A. Patients who are anuric for 16 hours are classed as at risk of acute kidney injury
B. Patients with loss of kidney function 6 weeks after the original injury would be classed as having end-stage kidney disease
C. Baseline creatinine is required to fully classify patients using the RIFLE criteria
D. Patients who fall into RIFLE class R have an increased mortality compared to those who maintain normal function
E. Patients with a creatinine level twice their baseline level are classified as having acute kidney injury

Question B9

The Simplified Acute Physiology Score II (SAPS II):

A. Can be used to predict mortality
B. Is calculated daily
C. Is based purely on physiological measurements and observations
D. Can be modified according to region of the world
E. Excludes burns and cardiac patients

Question B10

Regarding anaphylaxis:

A. Muscle relaxants are a more common precipitant of anaphylaxis than antibiotics
B. Hypotension is usually the first sign in critically ill patients
C. ST elevation may be a feature on the ECG
D. Epinephrine 50 μg IM is the first-line treatment
E. Gelatin or starch solutions may be used to correct distributive shock

Question B11

Which of the following are Gram-positive bacilli?

A. *Pseudomonas aeruginosa*
B. *Clostridium perfringens*
C. *Clostridium botulinum*
D. *Bacillus cereus*
E. *Listeria monocytogenes*

Question B12

In a case of convulsive status epilepticus:

A. Intravenous diazepam is the recommended first-line drug
B. Intravenous lorazepam can be administered before phenytoin
C. Phenytoin should not be given to patients who are already taking antiepileptic medication
D. Propofol is contraindicated for induction of anaesthesia, because of its epileptiform effects
E. Pre-existing antiepileptic medication should not be administered

Question B13

Regarding the pharmacological management of life-threatening asthma:

A. Aminophylline administration commonly causes a lactic acidosis
B. Helium is used to reduce bronchoconstriction
C. Hypotension during mechanical ventilation should be treated with fluids
D. β-Adrenergic receptor agonists increase ventilation/perfusion mismatch
E. β-Adrenergic receptor agonists increase diaphragmatic contractility

Question B14

The following drugs are used in the management of atrial fibrillation:

A. Metoprolol
B. Verapamil
C. Sotalol
D. Flecainide
E. Isosorbide mononitrate

Question B15

Complications of positive-pressure ventilation include:

A. Cardiovascular collapse
B. Bronchopleural fistula
C. Increased carbon monoxide transfer factor
D. Deranged liver function tests (LFTs)
E. Dysphagia

Question B16

Regarding lactic acidosis in critically ill patients:

A. Metformin is associated with type B lactic acidosis
B. Lactate levels of > 10 mmol/l are associated with > 80% mortality
C. There is evidence that bicarbonate infusions reduce mortality in lactic acidosis
D. Venous blood samples can be used to monitor lactate levels
E. Lactate is removed efficiently by continuous venovenous haemofiltration

Question B17

During cardiopulmonary resuscitation, recommended drug dosages and regimens are as follows:

A. Epinephrine as soon as access is achieved in asystole
B. Epinephrine 3 mg via endotracheal tube for PEA/asystole if no IV access
C. Amiodarone 300 mg before the third shock in VF/VT
D. Atropine 3 mg for PEA at a rate of < 60 bpm
E. Epinephrine 1 mg after the second shock in VF/VT

Question B18

Complications of blood transfusion include:

A. Prolonged QT interval on ECG
B. Increase in cancer recurrence
C. Metabolic alkalosis
D. Incompatibility reactions due to IgG anti-A or anti-B antibodies
E. Anaphylaxis

Question B19

Regarding emergency cardiac pacing in a periarrest patient:

A. The QRS complex in complete heart block is > 0.12 seconds
B. Pacing should be routinely used in P-wave asystole
C. In percussion pacing, the fist should hit the lower third of the sternum
D. The preferred paddle position for transcutaneous pacing is right pectoral–apical
E. The average current required during transcutaneous pacing is 50–100 μA

Question B20

The following therapeutic options have been shown in a multicentre RCT to reduce mortality in acute respiratory distress syndrome (ARDS):

A. Lung-protective ventilation (LPV) at < 6 ml/kg actual body weight
B. Prone positioning
C. High-frequency oscillatory ventilation (HFOV)
D. Recruitment manoeuvres of 40 seconds at 40 cmH_2O
E. Ventilator care bundles

Question B21

Regarding the effects of hypothermia, which of the following are correct?

A. Metabolism reduces by 25% for every 1 °C reduction in core body temperature below 36 °C
B. Tissue oxygen delivery increases due to a reduction in haemoglobin affinity for oxygen
C. Drug metabolism is unaltered until core temperature falls below 35 °C
D. Osborn waves are commonly seen on the ECG of patients with core temperature below 32 °C
E. The QT interval is often increased in hypothermic patients

Question B22

Regarding the mechanism of action of antibiotics:

A. Benzylpenicillin is bacteriostatic
B. Clindamycin is bactericidal
C. Cephalosporins are bactericidal
D. Chloramphenicol is bacteriostatic
E. Macrolides are bacteriostatic

Question B23

Capnography (end-tidal CO_2 monitoring) can help diagnose the following:

A. Obstructive airways disease
B. Endobronchial intubation
C. Tricyclic antidepressant (TCA) overdose
D. Pulmonary embolus
E. Effective CPR

Question B24

The Parkland formula for fluid management in the treatment of burns:

A. Is not necessary for burns of less than 10% TBSA
B. Includes factors for size and thickness of burn, age and weight
C. Prevents over-administration of fluid
D. Does not include maintenance fluids
E. Starts from the time of admission to hospital

Question B25

Which of the following would you expect to be associated with a plasma sodium < 136 mmol/l?

A. Addison's disease
B. Acute tubular necrosis
C. Primary hyperaldosteronism
D. Cerebral salt wasting syndrome
E. Nephrogenic diabetes insipidus

Question B26

Suitable ventilator modes for a patient following intubation for life-threatening acute asthma include:

A. Synchronised intermittent mandatory ventilation (SIMV)
B. Bilevel ventilation (BIPAP)
C. Airway pressure-release ventilation (APRV)
D. Continuous positive airway pressure (CPAP)
E. Pressure-support ventilation (PSV)

Question B27

Regarding arterial blood gas (ABG) analysis:

A. Oxygen is measured with an oxygen fuel cell
B. Carbon dioxide is measured by change of pH of a bicarbonate buffer solution
C. pH is directly proportional to hydrogen ion concentration
D. Base excess is measured using a selectively permeable glass electrode
E. The standard bicarbonate is the amount of HCO_3^- in the plasma

Question B28

Regarding electroencephalogram (EEG) use in critical care:

A. The amplitude of most EEG signals is 20–200 mV
B. Alpha activity is increased with eye opening after hypoxic brain injury
C. The presence of N20 median nerve somatosensory evoked potentials (SSEPs) after cardiac arrest is associated with a good outcome
D. Burst suppression on an EEG trace is 1–2 spikes per minute
E. An isoelectric EEG is a requirement for brainstem death diagnosis

Question B29

Indications for not starting a resuscitation attempt, or for ceasing one, include:

A. Next-of-kin refusal for cardiopulmonary resuscitation
B. Fixed dilated pupils
C. Ventricular fibrillation after 10 shocks (about 20 minutes of resuscitation)
D. Asystole for over 20 minutes in a hypothermic patient
E. A valid advance directive written by the patient

Question B30

Concerning flexible bronchoscopy on ICU:

A. It rarely requires extra sedation in intubated patients
B. It is required for accurate diagnosis of ventilator-associated pneumonia (VAP)
C. A post-procedure chest radiograph (CXR) is only required if biopsies have been taken
D. It should not be performed in patients with haemoptysis
E. Intubated patients should be ventilated with volume-control ventilation (VCV)

Question B31

The following may be measured by pulmonary artery (PA) catheters:

A. Cardiac output (CO)
B. Right atrial pressure (RAP)
C. Stroke volume variation (SVV)
D. Real-time cardiac output changes to fluid boluses
E. Left ventricular end-diastolic pressure (LVEDP)

Question B32

The following are recognised causes of prolonged QT and torsades de pointes

A. Hypokalaemia
B. Amiodarone
C. Hypercalcaemia
D. Clarithromycin
E. Pineapple juice

Question B33

Extended-spectrum β-lactamase (ESBL) producing organisms:

A. Are effectively treated with third-generation cephalosporins, e.g. ceftazidime
B. Are most commonly *Enterobacter* species
C. Are resistant to meropenem
D. Are resistant to gentamicin
E. Have plasmid-mediated resistance mechanisms

Question B34

Vasopressin:

A. Causes vasoconstriction by action on V_2 receptors
B. Endogenous levels are low in all types of shock
C. Decreases plasma osmolality

D. Should be used instead of norepinephrine in septic shock
E. Acts on vasoconstrictor receptors that are heterogeneously distributed in the body

Question B35

Regarding urinary catheters in the intensive care unit:

A. There is evidence that silver alloy catheters may reduce the risk of catheter-related urinary tract infection (UTI)
B. Bladder irrigation and washouts should not be used to prevent catheter-associated infection
C. Catheterisation should be an aseptic procedure
D. The indication for catheterisation should be documented
E. The largest-gauge catheter possible for the patient should be used, to encourage urinary flow

Question B36

The following are causes of hyperkalaemia:

A. Metabolic acidosis
B. Suxamethonium
C. Malignant hyperthermia
D. Conn's syndrome
E. Digoxin overdose

Question B37

Regarding the use of scoring systems in critical care:

A. The Standardised Mortality Ratio (SMR) is the ratio of expected to observed mortality
B. Expected mortality for the SMR can come from APACHE, SAPS or MPM scores
C. Predicted mortality scores are useful as part of a critcal care unit's clinical audit programme
D. An ICU with an SMR > 1.0 is performing above expectations
E. Predicted mortality should not be used to make clinical decisions

Question B38

Regarding influenza:

A. Influenza epidemics occur due to antigenic drift of the influenza virus
B. Vomiting and diarrhoea are commoner in seasonal influenza than in pandemic influenza
C. Non-invasive ventilation is the optimal treatment for viral pneumonia
D. High-frequency oscillation ventilation (HFOV) is the treatment of choice for refractory hypoxia
E. Severity scoring should be used to triage patients for extracorporeal membrane oxygenation (ECMO) treatment

Question B39

Regarding intracranial pressure (ICP) monitoring:

A. ICP monitoring is indicated in closed head injury unless the CT is normal
B. Monitors can be extradural, subarachnoid, intraventricular or intraparenchymal
C. Intraventricular monitors can be therapeutic devices
D. ICP monitoring is contraindicated in coagulopathy, sepsis and severe hydrocephalus
E. Risk of infection is highest for the most accurate monitoring method

Question B40

The following are recognised direct causes of acute respiratory distress syndrome (ARDS):

A. Trauma
B. Fat embolism
C. Pancreatitis
D. Smoke inhalation
E. Sepsis

Question B41

According to the Spaulding classification:

A. A blood pressure cuff is a non-critical item and should be cleaned at the bedside
B. Surgical instruments should be sterilised
C. Endoscopes are critical items and should be sterilised
D. Laryngoscopes are non-critical items and should be disinfected
E. Semi-critical items should be disinfected to remove spores

Question B42

The Fick method for estimating cardiac output:

A. Can use oxygen or CO_2 levels
B. Requires measurement of oxygen consumption (VO_2) or CO_2 production
C. Gives the most accurate results when based on oxygen content in the pulmonary artery and vein
D. Estimates cardiac output by dividing VO_2 by the area under the concentration/time curve
E. Commonly assumes no intracardiac shunt

Question B43

Which of the following are associated with increased disease severity in adults with community-acquired pneumonia (CAP), according to CURB65?

A. Age > 60
B. Urea > 7 mmol/l
C. Mini-mental test score ≤ 8/10
D. Respiratory rate > 25 breaths/minute
E. Heart rate > 110 bpm

Question B44

Concerning acute subarachnoid haemorrhage (SAH):

A. Grading of severity is based solely on the Glasgow Coma Scale
B. Patients with suspected SAH should have a lumbar puncture
C. Control of the bleeding aneurysm should be undertaken at the earliest feasible opportunity
D. Systolic blood pressure should be kept low (< 140 mmHg) to prevent rebleeding
E. Corticosteroids should be administered to reduce cerebral oedema

Question B45

The definitions of acute kidney injury (AKI) and its severity include:

A. Urine volume < 0.5 ml/kg/h for 6 hours
B. Increase in serum creatinine by > 26.5 μmol/l within 48 hours
C. Increase in serum creatinine to > 1.5 times baseline in 7 days
D. Stage 3 AKI: eGFR < 35 ml/min per 1.73 m^2 in patients aged 18 years or over
E. Stage 3 AKI: anuria for > 12 hours

Question B46

The following therapies are recommended for patients with severe sepsis, according to the Surviving Sepsis guidelines (2012):

A. Antimicrobial therapy must not start until two sets of blood cultures have been taken
B. Effective intravenous antimicrobials within 1 hour of recognition of severe sepsis
C. Surgical intervention for source control within 12 hours
D. The use of albumin in patients requiring large volumes of crystalloid resuscitation
E. Continuous infusion of hydrocortisone in vasopressor-refractory septic shock

Question B47

Regarding refeeding syndrome:

A. Thiamine deficiency is the most clinically significant vitamin deficiency seen
B. Feed should be introduced at a rate to meet the patient's full nutritional requirements
C. Refeeding syndrome causes hyperglycaemia
D. Potassium deficiency is the most common finding
E. Refeeding syndrome is more common in patients on diuretics

Question B48

Risk factors for invasive candidiasis include:

A. Renal replacement therapy
B. Oral fluconazole
C. Oesophageal surgery
D. Perforated duodenal ulcer
E. Proton-pump inhibitors

Question B49

Light's criteria for the diagnosis of pleural effusions state that:

A. Pleural fluid protein divided by serum protein > 0.5 suggests an exudate
B. Pleural fluid lactate dehydrogenase (LDH) divided by serum LDH < 0.6 suggests an transudate
C. Pleural fluid glucose < 2/3 of plasma glucose suggests an exudate
D. Pleural fluid pH < 7.2 suggests empyema
E. Pleural fluid LDH > 2/3 the upper limit of the laboratory normal value for serum LDH suggests a transudate

Question B50

Central venous catheter-related bloodstream infection (CRBSI):

A. Is an opportunistic infection if the pathogen is methicillin-resistant *Staphylococcus aureus* (MRSA)
B. Is an opportunistic infection if the pathogen is a coagulase-negative *Staphylococcus*
C. Occurs in up to 25% of patients with central venous catheters
D. Is a greater risk with pulmonary artery catheters than with dialysis catheters
E. Occurs less frequently with subclavian vein cannulation than with cannulation of the femoral or internal jugular vein

Question B51

Regarding ICU delirium, which of the following are correct?

A. Morbidity and mortality is increased in patients with ICU delirium
B. Persisting cognitive impairment is common in patients with ICU delirium
C. Patients with ICU delirium cost more to treat
D. Hypoactive delirium is common in patients on ICU
E. Patients with hyperactive delirium are at a higher risk of long-term memory problems

Question B52

Regarding *Clostridium difficile*-associated diarrhoea:

A. Prior use of penicillins or macrolides is not a risk factor
B. Probiotics have been shown to reduce mortality from *C. difficile* in critical care
C. Meticulous use of alcohol-based hand gels reduces *C. difficile* transmission
D. Surgical resection of infected colon may be required
E. A toxin produced by the bacillus is responsible for the disease

Question B53

With regards to the pathophysiology of burns, which of the following are correct?

A. The depth of the burn is related only to the temperature to which the skin is exposed
B. Scalds are an unusual cause of burns in children
C. Flame burns are often deep or full-thickness burns

D. The severity of electrical burns is mainly related to the voltage applied
E. Coagulative necrosis occurs at the site of burn injury

Question B54

The following are signs of cardiac tamponade:

A. Enlarged cardiac silhouette on chest radiograph (CXR) with clear lung fields
B. A drop in diastolic blood pressure of > 10 mmHg during inspiration
C. Muffled heart sounds on auscultation
D. Diastolic collapse of heart chambers on echocardiography
E. Absent or reduced *x* descent on CVP trace

Question B55

Regarding anaemia:

A. Anaemia shifts the oxyhaemoglobin dissociation curve to the left
B. Haemolysis causes a microcytic anaemia
C. There is a reduced response to erythropoietin
D. Increased hepcidin synthesis is responsible for the fall in serum iron
E. Ferritin concentrations are decreased in the critically ill

Question B56

Regarding airway pressure-release ventilation (APRV)

A. Peak pressures are higher than with BIPAP for a given tidal volume
B. T_{high} is usually a minimum of 4 seconds
C. Neuromuscular blockade is often required to prevent patient/ventilator asynchrony
D. Hypercapnia is a contraindication to its use
E. Spontaneous breathing is sensed by the ventilator and mandatory breaths synchronised

Question B57

The P-POSSUM system

A. Is a modification of POSSUM with reductions in predicted mortality
B. Only applies to patients undergoing surgery
C. Uses categorised clinical and observational data
D. Relies on the results of blood tests
E. Can be used to predict preoperative risk of surgery

Question B58

The following are recognised causes of acute heart failure (AHF):

A. Pregnancy
B. Aortic stenosis
C. Sickle cell disease

D. Atrial fibrillation
E. Ventricular septal defect (VSD)

Question B59

With regards to paraquat poisoning, which of the following are correct?

A. It is commoner in the developing world
B. A patient who has ingested 10 mg paraquat ion per kg body weight is likely to make a full recovery
C. Oesophageal perforation has a mortality rate of around 100%
D. Paraquat is mostly metabolised to toxic metabolites that are excreted by the kidney
E. Concentrations are lowest in the lung due to reduced uptake into cells

Question B60

Concerning critical illness neuromyopathy (CINM):

A. CINM affects up to 30% of all ventilated patients on ICU
B. It is diagnosed by clinical examination
C. The risk is increased by hyperglycaemia
D. Development of CINM is an independent risk factor for ICU mortality
E. Steroid use is an independent risk factor for the development of CINM

Question B61

Brainstem reflex tests for diagnosis of neurological death include:

A. Tests of cranial nerves II to X inclusive
B. Doll's eye movements
C. Response to central and peripheral painful stimuli
D. Carinal stimulation
E. Consensual pupillary reaction to light

Question B62

Regarding hypermagnesaemia, which of the following are correct?

A. Diuretics are a common cause
B. Magnesium crosses the placenta
C. Levels over 5 mmol/l lead to cardiac arrest
D. Higher doses of non-depolarising muscle relaxants are required
E. Hypermagnesaemia leads to loss of deep tendon reflexes

Question B63

The following are recognised causes of acute pancreatitis:

A. Choledocholithiasis
B. Protozoal infection
C. Hypocalcaemia
D. Hypothermia
E. Corticosteroids

Question B64

Concerning blood products:

A. Human albumin solution contains some clotting factors
B. Fresh frozen plasma (FFP) should be ABO-compatible with the recipient
C. AB-negative patients are universal recipients
D. Fresh frozen plasma (FFP) should be rhesus-compatible with the recipient
E. Fresh frozen plasma (FFP) should be stored at −18 °C

Question B65

Which of the following treatments have been shown to improve survival after cardiac arrest?

A. Amiodarone 300 mg after the third shock for ventricular fibrillation
B. Epinephrine 1 mg IV
C. Untrained bystander CPR
D. Bipolar defibrillation
E. Airway maintenance with a laryngeal mask airway or endotracheal tube

Question B66

With regards to acute colonic pseudo-obstruction, which of the following are correct?

A. There must be clinical and radiological evidence of large bowel obstruction for diagnosis
B. It is also known as Ogilvie's syndrome
C. Ischaemia and perforation rarely occur
D. Oral neostigmine has been shown to be effective in up to 80% of patients
E. Endoscopic decompression can be performed as an alternative to surgery

Question B67

Regarding tetanus:

A. The clinical effects are due to the endotoxin tetanospasmin
B. Tetanus spores are eradicated by autoclaving
C. The neurotoxin enters the nervous system via synapses
D. Diagnosis is confirmed by culture of *Clostridium tetani*
E. *Clostridium tetani* is an aerobic Gram-positive coccus

Question B68

Patients with severe acute liver failure (ALF) should receive:

A. *N*-acetyl-cysteine (NAC) regardless of paracetamol level
B. Hypertonic saline for cerebral oedema
C. Correction of coagulopathy with fresh frozen plasma (FFP) if INR > 4.0
D. Ornithine aspartate to reduce ammonia levels
E. Prophylactic parenteral antibiotics

Question B69

Concerning donation after circulatory death (DCD):

A. DCD should not be considered if life-sustaining care is to be withdrawn
B. DCD does not apply to patients diagnosed as brainstem dead
C. DCD can be considered and organised after the death of a patient
D. The time between withdrawal and death can determine which organs are retrieved
E. DCD is only possible for liver, kidneys and pancreas

Question B70

In the management of a patient with acute spinal cord injury, which of the following are correct?

A. Pharmacological thromboprophylaxis should be commenced as early as possible following the injury
B. Intravenous methylprednisolone should be commenced as soon as possible
C. Stabilisation of unstable vertebral injuries should be performed within 24 hours
D. Patients with unstable vertebral injuries and spinal cord damage should be immobilised on a hard spinal board until definitive surgery
E. Rapid sequence induction and intubation is commonly indicated for patients with high cervical spine injuries within the first 72 hours

Question B71

Which of the following apply to thyroid storm?

A. The commonest precipitant is infection
B. Iodine should be administered before antithyroid treatment is given
C. Administration of steroids is recommended
D. Thyroid surgery is a common cause of thyroid storm
E. Atrial fibrillation is the commonest arrhythmia seen

Question B72

Features of systemic inflammatory response syndrome (SIRS) include:

A. Heart rate > 100 bpm
B. Respiratory rate > 20/minute
C. Temperature < 35 °C or > 38 °C
D. > 10% immature neutrophils
E. $PaCO_2$ < 32 mmHg (4.3 kPa)

Question B73

Which of the following are methods used to reduce raised intracranial pressure (ICP)?

A. Hypertonic saline
B. Suxamethonium
C. Hypothermia
D. Vecuronium
E. Hypoventilation

Question B74

Causes of a high anion gap acidosis include:

A. Short gut syndrome
B. Chronic paracetamol (acetaminophen) ingestion
C. Resuscitation with 0.9% sodium chloride
D. Urine reabsorption from ileal conduit
E. Acetazolamide

Question B75

With regards to the presentation and management of patients with a history of submersion in water or drowning, which of the following are correct?

A. Pulmonary complications are unlikely if the PaO_2 is normal 1 hour after the episode
B. 'Secondary drowning' occurs with aspiration of salt water into the alveoli, but not with fresh water
C. Cervical spine immobilisation should be considered in all patients
D. Exogenous surfactant can improve outcome in patients with progressive respiratory distress
E. Immersion in cold water results in hyperventilation and reduced breath-hold time

Question B76

Regarding intercostal chest drains (ICDs):

A. Wide-bore ICDs are more likely to cause pleural infection than Seldinger ICDs
B. Trocars should only be used under direct vision, to prevent complications
C. Seldinger ICDs should not be used in acute haemothorax
D. Chest-drain tubing should be clamped prior to transfer
E. ICDs should be secured with 'purse-string' sutures, gauze and tape

Question B77

With regards to the management of patients with lithium toxicity, which of the following are correct?

A. The presence of a goitre suggests acute intoxication
B. Oral bioavailability of lithium is poor
C. ACE inhibitors promote the excretion of lithium from the kidneys
D. A plasma lithium concentration above 3.5 mEq/l is classed as severe toxicity
E. Lithium is the most dialysable common toxin known

Question B78

Which of the following statements correctly describe the uses of hyperbaric oxygen therapy?

A. It can be useful in the management of patients with ARDS following chest trauma
B. It is usually administered at 8–10 times atmospheric pressure at sea level
C. Charles's law governs the increase in oxygen partial pressure of the blood

D. Necrotising fasciitis is an indication for the use of hyperbaric oxygen therapy
E. Seizures are common and often prolonged and may lead to permanent neurological disability

Question B79

Regarding notifiable diseases in the UK, which of the following are correct?

A. Responsibility for notification lies with the patient's general practitioner
B. Acute infective hepatitis of any cause is a notifiable disease
C. Notification of certain infectious diseases first came into practice in the 1800s
D. Acute meningitis of any cause is a notifiable disease
E. Microbiological confirmation via microscopy or culture is required for official notification

Question B80

In a case of massive obstetric haemorrhage, which of the following are correct?

A. It can be defined as blood loss > 500 ml following caesarean section
B. The commonest cause of secondary post-partum haemorrhage is uterine atony
C. Administration of recombinant activated factor VII is contraindicated
D. Carboprost 250 μg boluses can be repeated up to a total of 2 mg
E. First-line medical management for post-partum haemorrhage is intramuscular ergometrine

Question B81

Indications for percutaneous tracheostomy insertion include:

A. A contraindication to surgical tracheostomy placement
B. Insertion by day 4 in patients expected to be ventilated for more than 14 days
C. Irreversible brain injury
D. Failure of needle cricothyroidotomy
E. Excessive respiratory secretions

Question B82

Parenteral nutrition:

A. Should be started as soon as enteral nutrition is deemed unsuitable
B. Should not overlap with enteral feeding
C. Should meet at least 66% of a patient's nutritional needs
D. Is a recognised cause of lipolysis
E. Should be adjusted to take account of propofol sedation

Question B83

Sengstaken–Blakemore tubes:

A. Have three lumens – gastric balloon, oesophageal balloon and oesophageal aspiration port
B. Control around 90% of cases of variceal bleeding
C. When correctly sited, should be attached to 5 kg of traction

D. Usually have the oesophageal balloon inflated before the gastric balloon
E. Should only be left in for 12 hours

Question B84

Norepinephrine:

A. Is a weak base
B. Stimulates β-adrenergic receptors to cause coronary vasodilatation
C. Must not be infused into a peripheral vein
D. Should be used with caution in patients taking linezolid, amitriptyline or atenolol
E. Increases platelet aggregation and GI tract relaxation

Question B85

With regards to the use of intravenous immunoglobulin use in critically ill adult patients, which of the following are correct?

A. The most widely practised use of immunoglobulin is for group B streptococcal toxic shock syndrome
B. The recommended dose for severe sepsis is 1 mg/kg/day for 2 days
C. The Surviving Sepsis Campaign guidelines recommend its use in patients with septic shock who fail to respond to initial resuscitation measures
D. Intravenous immunoglobulin is a pooled blood product from over 1000 donors
E. IgM-enriched immunoglobulin is not routinely used in clinical practice

Question B86

Regarding the early management of the multiply injured patient:

A. If a serious head injury is suspected the patient should be cooled to a temperature of < 35 °C
B. Diaphragmatic rupture in blunt trauma is typically on the right
C. Laboratory clotting studies are helpful in guiding blood product administration to the multiply injured patient with ongoing blood loss
D. Around 10% of patients with cervical spine injury have another non-contiguous vertebral fracture
E. Chest wall subcutaneous emphysema is a worrying sign in a patient with normal chest x-ray

Question B87

In renal transplant patients:

A. ARDS frequently occurs early in the post-transplant period
B. The mortality rate on ICU is higher than in other patients
C. The incidence of critical care admission is higher than among liver transplant patients
D. The most common reason for ICU admission is the requirement for renal replacement therapy
E. Immunosuppression is a significant factor in the need for intensive care

Question B88

With regards to the management of patients with metabolic acidaemia, which of the following are correct?

A. Rapidity of correction of severe acidaemia on admission to ICU is inversely proportional to mortality
B. The administration of bicarbonate to patients with severe metabolic acidosis has been shown to improve prognosis
C. Bicarbonate administration can result in reduced ionised calcium levels and therefore arrhythmias
D. Bicarbonate administration to patients with chronic kidney disease is widely practised
E. It is recommended that bicarbonate be administered to patients with diabetic ketoacidosis if the pH is < 7.2

Question B89

In the treatment of patients with bites from venomous snakes, which of the following are correct?

A. Children and adults are affected similarly by adder bites
B. A tourniquet should be applied to the affected limb to prevent systemic spread of venom
C. Secondary cellulitis develops quickly, and prophylactic antibiotics should be commenced early
D. Antivenom is widely available, and the standard dose is the same for all patients
E. Blood transfusion may be required, but heparin should be avoided

Question B90

In a case of hyperkalaemia, which of the following ECG changes are seen?

A. The QRS complex is often narrowed
B. A prolonged PR interval is the first ECG change to be seen
C. The P wave is often absent
D. U waves are a late ECG sign
E. A normal ECG is incompatible with severe hyperkalaemia

Exam B: Answers

Question B1: Myocardial infarct localisation

Regarding the localisation of myocardial infarction (MI) and myocardial blood supply:

A. The left circumflex artery supplies the lateral and posterior walls of the left ventricle
B. The right coronary artery (RCA) usually supplies the sinoatrial node
C. ST elevation in leads I, II and aV_F usually indicates an inferior MI
D. ST elevation in V_6, I and aV_L suggests distal RCA occlusion
E. Proximal left anterior descending (LAD) artery occlusion causes extensive anterolateral infarction

Answer: TTFFT

Short explanation

ST elevation in inferior leads (II, III, aV_F) suggests RCA occlusion and an inferior MI. ST elevation in lateral leads (V_6, I and aV_L) suggests circumflex artery occlusion. The RCA supplies the right ventricle, parts of the left ventricle and (in 90% of people) the sinoatrial and atrioventricular nodes. The left coronary artery (LCA) supplies the anterior, lateral and posterior walls of the left ventricle.

Long explanation

The coronary arteries originate in the aortic sinuses at the root of the aorta. The left coronary artery (LCA) has two main branches. The left anterior descending (LAD) supplies the anterior interventricular septum and anterior wall of the left ventricle. The left circumflex artery supplies the lateral and posterior walls of the left ventricle.

The right coronary artery (RCA) supplies the sinoatrial node and the atrioventricular node (in 90% of people), the right ventricle, and usually the posterior and inferior parts of the left ventricle via the posterior descending artery (PDA). Roughly 15% of people have a dominant circumflex artery, which gives rise to the PDA instead.

Occlusion of coronary arteries leads to myocardial infarction (MI) in the territories they supply. It is possible to infer the location of the occlusion from the ECG and other aspects of the clinical picture, with the caveat that this may differ from the findings at angiography. Knowledge of the approximate location of the infarct helps pre-empt complications (e.g. arrhythmias) or guide treatment.

Artery occluded	Infarcted territory	Leads showing ECG changes
LCA/proximal LAD	Extensive anterolateral	V_1–V_6, I, aV_L
LAD (septal braches)	Septal	V_1–V_3
LAD	Anterior	V_2–V_5
Circumflex	Lateral	V_5, V_6, I, aV_L
Circumflex (dominant)	Inferolateral	II, III, aV_F, V_5, V_6, I, aV_L
RCA (proximal)	Right ventricle	V_1, V_4R, II, III, aV_F
RCA	Inferior	II, III, aV_F
RCA (dominant)	Inferoposterior	II, III, aV_F, V_7, V_8

Right ventricular and posterior wall infarcts may be difficult to spot with standard lead placement; a posterior MI may present with ST depression in V_1 and V_2 only. Alternative lead placement may help with diagnosis – V_4R is a right-sided chest lead (equivalent to V_4 on the left) that may show ST elevation in right ventricular infarcts; V_7 and V_8 are posterior left-sided leads (continuing the line of chest leads from V_6) that may show ST elevation in posterior wall infarcts.

Power B. Acute cardiac syndromes, investigations and interventions. In Bersten AD, Soni N. *Oh's Intensive Care Manual*, 6th edn. Edinburgh: Butterworth-Heinemann, 2009, pp. 155–78.

Question B2: Ventilator mechanics

Regarding the mechanics of ventilators:

A. Pressure-controlled ventilators are flow-cycled
B. Volume-controlled ventilators are time-cycled
C. Flow triggering is more sensitive than pressure triggering
D. Flow is constant with volume-controlled ventilation
E. Flow is constant with pressure-controlled ventilation

Answer: FFTTF

Short explanation

Pressure-controlled ventilators are time-cycled with a variable flow throughout the inspiratory phase to achieve a constant pressure. Volume-controlled ventilators are volume-cycled and flow is constant throughout inspiration.

Long explanation

Ventilator control describes how the breath is delivered to the patient. In volume-controlled ventilation, the volume to be delivered is static, so the rate of flow is constant until that volume is achieved. The pressure generated is therefore dependent on the compliance of the lung. Pressure-controlled ventilation delivers a breath by suppling a constant pressure to inflate the lung, with a flow that decelerates throughout inspiration. The tidal volume delivered is determined by the compliance of the lung.

Cycling describes how the ventilator switches from inspiration to expiration. Pressure-controlled ventilation is time-cycled with set inspiratory time and inspiratory:expiratory ratio (I:E ratio). Pressure-support ventilation is flow-cycled: when the ventilator senses a reduction in the peak inspiratory flow it switches to expiration. Volume-controlled ventilation may be either volume-cycled, with the ventilator switching between inspiration and expiration on delivery of the set volume; or time-cycled, with an inspiratory pause if the tidal volume is delivered in a shorter time.

Triggering refers to the ventilator's response to spontaneous patient breaths. Pressure triggering implies that the ventilator delivers a breath on sensing the negative pressure generated by the initiation of a spontaneous breath. Flow triggering has a background constant gas flow (flow-by) throughout the respiratory cycle. A flow sensor picks up the change in this flow from a patient breath. Flow triggering is more sensitive, as there is no need for an inspiratory valve to open, and it therefore improves patient–ventilator synchrony and reduces the work of breathing.

Gould T, de Beer JMA. Principles of artificial ventilation. *Anaesth Intensive Care Med* 2007; 8: 91–101.

Waldmann C, Soni N, Rhodes A. *Oxford Desk Reference: Critical Care*. Oxford: Oxford University Press, 2008; pp. 8–9.

Question B3: Cardiogenic pulmonary oedema

The following are features of acute cardiogenic pulmonary oedema on chest radiograph (CXR):

A. Enlarged upper-zone vessels
B. Cardiomegaly
C. Kerley B lines
D. Increased vascular pedicle width
E. Prominent horizontal fissure

Answer: TFTFT

Short explanation

The earliest CXR change is enlarged upper-zone vessels. Kerley B lines and prominent fissures develop at higher pulmonary venous pressures. Cardiomegaly indicates a chronic process. Increased vascular pedicle width is a measure of volume overload.

Long explanation

The chest radiograph (CXR) is a common investigation in patients with respiratory distress. It is therefore important to recognise the features of different diseases. Acute cardiogenic pulmonary oedema occurs when left atrial pressure increases, for example due to left ventricular failure or mitral regurgitation. The left atrial pressure is transmitted backwards to the pulmonary veins and capillaries. The formation of oedema is related to Starling forces; when the hydrostatic pressure difference pushing fluid out exceeds the osmotic pressure difference pulling it into the capillary, a net outward flow occurs. As capillary hydrostatic pressure is highest in the lower zones of the lung, oedema forms in the bases, which reduces vascular compliance and leads to redistribution of blood to the upper zones.

Oedema formed in this way is redirected to the circulation by way of the lymphatics, which become enlarged and visible as Kerley B lines. As the majority of the oedema is basal, Kerley B lines are seen just above the costodiaphragmatic angle. As pulmonary venous pressures increase, the production of oedema exceeds the capacity of the lymphatics to resorb the fluid, and alveolar oedema becomes visible on the CXR, first as a haziness and later as fluffy bilateral infiltrates. Interstitial oedema also results in thickening of the fissures, which become prominent on the CXR. Later, pleural effusions start to be seen as blunting of the costodiaphragmatic angles.

Cardiomegaly is defined as a cardiothoracic ratio of > 0.5 on a PA chest film; the widest horizontal dimension of the heart shadow is greater than half the widest horizontal distance of the basal lung fields. This is usually a sign of chronic heart failure or ventricular hypertrophy. An increased vascular pedicle width is a measure of the mediastinal silhouette of the great vessels, and is used as an indicator of fluid overload. While this is undoubtedly a useful measure, it is not a sign of acute pulmonary oedema.

Sutton D. *Textbook of Radiology and Imaging*, 7th edn. London. Churchill Livingstone, 2002.

Question B4: Veins of the leg

Regarding the venous drainage of the leg:

A. The great saphenous vein may be cannulated anterior to the medial malleolus
B. The short saphenous vein runs anterior to the lateral malleolus
C. The popliteal vein becomes the femoral vein at the inguinal ligament
D. The great saphenous vein runs from the arch of the foot to the femoral triangle
E. The short saphenous vein becomes the popliteal vein at the knee

Answer: TFFTF

Short explanation

The great saphenous vein, which runs from the arch of the foot to the femoral triangle, is commonly used for cannulation anterior to the medial malleolus. The short saphenous vein runs posterior to the lateral malleolus and empties into the popliteal vein in the popliteal fossa. This becomes the femoral vein at the adductor hiatus in the inferior thigh.

Long explanation

The dorsal venous arch of the foot is formed from digital veins of each toe. The medial end of the arch runs along the arch of the foot as the great saphenous vein; the lateral end of the arch runs posteriorly, forming the small saphenous vein at the lateral malleolus. The plantar venous arch is formed from the superficial veins of the sole of the foot, the medial and lateral ends of which empty into the great and small saphenous veins respectively. The muscles of the foot are drained by deep veins, which empty via perforating veins into the saphenous veins.

The short saphenous vein starts posterior to the lateral malleolus, runs just lateral to the Achilles tendon, and ascends on the posterior aspect of the leg, before perforating the deep fascia in the popliteal fossa, where it empties into the popliteal vein.

The great saphenous vein is formed on the medial aspect of the foot and runs anterior to the medial malleolus, where it is commonly used for cannulation, especially in infants. It runs superiorly on the medial aspect of the leg, passing medial to the knee into the thigh. In the thigh, the great saphenous vein runs superficially along the medial aspect before passing into the femoral triangle through the fascia lata, where it empties into the femoral vein.

The muscles of the leg are drained by deep veins, which perforate the fasciae to empty into the saphenous veins. The venae commitantes of the tibial arteries combine in the leg to form the popliteal vein. This ascends into the popliteal fossa alongside the popliteal artery and enters the adductor hiatus in the inferior thigh, where it becomes the femoral vein. This ascends through the femoral triangle with the femoral artery in the femoral sheath, initially deep and then medial to the artery. The profunda femoris vein (which drains the deep structures of the thigh) and the great saphenous vein empty into the femoral vein in the femoral triangle. The femoral vein passes under the inguinal ligament medial to the artery, becoming the external iliac vein.

Moore KL, Dalley AF, Agur AMR. *Clinically Oriented Anatomy*, 7th edn. Philadelphia, PA: Lippincott, Williams & Wilkins, 2013.

Question B5: Arterial pressure waveform

Estimates of the following may be derived from the arterial pressure waveform:

A. Stroke volume
B. Myocardial contractility
C. Systemic vascular resistance (SVR)
D. Intravascular filling
E. Arterial compliance

Answer: TTTTT

Short explanation

All these parameters may be estimated from aspects of the arterial pressure waveform: stroke volume from the area under the systolic pressure wave; contractility from the rate of change of pressure over time; SVR from the slope of the diastolic pressure drop; filling from pressure variation over the respiratory cycle ('swing'); arterial compliance from the dicrotic notch.

Long explanation

The arterial pressure waveform can impart a great deal of information. Most simply, the systolic and diastolic blood pressures are directly measured, and the heart rate simply calculated from the time between successive systolic peaks. The waveform is now commonly used to derive further physiological measures by minimally invasive cardiac output monitors.

The area under the curve of the systolic part of the pressure waveform is used to derive stroke volume and hence cardiac output. To do so, a measure or estimate of arterial compliance is required, which can be derived from the slope of the diastolic pressure decay and the position of the dicrotic notch. Patient demographic and physical data may be used to calibrate this. An estimate of myocardial contractility may be derived from the slope of the pressure waveform at the onset of systole, the rate of change of pressure over time, dP/dt.

Intravascular filling or volume status may be estimated from changes in the arterial pressure over the respiratory cycle. Changes in intrathoracic pressure, particularly with positive-pressure ventilation, affect venous return to the heart and lead to periodic increases and decreases in arterial blood pressure. These changes are more marked in hypovolaemia, so a measure of the degree of variability (pulse pressure or stroke volume variation) is a reliable indicator of fluid-responsiveness.

Many of these derived measures rely on assumptions or demographic data, and as such they may be inaccurate as measures of specific values. However, analysis of trends or response to interventions such as fluid challenges can yield very valuable information. The accuracy of these measures is increased by calibration, for example by indicator dilution methods.

Marik PE, Cavallazzi R, Vasu T, Hirani A. Dynamic changes in arterial waveform derived variables and fluid responsiveness in mechanically ventilated patients: a systematic review of the literature. *Crit Care Med* 2009; 37: 2642–7.

Question B6: Electrical safety

Regarding electrical safety, which of the following are correct?

A. Moist skin surfaces reduce the risk of microshock
B. Microshock is defined as current flow of less than 1 amp
C. Pulmonary artery catheters would are classed as type BF electrical equipment
D. Floating circuits improve the safety of operating theatres
E. UK mains electricity is supplied at 50 Hz 240 V alternating current

Answer: FFFTT

Short explanation

Moist skin surfaces increase the risk of microshock due to a reduction in impedance. Microshock is defined as current flow of less than 100 micro-amps (μA). Type BF equipment uses a floating circuit but is not appropriate for direct connection to the heart. Type CF electrical equipment can be directly connected to the heart.

Long explanation

Electrical safety is very important in critical care. Commonly we use multiple electrical appliances which are connected directly to the patient in the presence of fluids and moist surfaces. Mains electricity in the UK is supplied at a frequency of 50 Hz and a potential of 240 volts. Electrical current at this frequency is most likely to result in cardiac arrhythmias.

Electrical damage can be caused by electrocution, burns or ignition of a flammable material causing a fire or explosion. The amount of current that flows through the body will determine the amount of damage that is caused. Current is directly related to voltage and indirectly proportional to resistance or impedance. If there is moisture present on the skin surface, the impedance will be lowered and so the current flow will be greater. Current flow of 15 mA will cause tetany and muscle spasm leading to respiratory failure if not removed. Current flow of 75 mA will cause ventricular fibrillation.

Microshock occurs when much smaller currents are directly conducted through the heart. Current of less than 100 μA can induce ventricular fibrillation if it flows directly through the heart. This may occur via a pulmonary artery catheter or central line. Such equipment, which is connected to the heart, has special electrical safety limits and type designations. These are based on the maximum permissible leakage currents. Type B equipment has a maximum leakage current of 100 μA. It is not suitable for direct connection to the heart. Type BF equipment is similar to type B but has an isolated circuit. Type CF equipment provides the highest level of protection. The maximum permissible leakage current is less than 10 μA. It is suitable for direct connection to the heart and includes equipment such as ECG leads, pressure transducers and thermodilution computers. Floating circuits use an isolating transformer to prevent current flowing from source directly to earth. The patient is not earthed and is said to be floating. Entire operating theatres can be supplied with electricity by these means.

Boumphrey S, Langton J. Electrical safety in the operating theatre. *Br J Anaesth CEPD Rev* 2003; 3: 10–14.

Sanders D, McCormick B. Electricity and magnetism. *Update Anaesth* 2008; 24: 174–81.

Question B7: Septic shock

Septic shock:

A. Is defined as sepsis with hypotension
B. Has both pathogen and host aetiological factors
C. Invariably leads to an increase in cardiac output
D. Leads to multi-organ failure and death in up to 50% of cases
E. Is usually characterised by high levels of IL-1, IL-5 and TNF-γ

Answer: FTFTF

Short explanation

Septic shock is hypotension and tissue hypoperfusion secondary to infection despite adequate fluid resuscitation. Cardiac output is commonly but not universally increased. The pathophysiology is complex and involves multiple factors related to the pathogen, host defence and host physiology. Pro-inflammatory cytokines commonly implicated in septic shock are IL-1, IL-6 and TNF-α.

Long explanation

There are several definitions in the field of systemic infection:

- SIRS: systemic inflammatory response syndrome
- Sepsis: SIRS due to infection
- Severe sepsis: sepsis with organ dysfunction or tissue hypoperfusion
- Sepsis-induced hypotension (SIH): systolic blood pressure < 90 or mean arterial pressure < 70 mmHg secondary to sepsis
- Septic shock: SIH and hypoperfusion despite adequate fluid resuscitation

Septic shock is a major cause of intensive care admission and mortality. It commonly leads to multi-organ dysfunction, failure and death. Mortality rates from septic shock can be in excess of 50%.

The primary insult in septic shock is infection of a normally sterile tissue by a pathogen. The commonest cause of sepsis is bacterial infection, but viral and fungal infections can also lead to septic shock. Invading pathogens must evade early host defences to establish a significant infection, which depends on the number of organisms in the initial insult and various virulence factors allowing host defence avoidance.

The inflammatory immune response is responsible for the majority of the pathology in septic shock. It is triggered by detection of pathogen-released components or toxins (e.g. lipopolysaccharide, peptidoglycan, bacterial DNA) by pattern recognition receptors (e.g. toll-like receptors) on cells of the innate immune system, such as monocytes. A positive feedback system is activated, leading to the release of pro-inflammatory (e.g. IL-1, IL-6, TNF-α) and anti-inflammatory cytokines (e.g. IL-10, IL-4), and activation of complement, platelet aggregation and the coagulation cascade.

In severe sepsis and septic shock, an exaggerated response leads to cell, tissue and organ dysfunction. Neutrophils and lymphocytes undergo increased apoptosis and the coagulation system is abnormally activated, which can lead to microvascular occlusion and disseminated intravascular coagulation (DIC). Microcirculatory dysfunction, vasodilatation and increased capillary permeability lead to effective hypovolaemia and cardiovascular compromise. Cardiac output is usually increased but not universally, and sepsis-induced myocardial dysfunction is common.

Septic shock therefore shares some features with other distributive shocks, but also exhibits elements of hypovolaemic and cardiogenic shock. Management of this complicated condition should be goal-directed and flexible, encompassing both the shock syndromes and the underlying condition.

Dellinger RP, Levy MM, Rhodes A, *et al*. Surviving Sepsis Campaign. International guidelines for management of severe sepsis and septic shock: 2012. *Crit Care Med* 2013; 41: 580–637.

Question B8: RIFLE criteria for acute kidney injury

With regards to the assessment of acute kidney injury using the RIFLE criteria:

A. Patients who are anuric for 16 hours are classed as at risk of acute kidney injury
B. Patients with loss of kidney function 6 weeks after the original injury would be classed as having end-stage kidney disease
C. Baseline creatinine is required to fully classify patients using the RIFLE criteria
D. Patients who fall into RIFLE class R have an increased mortality compared to those who maintain normal function
E. Patients with a creatinine level twice their baseline level are classified as having acute kidney injury

Answer: FFFTT

Short explanation

Patients who are anuric for over 12 hours are classified as acute kidney injury. Patients with loss of kidney function beyond 3 months following the original injury are classified as having end-stage kidney disease. Urine output is sufficient to diagnose acute kidney injury according to the RIFLE criteria.

Long explanation

There have been recent efforts to classify acute kidney injury and failure in order to diagnose patients and prognosticate. Evidence suggests that small rises in creatinine can be significant and lead to further kidney damage if not addressed early. The Acute Dialysis Outcome Initiative group proposed the RIFLE criteria in 2004. This aims to achieve a standard means of diagnosis and classification of acute kidney injury.

There are three grades of severity – Risk, Injury and Failure – and two grades of outcome – Loss of kidney function and End-stage kidney disease. The severity grades are based on either the creatinine levels or the urine output or both. The severity grade is defined as the worst possible criterion that a patient achieves. Subsequent studies using these criteria have confirmed that they can be used as a predictive tool for hospital mortality.

Joannidis M, Metnitz B, Bauer P, *et al*. Acute kidney injury in critically ill patients classified by AKIN versus RIFLE using the SAPS 3 database. *Intensive Care Med* 2009; 35: 1692–702.

Question B9: SAPS II

The Simplified Acute Physiology Score II (SAPS II):

A. Can be used to predict mortality
B. Is calculated daily
C. Is based purely on physiological measurements and observations

D. Can be modified according to region of the world
E. Excludes burns and cardiac patients

Answer: TFFFT

Short explanation

SAPS II is a severity of illness score. It uses age, three measures of chronic health, type of admission and 12 weighted physiological variables to produce a numerical raw score and predicted mortality. It is calculated once, using the worst value of each physiological variable in the first 24 hours of admission. Burns, cardiac and juvenile patients are excluded from analysis.

Long explanation

The Simplified Acute Physiology Score II (SAPS II) was developed in 1993 as the successor to SAPS (1984). It is the most commonly used illness severity score in Europe. It was based on more than 13,000 European and North American patients, excluding burns patients, cardiology and cardiac surgery patients, and patients under 18 years of age. Its successor, SAPS 3, can be modified according to region of the world.

SAPS II uses weighted scores of 17 variables to give a numerical score between 0 and 163, with a sigmoid relationship to predicted mortality. Twelve of the variables are acute physiological measures (see below), with the worst value in the first 24 hours entered into the calculation. The other variables are age, type of admission (medical, expected surgical or unexpected surgical) and chronic condition (metastatic cancer, haematological malignancy, AIDS).

The physiological variables are as follows:

Observations	Investigations
Heart rate	Serum bicarbonate
Systolic BP	Serum bilirubin
Temperature	Serum urea
PaO_2/FiO_2 ratio	White blood cell count
Urine output	Serum potassium
Glasgow Coma Scale	Serum sodium

SAPS II differs from APACHE II in some of the physiological variables measured, but mainly in that SAPS II is able to give a predicted mortality without the admitting diagnosis being recorded. Both scoring systems have similar predictive value (area under ROC curve 0.86 for SAPS II, 0.85 for APACHE II). The APACHE II values should only be used for audits or studies, and not for prognostication in individual patients.

Le Gall JR, Lemeshow S, Saulnier F. A new Simplified Acute Physiology Score (SAPS II) based on a European/North American multicenter study. *JAMA* 1993; 270: 2957–63.

Palazzo M. Severity of illness and likely outcome from critical illness. In Bersten AD, Soni N. *Oh's Intensive Care Manual*, 6th edn. Edinburgh: Butterworth-Heinemann, 2009, pp. 17–30.

Question B10: Anaphylaxis

Regarding anaphylaxis:

A. Muscle relaxants are a more common precipitant of anaphylaxis than antibiotics
B. Hypotension is usually the first sign in critically ill patients
C. ST elevation may be a feature on the ECG
D. Epinephrine 50 μg IM is the first-line treatment
E. Gelatin or starch solutions may be used to correct distributive shock

Answer: TTTFF

Short explanation

Gelatin and starch solutions may be the precipitants for anaphylactic reactions, so their use in resuscitation is not advised. First-line treatment of anaphylaxis is epinephrine 500–1000 μg IM or 50–100 μg IV.

Long explanation

Anaphylaxis is a severe, life-threatening, generalised or systemic hypersensitivity reaction. Anaphylaxis may be classified into allergic anaphylaxis and non-allergic anaphylaxis, previously called 'anaphylactoid'. Allergic anaphylaxis occurs when exposure to a foreign antigen stimulates production of IgE antibodies which bind to mast cells and basophils. After further exposure to the antigen, IgE cross-linking results in mast-cell degranulation and release of histamine, slow-reacting substance A, leukotrienes, tryptase and prostaglandins. These substances lead to the clinical features of increased mucous secretion, bronchoconstriction, vasodilatation and increased vascular permeability. The clinical features may be identical in allergic and non-allergic anaphylaxis, but in the latter IgE is not part of the pathological process.

Common triggers in intensive care and anaesthesia include muscle relaxants, colloids, induction agents, antibiotics and contrast media. For this reason, amongst many others, gelatin and starch solutions are not suitable for the resuscitation of these patients as they may be the precipitant or worsen the condition.

The clinical features seen in the critically ill or anaesthetised patient may not be typical. Cardiovascular collapse or hypotension is a common first sign, followed by bronchospasm. Local release of mediators may cause coronary artery spasm with signs of myocardial ischaemia or acute left or right ventricular failure. Hypotension exacerbates myocardial ischaemia, and myocardial infarction is a possibility. Differential diagnosis should include tension pneumothorax, acute asthma, pulmonary embolus and tube displacement.

Management of anaphylaxis involves an 'ABC' approach with immediate administration of epinephrine. The dose of epinephrine is 500 μg IM or 50 μg IV. Further treatment includes intravenous steroids and antihistamines, crystalloid fluid resuscitation, salbutamol nebulisers or infusion for bronchospasm, and occasionally epinephrine infusions for refractory shock.

Anaphylaxis usually resolves in 2–8 hours, but the response may be biphasic, and therefore observation of the patient for 4–6 hours is recommended even in non-life-threatening episodes. Complications of anaphylaxis include myocardial ischaemia, hypoxic brain injury, coagulopathy and death.

Association of Anaesthetists of Great Britian and Ireland. *AAGBI Safety Guideline: Suspected Anaphylactic Reactions Associated with Anaesthesia*. London: AAGBI, 2009.

Ryder SA, Waldmann C. Anaphylaxis. *Contin Educ Anaesth Crit Care Pain* 2004; 4: 111–13.

Sim K, Webster N, Anaphylaxis. In Waldmann C, Soni N, Rhodes A. *Oxford Desk Reference: Critical Care*. Oxford: Oxford University Press, 2008; pp. 456–7.

Question B11: Gram-positive bacilli

Which of the following are Gram-positive bacilli?

A. *Pseudomonas aeruginosa*
B. *Clostridium perfringens*
C. *Clostridium botulinum*
D. *Bacillus cereus*
E. *Listeria monocytogenes*

Answer: FTTTT

Short explanation

Pseudomonas aeruginosa is a Gram-negative aerobic bacterium. Gram-positive bacilli are one of the smallest groups of bacteria. They are commonly motile and spore-forming. Spores often survive heat, drying, radiation and chemicals.

Long explanation

Gram-positive bacilli are a small group of bacteria, many of which have significant clinical importance for critical care clinicians. Some of these bacteria may cause life-threatening infections. *Bacillus anthracis* causes cutaneous anthrax, pulmonary anthrax (which may be fatal within hours) and gastrointestinal anthrax. Its endospore can disperse widely in dust and water and causes outbreaks among humans and cattle. *Bacillus cereus* (and its endospores) causes severe gastrointestinal upset which usually self-terminates in 24 hours. It is often contracted from reheated rice.

The *Bacillus* microbes are aerobes. The *Clostridium* group of bacteria are anaerobes. *C. perfringens* causes gas gangrene, also known as anaerobic cellulitis. *C. difficile* causes antibiotic-associated diarrhoea and may lead to pseudomembranous colitis and toxic megacolon requiring emergency surgery. *C. botulinum* causes botulism, a serious condition where acetylcholine release at the neuromuscular junction is blocked. Difficulty swallowing and respiratory paralysis can occur. *C. tetani* produces an exotoxin which blocks interneuron inhibition of motor neuron activity. This leads to muscular spasm, affecting the jaw muscles (causing lockjaw), facial muscles (risus sardonicus) and paraspinal muscles (opisthotonus), amongst other effects.

Listeria monocytogenes can cause gastrointestinal upset but also causes meningitis in neonates and the elderly. This is not a spore-forming organism. *Corynebacterium diphtheriae* is also non-spore-forming and produces a toxin which can cause systemic sepsis and myocardial and neuronal effects. An effective vaccine is available. Bacteria of the genus *Propionibacterium* cause skin problems such as acne vulgaris.

Steinbach W, Shetty A. Use of the diagnostic laboratory: a practical review for the clinician. *Postgrad Med J* 2001; 77: 148–56.

Question B12: Status epilepticus

In a case of convulsive status epilepticus:

A. Intravenous diazepam is the recommended first-line drug
B. Intravenous lorazepam can be administered before phenytoin
C. Phenytoin should not be given to patients who are already taking antiepileptic medication

D. Propofol is contraindicated for induction of anaesthesia, because of its epileptiform effects
E. Pre-existing antiepileptic medication should not be administered

Answer: FTFFF

Short explanation

Diazepam 10 mg should be administered rectally and repeated after 10–15 minutes if the seizure continues. Buccal midazolam may be used as an alternative. Lorazepam is the intravenous drug of choice. Propofol has anticonvulsant effects. Phenytoin should be administered with caution in patients who are already taking it. Pre-existing antiepileptic medication should be reinstituted as soon as possible.

Long explanation

Status epilepticus is a medical emergency with a high mortality rate if not treated quickly and correctly. Status epilepticus has a number of definitions, including seizure activity lasting 30 minutes or more, or intermittent seizure activity lasting 30 minutes during which consciousness is not regained.

During the first phase of seizures the metabolic requirements of neurons are increased. This increased requirement is met by increased cerebral blood flow brought about by autonomic activation, hypertension and tachycardia. High blood glucose is also stimulated via the autonomic response. After prolonged seizure activity (around 30 minutes) the compensatory mechanisms begin to fail and adequate cerebral perfusion is not maintained. This leads to a failure of cerebral autoregulation, raised intracranial pressure, hypotension, hypoglycaemia and rising lactate levels. This can lead to electromechanical dissociation whereby there is little muscle twitching associated with ongoing seizure activity.

Emergency management should be based on an ABC resuscitation approach while also administering antiepileptic medication. Initial management focuses on establishing and securing the airway, administering oxygen and obtaining intravenous access. Glucose should be administered if hypoglycaemia is suspected or found. In a prehospital setting, the patient should receive 10 mg of PR diazepam, repeated after 15 minutes if still fitting; 10 mg buccal midazolam may be given as an alternative. Once intravenous access is established, lorazepam 0.1 mg/kg (usually 4 mg) may be given and repeated once after 10–20 minutes. If seizures continue, phenytoin 15–18 mg/kg should be administered at a rate of 50 mg per minute. Refractory status epilepticus should be treated with induction of general anaesthesia, using propofol, midazolam or thiopental and transfer to the intensive care unit.

National Clinical Guideline Centre. *Pharmacological Update of Clinical Guideline 20: The Epilepsies: the Diagnosis and Management of the Epilepsies in Adults and Children in Primary and Secondary Care*. London: National Clinical Guideline Centre, 2012.

National Institute for Health and Care Excellence. *CG137: The Epilepsies: the Diagnosis and Management of the Epilepsies in Adults and Children in Primary and Secondary Care*. London: NICE, 2012. http://www.nice.org.uk/cg137 (accessed June 2014).

Question B13: Life-threatening asthma

Regarding the pharmacological management of life-threatening asthma:

A. Aminophylline administration commonly causes a lactic acidosis
B. Helium is used to reduce bronchoconstriction
C. Hypotension during mechanical ventilation should be treated with fluids

D. β-Adrenergic receptor agonists increase ventilation/perfusion mismatch
E. β-Adrenergic receptor agonists increase diaphragmatic contractility

Answer: FFFTF

Short explanation

β-Adrenergic receptor agonists increase V/Q mismatch and may cause a lactic acidosis. Aminophylline increases diaphragmatic contractility. Helium reduces the work of breathing. Hypotension during mechanical ventilation may be due to dynamic hyperinflation.

Long explanation

Asthma is a chronic inflammatory disease of the airways characterised by variable bronchoconstriction and airflow limitation. Treatment includes a stepwise management approach with short-acting β-adrenergic receptor agonists, inhaled corticosteroids, long-acting β-adrenergic receptor agonists and adjunctive agents including leukotriene receptor antagonists, chromoglycates and theophylline.

Life-threatening asthma is a reason for critical care admission, and one should be alerted to its presence if one or more of the following features are present:

(1) peak expiratory flow rate (PEFR) < 33% best or predicted
(2) SpO_2 < 92% or PaO_2 < 8 kPa
(3) normal $PaCO_2$
(4) silent chest
(5) cyanosis
(6) poor respiratory effort or exhaustion
(7) cardiac arrhythmias
(8) altered conscious level

Acute severe or life-threatening asthma is initially treated with continuous nebulised β-adrenergic receptor agonists. These reduce bronchoconstriction and therefore increase V/Q mismatch, but this may be offset with supplementary oxygen. High-dose inhaled or intravenous β-adrenergic receptor agonists may cause a lactic acidosis. Aminophylline is used as a bronchodilator. It also increases diaphragmatic contractility, although toxicity is a problem. Helium reduces the work of breathing only; it has no effect on bronchoconstriction. Hypotension during mechanical ventilation is common in asthmatic patients. These patients may be hypovolaemic prior to intubation due to insensible losses, so fluid loading may be appropriate before induction. After induction, gas trapping and dynamic hyperinflation are causes of hypotension that need to be excluded.

British Thoracic Society, Scottish Intercollegiate Guidelines Network. *British Guideline on the Management of Asthma: A National Clinical Guideline*. May 2008, revised January 2012. Edinburgh & London: BTS & SIGN, 2012.

Question B14: Atrial fibrillation management

The following drugs are used in the management of atrial fibrillation:

A. Metoprolol
B. Verapamil
C. Sotalol
D. Flecainide
E. Isosorbide mononitrate

Answer: TTTTF

Short explanation

All of these drugs, with the exception of isosorbide mononitrate (used for prophylaxis of angina and as an adjunct in the treatment of congestive cardiac failure) can be used in the management of atrial fibrillation. Some of the drugs have slightly different indications for use. Atrial fibrillation can occur acutely with cardiovascular compromise, as a chronic condition or as paroxysmal episodes. In addition to rate and/or rhythm control, it is important to reduce the risk of embolic events in these patients. Antiplatelet agents or anticoagulants are used for this reason.

Long explanation

The pharmacological management of atrial fibrillation (AF) sometimes appears to be quite complicated. When approaching a patient with AF it is important to start with the basic principles before considering what drugs may be used.

In critical care patients, AF may be a new diagnosis or a pre-existing condition, and this should be elucidated. Some patients have chronic AF, either continuously or as paroxysmal episodes. These patients are at a higher risk of acute episodes of fast AF when they are critically ill. Other patients may experience their first episode while on the intensive care unit. This can be precipitated by many factors, including sepsis, hypovolaemia, electrolyte disturbances such as hypomagnesaemia, or administration of pro-arrhythmic agents such as inotropes.

An assessment of the cardiovascular status of the patient should be made as soon as possible. If there is significant cardiovascular instability in an episode of new-onset AF, then electrical DC cardioversion must always be considered. If the cardiovascular compromise is not considered life-threatening, then pharmacological agents may be required. The clinician needs to decide whether rhythm and rate or just rate control is required. In the acute setting where rate control is required, then either an oral β-blocker or a non-dihydropyridine calcium-channel antagonist should be given. If the intravenous route is preferred for faster onset then intravenous metoprolol or verapamil should be given. In patients with severely impaired left ventricular function, amiodarone may be used as an alternative. If the patient is haemodynamically compromised and pharmacological cardioversion is preferred, then the recommended agents are flecainide or propafenone, which work quicker than amiodarone. Digoxin is ineffective for AF termination and is not recommended.

Long-term treatment of AF is tailored to individual patients and will require specialist advice. Stroke prevention is particularly important and must be considered early in the diagnosis.

European Society of Cardiology (ESC) Task Force for the Management of Atrial Fibrillation. Guidelines for the management of atrial fibrillation. *Eur Heart J* 2010; 31: 2369–429.

Question B15: Positive-pressure ventilation complications

Complications of positive-pressure ventilation include:

A. Cardiovascular collapse
B. Bronchopleural fistula
C. Increased carbon monoxide transfer factor
D. Deranged liver function tests (LFTs)
E. Dysphagia

Answer: TTFTT

Short explanation

Positive pressure ventilation, while often a necessity as part of the management of the critically ill patient is associated with a number of complications. Carbon monoxide transfer factor is usually reduced as a consequence of damage to lung parenchyma.

Long explanation

Short-term complications of positive-pressure ventilation include hypotension and reduced cardiac output due to the reduced venous return from increased intrathoracic pressures. This may be sufficient to cause cardiac arrest in patients with very high intrathoracic pressures (e.g. asthmatics), especially if there is pre-existing uncorrected hypovolaemia. Reduced cardiac output may compromise liver perfusion and lead to deranged liver function tests and hyperlactataemia.

Pneumothoraces are a risk throughout the period of ventilation, and a bronchopleural fistula may be the end result.

Medium-term complications of ventilation include ventilator-induced lung injury, including atelectasis and parenchymal damage from exposure to high oxygen concentrations. This may reduce the carbon monoxide transfer factor. The risk of ventilator-associated pneumonia increases with time and may further damage the lungs.

Long-term complications of ventilation are usually upper airway problems related to intubation, e.g. tracheal stenosis, dysphonia, dysphagia and laryngeal swelling. Dysphagia may also be of relevance in patients with tracheostomies, particularly with the cuff inflated. Regular swallow assessment is necessary, and dietary modifications may be required.

Strategies to avoid complications of positive-pressure ventilation include fluid resuscitation, minimisation of ventilator pressures, and regular assessments of the patient's ability to wean from the ventilator.

Gould T, de Beer JMA. Principles of artificial ventilation. *Anaesth Intensive Care Med* 2007; 8: 91–101.

Waldmann C, Soni N, Rhodes A. *Oxford Desk Reference: Critical Care*. Oxford: Oxford University Press, 2008; pp. 6–7.

Question B16: Lactic acidosis

Regarding lactic acidosis in critically ill patients:

A. Metformin is associated with type B lactic acidosis
B. Lactate levels of > 10 mmol/l are associated with > 80% mortality
C. There is evidence that bicarbonate infusions reduce mortality in lactic acidosis
D. Venous blood samples can be used to monitor lactate levels
E. Lactate is removed efficiently by continuous venovenous haemofiltration

Answer: TTFTF

Short explanation

Bicarbonate has not been shown to improve outcome in lactic acidosis. Lactate is not removed efficiently by continuous venovenous haemofiltration, and treatment of lactic acidosis is of the underlying cause.

Long explanation

Lactate is a by-product of anaerobic glycolysis. Hyperlactataemia is defined as a plasma lactate > 2 mmol/l, with lactic acidosis defined as hyperlactataemia plus acidosis. Lactic acidosis may be subdivided into two types according to aetiology, but this is of minimal significance clinically as the two types often co-exist in the critically ill patient. Type A lactic acidosis is due to tissue hypoxia, e.g. shock, hypoxia, cardiac failure. Type B is due to impaired lactate clearance and the patients do not show overt signs of tissue hypoxia, e.g. hepatic failure, diabetes mellitus, drugs including metformin, and inborn errors of metabolism.

Lactate may be measured in arterial or venous blood samples, as there is very little difference between the two.

Lactic acidosis is of significance in intensive care patients because it is associated with a high mortality in general ICU patients, and may be predictive of adverse outcomes in trauma patients. Lactate levels of > 10 mmol/l are associated with > 80% mortality in general ICU patients, and a lactate > 2 mmol/l 48 hours after injury in trauma patients has a mortality of 86%.

Treatment of lactic acidosis is mainly that of the underlying cause with supportive treatment of organ systems. Continuous venovenous haemofiltration is inefficient at reducing plasma lactate. Bicarbonate infusion remains controversial as it may cause hypocalcaemia and acute hypercapnia, and may shift the oxyhaemoglobin dissociation curve to the right, thereby actually reducing oxygen delivery to the tissues. There is no evidence of clinical benefit from bicarbonate administration.

Abramson D, Scalea TM, Hitchcock R, *et al*. Lactate clearance and survival following injury. *J Trauma* 1993; 35: 584–8.

Cooper DJ, Nichol AD. Lactic acidosis. In Bersten AD, Soni N. *Oh's Intensive Care Manual*, 5th edn. Edinburgh: Butterworth-Heinemann, 2003; pp. 173–4.

Phypers B, Pierce JMT. Lactate physiology in health and disease. *Contin Educ Anaesth Crit Care Pain* 2006; 6: 128–32.

Stacpoole PW, Wright EC, Baumgartner TG, *et al*. Natural history and course of acquired lactic acidosis in adults. DCA-Lactic Acidosis Study Group. *Am J Med* 1994; 97: 47–54.

Question B17: Drug administration during CPR

During cardiopulmonary resuscitation, recommended drug dosages and regimens are as follows:

A. Epinephrine as soon as access is achieved in asystole
B. Epinephrine 3 mg via endotracheal tube for PEA/asystole if no IV access
C. Amiodarone 300 mg before the third shock in VF/VT
D. Atropine 3 mg for PEA at a rate of < 60 bpm
E. Epinephrine 1 mg after the second shock in VF/VT

Answer: TFFFF

Short explanation

Epinephrine 1 mg is given after the third shock in VF/VT. The endotracheal route is no longer recommended; intraosseous access is used if IV access is not possible. Amiodarone is given after the third shock for refractory VF/VT. Atropine is not longer recommended for PEA or asystole.

Long explanation

Epinephrine 1 mg is given after the third shock in VF/VT, and as soon as venous access is established in non-shockable rhythms. Amiodarone is also given after the third shock for refractory VF/VT. Atropine is no longer recommended for the treatment of pulseless electrical activity (PEA) or asystole.

The endotracheal route is no longer recommended for drug administration; intraosseous (IO) access is preferred if intravenous (IV) access is not possible. This is because unpredictable plasma concentrations are achieved when drugs are given via a tracheal tube, and therefore the tracheal dose of most drugs is unknown; it could be 3–10 times the IV dose. Drug delivery via a supraglottic airway device is even less reliable and should not be attempted. There is now an increased availability and simplicity of intraosseous devices, and evidence that intraosseous injection of drugs achieves adequate plasma concentrations in a time comparable with injection through a central venous catheter.

Atropine is an acetylcholine antagonist at muscarinic receptors blocking the effect of the vagus nerve on both the sinoatrial (SA) node and the atrioventricular (AV) node, increasing sinus automaticity and facilitating AV node conduction. However, studies have shown no benefit from administration of atropine during cardiac arrest, probably because asystole during cardiac arrest is usually due to primary myocardial pathology rather than excessive vagal tone. Routine use of atropine for asystole or PEA is therefore no longer recommended. Atropine is indicated in sinus, atrial or nodal bradycardias with haemodynamic compromise.

Resuscitation Council (UK). Advanced life support algorithm. In *Advanced Life Support*, 6th edn. London: Resuscitation Council, 2011; Chapter 6.

Deakin CD, Nolan JP, Soar J, *et al.* European Resuscitation Council Guidelines for Resuscitation 2010. Section 4: Adult advanced life support. *Resuscitation* 2010; 81: 1305–52.

Waldmann C, Soni N, Rhodes A. *Oxford Desk Reference: Critical Care*. Oxford: Oxford University Press, 2008; pp. 240–1.

Question B18: Blood transfusion complications

Complications of blood transfusion include:

A. Prolonged QT interval on ECG
B. Increase in cancer recurrence
C. Metabolic alkalosis
D. Incompatibility reactions due to IgG anti-A or anti-B antibodies
E. Anaphylaxis

Answer: TTTFT

Short explanation

Antibodies to ABO are IgM. Anti-rhesus D antibodies are IgG.

Long explanation

Adverse reactions to blood transfusions may be divided into immune and non-immune.

Non-immune reactions include a dilutional coagulopathy, disseminated intravascular coagulation (DIC), circulatory overload, air embolism, thrombophlebitis, hyperkalaemia, citrate toxicity, hypothermia and transmission of infection.

Citrate is used as an anticoagulant when blood is donated and remains in the plasma fraction which is present in fresh frozen plasma (FFP) and to a lesser extent in platelets and cryoprecipitate. There is virtually no citrate in red cell concentrate transfusions, as these are stored in SAG-M (saline adenine, glucose and mannitol). Citrate will bind plasma calcium unless it is first metabolised by the liver to bicarbonate. Excessive citrate administration will cause a metabolic alkalosis, although in practice patients requiring a blood transfusion of this size are usually shocked and have a metabolic acidosis masking any effect of the citrate. If the patient is hypothermic, citrate metabolism is reduced and hypocalcaemia may be clinically significant. It may result in hypotension, flat ST segments and prolonged QT interval on an ECG.

Immune reactions to blood transfusion include immediate and delayed haemolytic reactions, non-haemolytic febrile reactions, transfusion-related lung injury (TRALI), anaphylaxis, graft-versus-host disease and immune sensitisation (rhesus D antigen leading to haemolytic disease of the newborn).

ABO incompatibility is the leading cause of immediate haemolytic reactions. Antibodies to ABO are IgM. Anti-rhesus D antibodies are IgG and can therefore cross the placenta to cause haemolytic disease of the newborn.

Anaphylaxis is a rare complication of transfusion. It occurs most often in patients with a hereditary IgA deficiency and pre-existing anti-IgA antibodies. It is not dose-related, and treatment is the same as for anaphylaxis from other causes. It is prevented by the use of washed red blood cells (residual plasma and therefore IgA removed).

There is increasing evidence implicating blood transfusions as a factor in poorer outcomes seen in some patients undergoing major surgery, particularly for cancer. Transfusion-related immunomodulation is the term describing the immunosuppression seen after blood transfusion that may play a role in increased susceptibility to infection as well as the increased incidence of cancer recurrence.

Isbister JP. Blood transfusion. In Bersten AD, Soni N. *Oh's Intensive Care Manual*, 6th edn. Edinburgh: Butterworth-Heinemann, 2009; pp. 995–1010.

Maxwell MJ, Wilson MJA. Complications of blood transfusion. *Contin Educ Anaesth Crit Care Pain* 2006; 6: 225–9.

Question B19: Temporary cardiac pacing

Regarding emergency cardiac pacing in a periarrest patient:

A. The QRS complex in complete heart block is > 0.12 seconds
B. Pacing should be routinely used in P-wave asystole
C. In percussion pacing, the fist should hit the lower third of the sternum
D. The preferred paddle position for transcutaneous pacing is right pectoral–apical
E. The average current required during transcutaneous pacing is 50–100 μA

Answer: FTFTF

Short explanation

The QRS complex in complete heart block may be narrow or broad depending on the level of the block. In percussion pacing the fist should aim lateral to the lower left sternal edge. The average current required during transcutaneous pacing is 50–100 mA.

Long explanation

Temporary pacing is used in patients with a bradycardia that is insufficient to maintain adequate cardiac output and that has not responded to medical treatment such as atropine. Pacing may be non-invasive (percussion pacing or transcutaneous) or invasive (temporary or permanent transvenous pacing).

The QRS complex in complete heart block may be broad or narrow, depending on the level of the block. If the block is at the level of the atrioventricular (AV) node the escape rhythm will be produced in the cells immediately below the node and will travel down the His–Purkinje system resulting in a narrow QRS complex.

If all the fibres of the conducting system are affected by the myocardial infarction/disease process affecting conduction, then automaticity will be generated by the ventricular cells themselves. This is slow, unstable, broad complex and prone to further arrhythmias or asystole. The occurrence of significant or symptomatic pauses implies a risk of asystole, and temporary pacing should be initiated as soon as possible.

Percussion pacing is used in the periarrest situation or where there is P-wave asystole. It is less traumatic to the patient than CPR so should be considered in bradycardia or P-wave asystole. It is unlikely to be successful in true asystole and should not be attempted in this situation. The impulse should be delivered with the side of a closed fist from a height of approximately 10 cm onto the precordium at the lower left sternal edge. If initial blows do not produce a QRS complex, the site of the blow and its power may be altered. Should percussion pacing fail to produce an output, CPR should be started immediately.

Transcutaneous pacing can be established quickly in the periarrest/arrest situation, and should be continued until a natural rhythm is restored or transvenous pacing can be established. The preferred paddle position is right pectoral–apical, but anterior–posterior placement is also effective. The current should be gradually increased until there is electrical and mechanical capture. The average current required during transcutaneous pacing is 50–100 mA. Sedation/analgesia will usually be required for the discomfort associated with the procedure.

Transvenous pacing requires expertise and specialist equipment. If it is required, therefore, help should be requested early.

Resuscitation Council (UK). Cardiac pacing. In *Advanced Life Support*, 6th edn. London: Resuscitation Council, 2011; Chapter 10.

Question B20: Acute respiratory distress syndrome

The following therapeutic options have been shown in a multicentre RCT to reduce mortality in acute respiratory distress syndrome (ARDS):

A. Lung-protective ventilation (LPV) at < 6 ml/kg actual body weight
B. Prone positioning
C. High-frequency oscillatory ventilation (HFOV)
D. Recruitment manoeuvres of 40 seconds at 40 cmH_2O
E. Ventilator care bundles

Answer: FTFFF

Short explanation

LPV has been shown to reduce mortality in ARDS by using tidal volumes of < 6 ml/kg predicted body weight. Prone positioning reduces mortality in ARDS with P/F ratio ≤ 150 mmHg. There has not been multicentre RCT evidence of mortality benefit for the use of HFOV or regular recruitment manoeuvres. Ventilator care bundles aim to reduce ventilator-associated pneumonia, but do not reduce mortality in ARDS.

Long explanation

Acute respiratory distress syndrome (ARDS) is a common cause of morbidity and mortality in the critically ill patient. Many different treatments, ventilator strategies and general approaches have been tried over the years, although very few have shown mortality benefits in large multicentre RCTs.

The ARDSNet study in 2000 was a multicentre RCT in North America that compared standard ventilation at the time (12 ml/kg predicted body weight (PBW), plateau pressures ≤ 50 cmH_2O) with LPV at 6 ml/kg PBW and plateau pressures ≤ 30 cmH_2O. The trial was stopped early as there was significantly reduced mortality in the LPV group (31% vs. 40%). This finding has been repeatedly replicated and is now at the heart of many international guidelines.

Prone positioning was the subject of a French multicentre RCT published in 2013. ARDS patients with P/F ratio < 150 mmHg were randomised to prone positioning for 16 hours per day until oxygenation improved or complications arose. Mortality at 28 days was significantly reduced in the prone group (16% vs. 33%).

The OSCAR and OSCILLATE trials were two multicentre RCTs comparing HFOV with standard (LPV) care, in the UK and Canada respectively, both published in 2013. The OSCAR trial showed no benefit of HFOV in ARDS, whereas the OSCILLATE trial showed increased mortality in the HFOV group and was stopped after recruitment of less than half the proposed number of patients.

Recruitment manoeuvres have been widely studied and have been shown to improve measures of oxygenation, but no reduction in mortality has been demonstrated. Ventilator care bundles are important for the reduction in rates of ventilator-associated pneumonia (VAP), but have not been shown to reduce mortality in ARDS.

Guérin C, Reignier J, Richard JC, *et al.* Prone positioning in severe acute respiratory distress syndrome. *N Engl J Med* 2013; 368: 2159–68.

Pelosi P, Gama de Abreu M, Rocco PRM. New and conventional strategies for lung recruitment in acute respiratory distress syndrome. *Crit Care* 2010; 14: 210.

Sud S, Sud M, Friedrich JO, *et al.* High-frequency ventilation versus conventional ventilation for the treatment of acute lung injury and acute respiratory distress syndrome: a systematic review and. *Cochrane Database Syst Rev* 2013; (2): CD004085.

Question B21: Hypothermia

Regarding the effects of hypothermia, which of the following are correct?

A. Metabolism reduces by 25% for every 1 °C reduction in core body temperature below 36 °C
B. Tissue oxygen delivery increases due to a reduction in haemoglobin affinity for oxygen
C. Drug metabolism is unaltered until core temperature falls below 35 °C
D. Osborn waves are commonly seen on the ECG of patients with core temperature below 32 °C
E. The QT interval is often increased in hypothermic patients

Answer: FFFTT

Short explanation

Metabolism reduces by around 10% for every 1 °C reduction in core temperature below 36 °C. Tissue oxygen delivery is reduced due to increased haemoglobin affinity for oxygen. Drug metabolism is slowed in hypothermia.

Long explanation

Hypothermia, defined as temperature less than 35 °C, can be either accidental or medically induced. Induced or therapeutic hypothermia has evidence of benefit in survivors of cardiac arrest, although it may be used in patients with traumatic brain injury or raised intracranial pressure.

In the winter months elderly patients are commonly admitted to the emergency department with hypothermia. The effects of hypothermia can be significant and affect many organ systems.

Cardiovascular changes seen will depend on the actual temperature. Initially peripheral vasoconstriction and tachycardia is seen. As the temperature falls, a progressive bradycardia occurs, due to reduced spontaneous depolarisation of the pacemaker cells. Increased systemic vascular resistance may maintain the blood pressure. Repolarisation abnormalities are also seen, and this is the cause of Osborn waves (also known as J waves), usually best observed in the lateral leads on the ECG. Progressive changes include broadening of the QRS complex, ST changes, T-wave inversion, increased PR interval, second- or third-degree heart block and prolonged QT interval. At temperatures below 24 °C there is a high risk of asystole. It is important to be aware that these changes can be seen even after rewarming, and so patients should remain on a cardiac monitor until they are fully resolved. Ventricular fibrillation is also a risk and may be brought about by physical manipulation, tracheal intubation or rewarming. Unfortunately most antiarrhythmic drugs and inotropes and chronotropes are ineffective at temperatures below 30 °C.

Other effects of hypothermia include increased bleeding risk due to reduced function of coagulation cascade enzymes, pancreatitis and tissue hypoxia due to a higher affinity of haemoglobin for oxygen. The latter results in reduced delivery of oxygen to the tissues at the cellular level.

Mallett M. Pathophysiology of accidental hypothermia. *Q J Med* 2002; 95: 775–85.
Ramaswamy K. Perioperative hypothermia. *Prevention and Management Tutorial of the Week* 2008; 117. http://www.frca.co.uk/Documents/117%20-%20perioperative%20hypothermia.pdf (accessed June 2014).

Question B22: Antibiotic mechanisms

Regarding the mechanism of action of antibiotics:

A. Benzylpenicillin is bacteriostatic
B. Clindamycin is bactericidal
C. Cephalosporins are bactericidal
D. Chloramphenicol is bacteriostatic
E. Macrolides are bacteriostatic

Answer: FFTTT

Short explanation

Penicillins and cephalosporins are bactericidal. Clindamycin, chloramphenicol and the macrolides are all bacteriostatic.

Long explanation

In general, antibacterial drugs either suppress the growth of (bacteriostatic) or kill (bactericidal) bacteria. They all have different mechanisms for achieving this.

Bactericidal antibiotics

- β-lactams (penicillins, cephalosporins, carbepenems and monobactams): inhibit cell-wall synthesis
- nitroimidazoles (metronidazole): affect bacterial DNA synthesis
- rifampicin: inhibits DNA-dependent RNA polymerase
- aminoglycosides: inhibit bacterial protein synthesis, inhibit bacterial ribosomal translocation and disrupt the integrity of the bacterial cell membrane

- fluoroquinolones (ciprofloxacin): inhibit DNA gyrase and topoisomerase 4
- glycopeptides: inhibit cell wall synthesis

Bacteriostatic antibiotics

- macrolides: inhibit bacterial protein synthesis
- tetracyclines: inhibit bacterial protein synthesis
- lincosamides (clindamycin): inhibit bacterial protein synthesis
- fuscidic acid: blocks RNA-transferase
- chloramphenicol: binds to 50S ribosomal subunit of bacteria

Peck TE, Hill SA, Williams M. Antimicrobials. In *Pharmacology for Anaesthesia and Intensive Care*, 2nd edn. Cambridge: Cambridge Press, 2006; pp. 311–35.

Thirunavakkarasu S, Lynch G. Antibiotics in critical care: an introduction. *Anaesthesia Tutorial of the Week* 2010; 168. http://www.aagbi.org/sites/default/files/168-Antibiotics-in-Critical-Care-an-introduction.pdf (accessed June 2014).

Question B23: Capnography

Capnography (end-tidal CO_2 monitoring) can help diagnose the following:

A. Obstructive airways disease
B. Endobronchial intubation
C. Tricyclic antidepressant (TCA) overdose
D. Pulmonary embolus
E. Effective CPR

Answer: TFFTT

Short explanation

A sloping upstroke on the capnograph suggests severe asthma or COPD. Oesophageal intubation can be ruled out by capnography, but not an endobronchial intubation. TCA overdose is monitored with ECG and blood gas analysis. Pulmonary emboli cause V/Q mismatch and reduce cardiac output, thus reducing end-tidal CO_2. Effective CPR leads to increased CO_2 delivery to the lungs and hence may be monitored with capnography.

Long explanation

End-tidal CO_2 monitoring forms part of universal monitoring for anaesthesia and should also be used for all intubations and transfers in ICU, emergency departments and elsewhere. Capnography, which measures and graphically displays CO_2 partial pressure over time, should be used in preference to capnometry (simple measurement of CO_2 partial pressure). The presence or absence of CO_2, the value of its partial pressure and the shape of the waveform can give valuable information for the diagnosis of many conditions.

The primary use of capnography in ICU is to quickly and accurately determine whether an attempt to intubate the trachea has been successful. The oesophagus and stomach may contain very small amounts of CO_2, but sustained levels of CO_2 from two or more ventilations confirms endotracheal intubation. Endobronchial intubation cannot be ruled out by capnography, which requires clinical examination, radiography or endoscopic bronchoscopy.

CO_2 monitoring can be used as a guide to effective CPR and to detect return of cardiac output following cardiac arrest. Similarly, a drop in end-tidal CO_2 levels suggests a significant reduction in cardiac output. Pulmonary embolisms cause V/Q mismatch and reduced cardiac output, and may therefore be detected by a sudden fall in end-tidal CO_2. This applies to all embolic material (air, fat, amniotic fluid etc.).

The shape of the capnography trace may also guide diagnosis. In severe asthma or chronic obstructive pulmonary disease (COPD), the normal, square-wave shape is replaced by a sloping upstroke. A ventilator leak will lead to a narrower, smaller CO_2 trace.

Resuscitation Council (UK). *Advanced Life Support*, 6th edn. London: Resuscitation Council, 2011.

Question B24: Burns – the Parkland formula

The Parkland formula for fluid management in the treatment of burns:

A. Is not necessary for burns of less than 10% TBSA
B. Includes factors for size and thickness of burn, age and weight
C. Prevents over-administration of fluid
D. Does not include maintenance fluids
E. Starts from the time of admission to hospital

Answer: TFFTF

Short explanation

The Parkland formula calculates resuscitation fluid requirements for burns > 15% total body surface area (TBSA) (10% in children and the elderly) for 24 hours from the time of the burn:

$$\text{Fluid requirement (ml)} = 4 \times \text{weight (kg)} \times \%\ \text{TBSA burned}$$

Measures of fluid status and perfusion (e.g. urine output) should inform increases and decreases in fluid administration.

Long explanation

The Parkland formula for fluid management in burns was developed in the 1960s by Charles R. Baxter at the Parkland Hospital Burns Unit in Dallas, Texas. It is used to calculate the amount of fluid required for resuscitation in the first 24 hours after a burn. It is the the most widely used burns fluid requirement calculator and has been adopted into ATLS guidelines. It applies to all burns of over 15% TBSA (10% in children and the elderly) as calculated by the rule of nines (or a Lund–Browder chart in paediatric burns).

$$\text{Fluid requirement (ml)} = 4 \times \text{weight (kg)} \times \%\ \text{TBSA burned}$$

Half of the fluid should be administered within the first 8 hours, and the remainder over the following 16 hours. The period of 24 hours starts from the time of the burn, and so an initial catch-up bolus is often required. The original specification was for Ringer's lactate, but Hartmann's solution and 0.9% saline can also be used.

The Parkland formula often leads to over-prescription of fluids, and it should only be used as a guide. Some centres use a formula of 50–75% of Parkland fluid requirement to prevent this. Over-administration of fluids is common and can be as dangerous as under-resuscitation in burns patients. Therefore, regular assessment of fluid status informed by markers of end-organ perfusion is the key to appropriate fluid management. Vital signs and lactate levels should be monitored and urine output of 0.5–1 ml/kg/h (1–2 ml/kg/h in children) should be maintained.

Bersten AD, Soni N. *Oh's Intensive Care Manual*. 6th ed. Edinburgh: Butterworth-Heinemann, 2009.

Question B25: Hyponatraemia

Which of the following would you expect to be associated with a plasma sodium < 136 mmol/l?

A. Addison's disease
B. Acute tubular necrosis
C. Primary hyperaldosteronism
D. Cerebral salt wasting syndrome
E. Nephrogenic diabetes insipidus

Answer: TTFTF

Short explanation

Primary hyperaldosteronism causes hypertension, hypokalaemia, metabolic alkalosis and a high or high normal sodium level. Nephrogenic diabetes insipidus is associated with hypernatraemia from dehydration.

Long explanation

Hyponatraemia is defined as a serum sodium < 136 mmol/l. Above 120 mmol/l, patients may be asymptomatic, but this depends largely on the rate of reduction of the sodium level. Below 120 mmol/l, patients are often lethargic, and complain of nausea and vomiting, anorexia and muscle cramps. Below 110 mmol/l patients exhibit delirium, coma and seizures.

The cause of hyponatraemia may be classified by whether the patient has a high, normal or low serum osmolality with the hyponatraemia. The latter is the commonest, as sodium contributes approximately 90% of the osmolality of the serum.

Causes of hyperosmolar hyponatraemia are hyperglycaemia or retained mannitol or glycine. Iso-osmolar hyponatraemia or pseudohyponatraemia is due to raised levels of triglycerides or paraproteins in the blood increasing the solid phase of the plasma.

Hypo-osmolar hyponatraemia is further subdivided into whether the patient is hypovolaemic, euvolaemic or hypervolaemic.

Hypovolaemic hypo-osmolar hyponatraemia is caused by renal sodium loss (diuretics, severe adrenal insufficiency including Addison's disease, and cerebral salt wasting syndrome). It may also be due to extrarenal sodium loss from diarrhoea, burns or pancreatitis.

Euvolaemic hypo-osmolar hyponatraemia is caused by mild adrenal insufficiency, hypothyroidism, thiazide diuretics, renal failure, polydipsia and the syndrome of inappropriate antidiuretic hormone secretion (SIADH).

Hypervolaemic hypo-osmolar hyponatraemia is due to combined sodium and water retention and is seen in congestive cardiac failure, renal failure and nephrotic syndrome.

Primary hyperaldosteronism causes hypertension, hypokalaemia, metabolic alkalosis and a high or high normal sodium level. Nephrogenic diabetes insipidus is associated with hypernatraemia from dehydration.

Bradshaw K, Smith M. Disorders of sodium balance after brain injury. *Contin Educ Anaesth Crit Care Pain* 2008; 8: 129–33.
Bergmans DC. Hyponatraemia. In Waldmann C, Soni N, Rhodes A. *Oxford Desk Reference: Critical Care*. Oxford: Oxford University Press, 2008; p. 414.

Question B26: Ventilation in acute asthma

Suitable ventilator modes for a patient following intubation for life-threatening acute asthma include:

A. Synchronised intermittent mandatory ventilation (SIMV)
B. Bilevel ventilation (BIPAP)
C. Airway pressure-release ventilation (APRV)
D. Continuous positive airway pressure (CPAP)
E. Pressure-support ventilation (PSV)

Answer: FTFFF

Short explanation

Ventilator mode should minimise airway pressures, allow a long expiratory time and minimise gas trapping. The only suitable mode among those listed is BIPAP.

Long explanation

Life-threatening acute asthma is characterised by a silent chest, little air movement and significant gas trapping from obstruction to expiration. These patients are notoriously difficult to ventilate.

The aims are to:

- reduce the work of breathing
- minimise gas trapping
- minimise airway pressures
- facilitate gas exchange by encouraging air movement

SIMV is a form of volume-controlled ventilation with the addition of synchrony or pressure support for the patient's own breaths. The pressure waveform in SIMV shows a linear pressure increase to a peak with an exponential decrease in expiration representing constant inspiratory flow. This may lead to extremely high airway pressures in asthma, as the ventilator takes no account of the volume of air in the lungs at the start of inspiration, leading to gas trapping and an increase in intrinsic PEEP.

APRV is similar to BIPAP in that it cycles between two levels of pressure to allow carbon dioxide clearance, but it is a mode designed primarily for lung recruitment and lung-protective ventilation in a spontaneously breathing patient. As its objective is a high mean airway pressure it is unsuitable for use in severe asthma, where the short expiratory time would lead to hypercapnia.

CPAP is a spontaneous breathing mode with a background level of pressure throughout the respiratory cycle. It would not be used immediately following intubation, as deep sedation and paralysis are required in the early stages for ventilatory control. The same is true for PSV, which is a mode of pressure-assisted spontaneous ventilation. Although this might reduce the work of breathing in the longer term, in the acute setting it is unlikely to be successful.

BIPAP is really the only option in asthmatic patients acutely, and careful consideration needs to be given to the settings. In general, aim for:

- tidal volume 6 ml/kg ideal body weight
- respiratory rate 10–14 breaths/minute
- permissive hypercapnia
- prolonged expiratory phase, e.g. I:E 1:4
- low PEEP (up to 80% of measured intrinsic PEEP)
- peak airway pressure < 30 cmH_2O

Gould T, de Beer JMA. Principles of artificial ventilation. *Anaesth Intensive Care Med* 2007; 8: 91–101.

Waldmann C, Soni N, Rhodes A. *Oxford Desk Reference: Critical Care.* Oxford: Oxford University Press, 2008; pp. 264–5.

Question B27: Arterial blood gas analysis

Regarding arterial blood gas (ABG) analysis:

A. Oxygen is measured with an oxygen fuel cell
B. Carbon dioxide is measured by change of pH of a bicarbonate buffer solution
C. pH is directly proportional to hydrogen ion concentration
D. Base excess is measured using a selectively permeable glass electrode
E. The standard bicarbonate is the amount of HCO_3^- in the plasma

Answer: FTFFF

Short explanation

Oxygen is measured with a Clark electrode. pH is the negative logarithm (base 10) of the hydrogen ion concentration. Base excess is derived, not measured. Actual bicarbonate is the amount of HCO_3^- in the plasma; standard bicarbonate is the concentration of HCO_3^- in fully oxygenated blood equilibrated with PCO_2 of 40 mmHg at 37 °C.

Long explanation

Arterial blood gas (ABG) analysis is ubiquitous and of huge importance in critical care. Arterial blood is sampled from indwelling catheters or directly form an artery (usually radial). Samples should be heparinised to prevent coagulation within the ABG analyser. ABG analysers consist of multiple electrodes for measurement of individual gases and ions and a computer to derive other useful values.

pH is defined as the negative logarithm (base 10) of the hydrogen ion concentration. It is measured with a pH electrode, which consists of two electrodes (Ag/AgCl and Hg/Hg_2Cl_2), a buffer solution and a membrane selectively permeable to H^+ ions. Any difference in the pH between the sample and the reference buffer solution is translated into a change of voltage between the electrodes.

Oxygen is measured with a Clark electrode, which consists of a platinum cathode and a silver/silver chloride anode. Reduction of oxygen at the cathode generates a current, which is measured with reference to two calibrator gases.

Carbon dioxide is measured by detection of changes in the pH of a bicarbonate buffer solution separated from the blood sample by a membrane permeable to CO_2 but not ions, cells or plasma. pH change is proportional to changes in PCO_2 and is calibrated with two gases of known CO_2 concentration.

Base excess is not measured, but is a derived value defined as the amount of strong acid or base required to restore a litre of blood to pH 7.4 at 37 °C with PCO_2 of 40 mmHg (5.3 kPa).

Actual bicarbonate is the measured or calculated concentration of HCO_3^- ions in the plasma. Standard bicarbonate is the concentration of HCO_3^- in fully oxygenated blood equilibrated with PCO_2 of 40 mmHg at 37 °C.

Davis PD, Kenny GNC. *Basic Physics and Measurement in Anaesthesia*, 5th edn. London: Elsevier, 2005.

Question B28: EEG

Regarding electroencephalogram (EEG) use in critical care:

A. The amplitude of most EEG signals is 20–200 mV
B. Alpha activity is increased with eye opening after hypoxic brain injury
C. The presence of N20 median nerve somatosensory evoked potentials (SSEPs) after cardiac arrest is associated with a good outcome
D. Burst suppression on an EEG trace is 1–2 spikes per minute
E. An isoelectric EEG is a requirement for brainstem death diagnosis

Answer: FFFFF

Short explanation

The amplitude of most EEG signals is 20–200 μV. Alpha activity is decreased with eye opening, and the presence of SSEPs has no prognostic significance. Burst suppression is 1–2 spikes of activity per screen. An isoelectric EEG is an additional test but not a requirement for a diagnosis of brainstem death.

Long explanation

The EEG is a summation of cortical electrical activity in the brain recorded by scalp electrodes. It is used to evaluate brain function, and specific abnormalities may help in the diagnosis of certain conditions such as Creutzfeldt–Jakob disease. The criteria for EEG interpretation are based on frequency (alpha, beta, delta and theta waves), amplitude (usually 20–200 μV), location and paradoxical activity (abnormal bursts of activity). Alpha waves are seen in the occipital cortex in awake patients with their eyes closed. Generalised alpha waves unrelated to stimulation are associated with hypoxic or brainstem lesions. Beta waves are dominant in awake patients or those in drug-induced comas. Theta waves are seen mainly in children. High-voltage delta waves are seen in metabolic encephalopathies of any cause.

EEGs may be used on ICU in the treatment of status epilepticus, a medical emergency with a mortality approaching 10%, commonly requiring the administration of general anaesthetic agents to terminate seizure activity. Subclinical seizures may continue despite sedation, and an EEG is useful to titrate sedation and anticonvulsant agents, or in the diagnosis of pseudoseizures.

EEGs are also used in the evaluation of comatose patients, commonly hypoxic brain injury post cardiac arrest. An EEG may be performed at any time post arrest but is generally used at 72 hours after rewarming from therapeutic hypothermia and after sedative agents have been stopped. To date, no EEG appearance has been unequivocally associated with either good or poor outcomes, and it should be used with all other available information when used for prognostication. In general, status epilepticus, including myoclonic status epilepticus, or an unreactive EEG background are strongly predictive of poor outcome after cardiac arrest.

A variant of the EEG is the somatosensory evoked potential (SSEP). The commonest modality used is the N20 median nerve response, which is the cortical response to a stimulus in the median nerve distribution. SSEPs have been shown to provide some level of prognostication in comatose patients post cardiac arrest. Bilaterally absent

SSEPs are strongly predictive of a poor outcome; however, the presence of SSEPs does not necessarily indicate a good outcome.

Eynon A. EEG and CFAM monitoring. In Waldmann C, Soni N, Rhodes A. *Oxford Desk Reference: Critical Care*. Oxford: Oxford University Press, 2008; pp. 134–6.
Oddo M, Rossetti AO. Predicting neurological outcome after cardiac arrest. *Curr Opin Crit Care* 2011; 17: 254–9.

Question B29: Resuscitation attempts

Indications for not starting a resuscitation attempt, or for ceasing one, include:

A. Next-of-kin refusal for cardiopulmonary resuscitation
B. Fixed dilated pupils
C. Ventricular fibrillation after 10 shocks (about 20 minutes of resuscitation)
D. Asystole for over 20 minutes in a hypothermic patient
E. A valid advance directive written by the patient

Answer: FFFFT

Short explanation

Unless next of kin have been appointed as the patient's legal representative under the Mental Capacity Act 2005, they cannot make decisions on behalf of the patient. Resuscitation attempts should not cease until all reversible causes have been treated including hypothermia and ventricular arrhythmias. Fixed dilated pupils are attributable to other causes than death.

Long explanation

Cardiopulmonary resuscitation (CPR), although it is of benefit to many patients, must be balanced against the risks of subjecting a patient to futile invasive treatments that may prolong life in a fashion that is contrary to the patient's wishes. There are a number of factors that should influence the decision to resuscitate.

In hospital, the decision to stop CPR ultimately rests with the arrest team leader, but the opinion of the whole team should be sought. In general, a resuscitation attempt should not be terminated unless all reversible causes have been addressed and treated. This includes ventricular arrhythmias. Asystole that has not responded to good-quality CPR after 20 minutes is often accepted as irreversible, but if the patient is very hypothermic (e.g. submersion/exposure), then the resuscitation attempt should continue until the patient is warm, as hypothermia may be protective and increase the chance of a successful outcome.

Fixed dilated pupils have numerous causes, and are not a reliable sign of brainstem function in isolation. Other causes include atropine and epinephrine use, Guillain–Barré syndrome, blindness and prostheses. They should not therefore be used in a decision to stop CPR.

In hospital, it is preferable to make decisions regarding resuscitation attempts prior to the patient actually arresting. Under UK law, there is no obligation on the physician to offer futile treatments or to discuss this with the patient if it would provoke unnecessary distress. However, it is good practice to discuss all treatments with patients, including possible CPR. Adults who are deemed to have capacity may refuse CPR in the event of a cardiopulmonary arrest, although they cannot demand that CPR should be provided.

If the patient has an advance directive that is valid and applicable to the circumstance in which it is presented then that directive should be followed. This includes ceasing a resuscitation attempt once started if the directive is deemed to be valid.

There is no 'expiry date' on these directives, and therefore it is the physician's duty to decide whether the directive should stand. The directive must be witnessed, signed and dated to be valid for life-threatening decisions in England and Wales.

General Medical Council. *Treatment and Care Towards the End of Life: Good Practice in Decision Making*. London: GMC, 2010. http://www.gmc-uk.org/static/documents/content/Treatment_and_care_towards_the_end_of_life_-_English_1011.pdf (accessed June 2014).

Resuscitation Council (UK). Decisions relating to resuscitation. In *Advanced Life Support*, 6th edn. London: Resuscitation Council, 2011; Chapter 16.

Question B30: Flexible bronchoscopy

Concerning flexible bronchoscopy on ICU:

A. It rarely requires extra sedation in intubated patients
B. It is required for accurate diagnosis of ventilator-associated pneumonia (VAP)
C. A post-procedure chest radiograph (CXR) is only required if biopsies have been taken
D. It should not be performed in patients with haemoptysis
E. Intubated patients should be ventilated with volume-control ventilation (VCV)

Answer: FFFFF

Short explanation

Patients undergoing invasive procedures may require significantly more sedation than when at rest. VAP is preferentially diagnosed with blind sampling to reduce the risk of bronchial contamination. Any post-procedure deterioration in patient condition should be investigated, and CXR is a useful investigation. Haemoptysis is an indication for diagnostic and therapeutic bronchoscopy, with the appropriate expertise. Pressure-control ventilation (PCV) should be used to compensate for airway leaks around the bronchoscope.

Long explanation

Flexible bronchoscopy is an essential diagnostic and therapeutic tool on the intensive care unit. Indications for flexible bronchoscopy include:

- difficult intubation
- percutaneous tracheostomy
- assessing endotracheal tube position and patency
- sampling of sputum or tissue
- removal of unwanted material (blood, foreign bodies, etc.)
- endobronchial toilet (e.g. following inhalational injury)
- inspection of the lower airway

Haemoptysis is an indication for diagnostic and therapeutic flexible bronchoscopy, although appropriate expertise and support is mandatory. VAP is preferentially diagnosed with blind sampling to reduce the risk of bronchial contamination.

As with all unpleasant or invasive procedures, extra sedation is a humanitarian concern and is usually required for reasons of patient cooperation. Paralysis may also be required to prevent coughing (particularly in patients with raised intracranial pressure).

The procedure is usually performed on patients who are intubated. If not, emergency intubation equipment must be available. Pressure-control ventilation should be used to compensate for any leak around the bronchoscope during the procedure.

Following the procedure, any clinical deterioration should be urgently assessed and investigated with chest radiography. Common complications include:

- displacement or obstruction of the endotracheal tube
- derecruitment of the lung, impaired gas exchange
- cough or bronchospasm
- trauma to the lung tissues (pneumothorax, haemorrhage)
- infection

Du Rand I, Blaikley J, Booton R, *et al.* BTS guideline for diagnostic flexible bronchoscopy in adults. *Thorax* 2013; 68: i4–43.

Question B31: Pulmonary artery catheters

The following may be measured by pulmonary artery (PA) catheters:

A. Cardiac output (CO)
B. Right atrial pressure (RAP)
C. Stroke volume variation (SVV)
D. Real-time cardiac output changes to fluid boluses
E. Left ventricular end-diastolic pressure (LVEDP)

Answer: TFFFF

Short explanation

The pressures that may be measured by PA catheters are central venous pressure (CVP), right atrial pressure, right ventricular pressure, pulmonary artery pressure, and pulmonary capillary wedge pressure (PCWP). The latter may be used as an indicator of left arterial pressure (LAP) and hence LVEDP, but it is not a direct measure of LVEDP. CO may be measured by intermittent thermodilution, but continuous, real-time measurements of CO or SVV are not possible with the PA catheter.

Long explanation

The pulmonary artery (PA) catheter was developed by Swan and Ganz in 1970. It became very popular as a means of measuring physiological parameters that could not otherwise be measured in vivo, such as cardiac output, and estimating others, such as LVEDP. Various RCTs and meta-analyses have since been performed, which consistently failed to show an outcome benefit with the use of PA catheters and demonstrated a complication rate of up to 10%.

PA catheters are inserted into a central vein (internal jugular, subclavian or femoral) and advanced through the right atrium, tricuspid valve, right ventricle and pulmonary valve into the pulmonary artery. Pressure may be measured as it passes through these structures. Once sited in the pulmonary artery, a balloon is inflated to occlude the artery and obtain a PCWP distal to the occluding balloon. A continuous column of static blood then exists between the balloon and the left atrium, and so the PCWP is an indirect measure of LAP and hence LVEDP.

Cardiac output measurement are by intermittent thermodilution with cold saline, using the indicator dilution method. This method remains the gold standard of cardiac output measurement, against which all novel cardiac output monitors are judged. However, its intermittent nature means that real-time measurements such as SVV or responses to interventions (fluid challenge, leg raise) are not possible.

Bersten AD, Soni N. *Oh's Intensive Care Manual.* 6th ed. Edinburgh: Butterworth-Heinemann, 2009.

Rajaram SS, Desai NK, Kalra A, *et al.* Pulmonary artery catheters for adult patients in intensive care. *Cochrane Database Syst Rev* 2013; (2): CD003408.

Question B32: Prolonged QT and torsades de pointes

The following are recognised causes of prolonged QT and torsades de pointes

A. Hypokalaemia
B. Amiodarone
C. Hypercalcaemia
D. Clarithromycin
E. Pineapple juice

Answer: TTFTF

Short explanation

A prolonged QT interval can lead to torsades de pointes and sudden cardiac death. Causes include congenital ion channel abnormalities, electrolyte imbalance (hypokalaemia, hypomagnesaemia, hypocalcaemia), drugs (antiarrhythmics including amiodarone, macrolides, antihistamines, tricyclic antidepressants, etc.), cardiac disease (MI, bradycardia, mitral valve prolapse) and other causes (organophosphates, grapefruit juice, etc.).

Long explanation

The QT interval is a measure on the electrocardiogram (ECG) that reflects the time between the onset of ventricular depolarisation (QRS complex) and the onset of repolarisaton (T wave). The QT interval varies inversely with heart rate, and so a corrected measure, the QTc, is commonly used to assess the degree of QT prolongation. Patients with prolonged QT intervals are at risk of ventricular arrhythmias and death, notably torsades de pointes and ventricular fibrillation. There are many causes of prolonged QTc: congenital, electrolyte imbalance, drugs, cardiac disease and other causes.

Congenital prolonged QT results from genetic abnormalities of the sodium or potassium channels in cardiac tissue, resulting in abnormal repolarisation. These conditions are rare but are a significant cause of sudden cardiac death in otherwise healthy young people. Cardiac disease, such as myocardial infarction or mitral valve prolapse, can also increase the QT.

Medications are a common cause of prolonged QT. Many antiarrhythmics prolong the QT interval as part of their mode of action, such as amiodarone, procainamide, disopyramide, quinidine and sotalol. Many antipsychotics cause prolongation of the QT interval, particularly chlorpromazine, haloperidol, olanzipine and risperidone. Other types of drug linked to prolonged QT include anti-infectives (erythromycin, clarithromycin, fluconazole, levofloxacin, septrin), antidepressants (tricyclics, SSRIs, SNRIs), antiemetics (ondansetron, droperidol, domperidone) and others. Use of several such drugs has an additive effect, particularly in the presence of other risk factors.

Electrolyte abnormalities can cause prolongation of the QT interval, particularly in combination with another risk factor. Hypokalaemia, hypocalcaemia and hypomagnesaemia are all associated with prolonged QT and torsades de pointes. Other causes of prolonged QT include grapefruit juice, organophosphates and hypothyroidism.

Al-Khatib SM, Lapointe NM, Kramer JM, Califf RM. What clinicians should know about the QT interval, *JAMA* 2003; 289: 2120–7.

Montanez A, Ruskin J, Hebert P, Lamas G, Hennekens C. Prolonged QTc interval and risks of total and cardiovascular mortality and sudden death in the general population. *Arch Intern Med* 2004; 164: 943–8.

Yap G, Camm A. Drug induced QT prolongation and torsades de pointes. *Heart* 2003: 89: 1363–72.

Question B33: ESBL bacteria

Extended-spectrum β-lactamase (ESBL) producing organisms:

A. Are effectively treated with third-generation cephalosporins, e.g. ceftazidime
B. Are most commonly *Enterobacter* species
C. Are resistant to meropenem
D. Are resistant to gentamicin
E. Have plasmid-mediated resistance mechanisms

Answer: FFFTT

Short explanation

ESBL bacteria are resistant to all penicillins and cephalosporins. They may also be resistant to aminoglycosides. They are sensitive to carbapenems. The ESBL bacteria most commonly found are *Klebsiella* species.

Long explanation

Extended-spectrum β-lactamase (ESBL) producing organisms are Gram-negative organisms exhibiting resistance to β-lactam antibiotics. The commonest organism is *Klebsiella*, but *Serratia* and very highly resistant *Escherichia coli* and *Enterobacter* species have been isolated in recent years. These may cause outbreaks of resistant infections in the community as well as the hospital-acquired infections seen in susceptible individuals historically.

The mechanism for resistance with ESBL is plasmid-mediated. Plasmids are self-replicating circles of DNA that exist within the bacteria but are separate from the bacterial chromosome. They are the most common route of transmission of genetic information in bacteria seen in critical care.

ESBL organisms are best treated with carbapenems such as meropenem, because they are highly resistant to β-lactamase. ESBL bacteria may also exhibit resistance to aminoglycoside and quinolone antibiotics.

Varley AJ, Williams H, Fletcher S. Antibiotic resistance in the intensive care unit. *Contin Educ Anaesth Crit Care Pain* 2009; 9: 114–18.
Waldmann C, Soni N, Rhodes A. *Oxford Desk Reference: Critical Care*. Oxford: Oxford University Press, 2008; pp. 228–9.

Question B34: Vasopressin

Vasopressin:

A. Causes vasoconstriction by action on V_2 receptors
B. Endogenous levels are low in all types of shock
C. Decreases plasma osmolality
D. Should be used instead of norepinephrine in septic shock
E. Acts on vasoconstrictor receptors that are heterogeneously distributed in the body

Answer: FFTFT

Short explanation

Vasopressin, or ADH, acts on V_1 receptors to cause vasoconstriction in non-essential vascular beds. It also acts on V_2 receptors to increase water reabsorption, causing hypo-osmolality. Levels are high in cardiogenic shock, but inappropriately low in septic shock. It is used in synergy with norepinephrine, rarely as a sole vasoconstrictor.

Long explanation

Vasopressin (or antidiuretic hormone, ADH) is an endogenous peptide synthesised in the hypothalamus and released from the posterior pituitary. It has two physiological roles, osmotic and vasoactive, mediated by two different cell-surface receptors. Its antidiuretic effects are mediated by V_2 receptors in the distal convoluted tubule of the kidney, where it results in reabsorption of water from the tubular filtrate. This leads to a concentrated urine, and conservation of water, reducing plasma osmolality in the process.

The second action of vasopressin is via V_1 receptors on vascular smooth muscle, leading to increased intracellular calcium levels, causing contraction and hence vasoconstriction. This effect is not apparent in normal circumstances, but forms part of the response to shock. V_1 receptors are not homogenously distributed and so blood flow is redirected to vital organs during the response to shock. Levels of vasopressin have been found to increase up to fivefold in some forms of shock (e.g. cardiogenic), but are relatively deficient in septic shock.

The use of vasopressin infusions in addition to catecholamines in septic shock has been shown to lead to short-term improvements in parameters such as reducing norepinephrine infusion requirements and improving renal perfusion and creatinine clearance. In other studies, a reduction in organ dysfunction score was demonstrated, mainly due to improved renal perfusion compared with norepinephrine. No mortality benefit was demonstrated.

A large multicentre study (VASST) was therefore conducted comparing vasopressin and norepinephrine infusions in septic shock. This was unable to demonstrate a difference in mortality, despite a trend towards reduced mortality in the vasopressin group. A predefined subgroup of less-severe shock (defined as norepinephrine infusion rate below 15 μg/minute) did show reduced mortality when treated with vasopressin, although the reason for this (and its clinical significance) is as yet unknown. Future studies aim to further clarify the role of vasopressin.

Gordon AC. Vasopressin in septic shock. *J Intensive Care Soc* 2011; 12: 11–14.

Russell JA, Walley KR, Singer J, *et al.* Vasopressin versus norepinephrine infusion in patients with septic shock. *N Engl J Med* 2008; 358: 877–87.

Question B35: Urinary catheters

Regarding urinary catheters in the intensive care unit:

A. There is evidence that silver alloy catheters may reduce the risk of catheter-related urinary tract infection (UTI)
B. Bladder irrigation and washouts should not be used to prevent catheter-associated infection
C. Catheterisation should be an aseptic procedure
D. The indication for catheterisation should be documented
E. The largest-gauge catheter possible for the patient should be used, to encourage urinary flow

Answer: TTTTF

Short explanation

The larger the gauge of the catheter used the greater the chance of causing urethral trauma, so smaller-gauge catheters are preferable. Gauge of catheter (within those commercially available) makes no significance difference to urinary flow.

Long explanation

epic3 guidelines for urinary catheterisation (2014) aim to reduce catheter-associated infections by standardising care and ensuring regular assessment of the patient and the need for catheterisation. Catheters should be avoided if possible, but if one is indicated, then the smallest-gauge catheter that will allow free urine flow should be used. 10 ml balloons should be used in adults.

Catheterisation is an aseptic procedure, using sterile normal saline to clean the meatus and sterile lubricant to minimise urethral trauma. The catheter should be connected to a sterile closed urinary drainage system, which should be changed according to manufacturer's recommendation. Bladder irrigation and washouts should not be used to prevent catheter-associated infection. The catheter material will depend on local practice and the patient's latex allergy status, but there is some evidence that silver alloy catheters may reduce the risk of catheter-related UTI.

Loveday HP, Wilson JA, Pratt RJ, *et al*. epic3: national evidence based guidelines for preventing healthcare-associated infections in NHS hospitals in England. *J Hosp Infect* 2014; 86 (Suppl 1): S1–70.

Waldmann C, Soni N, Rhodes A. *Oxford Desk Reference: Critical Care*. Oxford: Oxford University Press, 2008; pp. 464–5.

Question B36: Hyperkalaemia

The following are causes of hyperkalaemia:

A. Metabolic acidosis
B. Suxamethonium
C. Malignant hyperthermia
D. Conn's syndrome
E. Digoxin overdose

Answer: TTTFT

Short explanation

Conn's syndrome is hyperaldosteronism secondary to an aldosterone-secreting adenoma, and it causes hypernatraemia and hypokalaemia.

Long explanation

Hyperkalaemia is defined as a serum potassium > 5.0 mmol/l, but it is often asymptomatic until plasma levels are > 6.5 mmol/l. Symptoms are generally related to skeletal and cardiac muscle dysfunction, with muscle twitching, cramps and weakness and arrhythmias including bradycardia, asystole or ventricular fibrillation (VF). ECG findings include bradycardia, peaked T waves, PR interval prolongation, QRS widening, QT shortening and a sinusoidal pattern preceding VF.

Suxamethonium causes release of potassium from cells following depolarisation, leading to a rise in serum potassium of approximately 0.5 mmol/l. In the presence of renal failure or pre-existing hyperkalaemia this may be enough to precipitate arrhythmias, and the rise may be 3–4 mmol/l in the presence of burns, immobility or spinal cord injuries more than 48 hours old.

A metabolic acidosis causes potassium to move out of cells in order to reduce hydrogen ion concentration in the blood.

Malignant hyperthermia causes hyperkalaemia due to increased muscle activity and eventually muscle breakdown, rhabdomyolysis and renal failure.

Digoxin overdose causes inactivation of the Na/K-ATPase pump. Hyperkalaemia is a marker of the severity of the overdose and a predictor of mortality.

Conn's syndrome is hyperaldosteronism secondary to an aldosterone-secreting adenoma. This causes hypernatraemia and hypokalaemia.

O'Neil P, Webster N. Electrolyte disorders. In Waldmann C, Soni N, Rhodes A. *Oxford Desk Reference: Critical Care*. Oxford: Oxford University Press, 2008; pp. 410–11.

Question B37: Mortality scores in critical care

Regarding the use of scoring systems in critical care:

A. The Standardised Mortality Ratio (SMR) is the ratio of expected to observed mortality
B. Expected mortality for the SMR can come from APACHE, SAPS or MPM scores
C. Predicted mortality scores are useful as part of a critcal care unit's clinical audit programme
D. An ICU with an SMR > 1.0 is performing above expectations
E. Predicted mortality should not be used to make clinical decisions

Answer: FTTFT

Short explanation

The SMR is the ratio of observed to expected mortality, so SMR > 1.0 is higher than expected mortality. Expected mortality may come from any valid and relevant statistical source. The SMR may be used to compare different ICUs, but is best used in tracking the performance of an individual unit over time. Predicted mortality scores are audit and research tools that are not applicable to individual patients, but may help inform discussions.

Long explanation

The Standardised Mortality Ratio (SMR) is a measure of the performance of a healthcare provider. It is calculated as the ratio of observed mortality to expected mortality. The expected mortality must originate from an applicable, relevant and validated statistical source. In critical care, expected mortality can be calculated using one of several severity of illness scoring systems, provided they have the capacity to provide a validated expected mortality figure. Common examples include the Acute Physiology and Chronic Health Evaluation (APACHE) scoring systems, the Simplified Acute Physiology Score (SAPS) and the Mortality Prediction Model (MPM). In the UK, the expected mortality is derived from the Intensive Care National Audit and Research Centre (ICNARC) dataset.

Although a crude tool, the SMR provides some useful information. An SMR of 1.0 indicates satisfactory performance, higher than 1.0 indicates poor performance, and lower than 1.0 indicates better than expected performance. SMR may be used to compare the performance of ICUs, although many inter-hospital variations are not accounted for in the predicted mortality models, and so comparisons may be misleading (e.g. tertiary centres attract the most complex cases and patients, so may have higher than expected mortality despite better performance). A better use of the

SMR is to track the performance of an individual unit over time, as most confounding factors will remain unchanged.

Predicted mortality scores may also be used in other ways, particularly to audit performance and in research as a measure of heterogeneity between groups. The figures are not applicable to individual patients and do not equate to a chance of a particular patient surviving to discharge, and therefore they should not be used as a basis for clinical decisions. However, predicted mortality or severity of illness scores may have a role in informing discussions or decisions, and many ICU admission guidelines include aspects of severity of illness scoring systems.

Palazzo M. Severity of illness and likely outcome from critical illness. In Bersten AD, Soni N. *Oh's Intensive Care Manual*, 6th edn. Edinburgh: Butterworth-Heinemann, 2009, pp. 17–30.

Question B38: Influenza

Regarding influenza:

A. Influenza epidemics occur due to antigenic drift of the influenza virus
B. Vomiting and diarrhoea are commoner in seasonal influenza than in pandemic influenza
C. Non-invasive ventilation is the optimal treatment for viral pneumonia
D. High-frequency oscillation ventilation (HFOV) is the treatment of choice for refractory hypoxia
E. Severity scoring should be used to triage patients for extracorporeal membrane oxygenation (ECMO) treatment

Answer: TFFFF

Short explanation

Vomiting and diarrhoea are commoner in pandemic influenza. Most patients with viral pneumonia will require invasive ventilation with lung-protective strategies. ECMO is the treatment of choice for refractory hypoxia, and patients should be assessed on individual need.

Long explanation

There are two types of influenza virus of clinical significance: influenza A and influenza B. Influenza A usually causes a more severe illness than influenza B. Both virus types may result in seasonal epidemics, but only influenza A viruses have the ability to cause a pandemic.

Seasonal epidemics occur due to antigenic drift (minor random changes in the antigenic characteristics of the hemagglutinin and neuraminidase glycoproteins of the influenza viruses). Pandemics occur with antigenic shift – a major change in the surface glycoproteins of the virus as a result of reassortment of genes between different influenza viruses, or through direct transmission of an animal virus to humans. This is the reason that pandemic flu predominantly affects young people without prior exposure to other strains of the virus in their lifetime.

The clinical manifestations of influenza are headache, pyrexia, rigors, dry cough, sore throat, myalgia and anorexia. Vomiting and diarrhoea tend to be associated with pandemic flu. Primary or secondary pneumonia and acute respiratory distress syndrome (ARDS) are the most severe pulmonary manifestations of influenza. As well as routine blood tests, lactate dehydrogenase (LDH), creatine phosphokinase and creatinine levels may help identify those with severe disease.

Management of patients with influenza is largely supportive. Most patients with viral pneumonia will require invasive ventilation with lung-protective strategies. ECMO is the treatment of choice for refractory hypoxia, and patients should be assessed on individual need.

Health Protection Agency. Critical care management of adults with influenza with particular reference to H1N1 (2009). Version 3 (2011). http://www.hpa.org.uk/webc/HPAwebFile/HPAweb_C/1287148502205 (accessed June 2014).

Rello J, Pop-Vicas A. Clinical review: primary influenza viral pneumonia. *Crit Care* 2009; 13: 235.

Question B39: Intracranial pressure monitoring

Regarding intracranial pressure (ICP) monitoring:

A. ICP monitoring is indicated in closed head injury unless the CT is normal
B. Monitors can be extradural, subarachnoid, intraventricular or intraparenchymal
C. Intraventricular monitors can be therapeutic devices
D. ICP monitoring is contraindicated in coagulopathy, sepsis and severe hydrocephalus
E. Risk of infection is highest for the most accurate monitoring method

Answer: FTTFT

Short explanation

ICP monitoring may be indicated in closed head injury with a normal CT (e.g. GCS < 8, age > 40, posturing). Intraventricular catheters can be used for CSF drainage and administration of intraventricular therapy; they are the most accurate but carry the highest risk of infection. Coagulopathy should be reversed prior to ICP monitor insertion wherever possible. Sepsis may influence the choice of device. Hydrocephalus is an indication for ICP monitoring.

Long explanation

Monitoring of intracranial pressure (ICP) is used to identify patients at risk of life-threatening intracranial hypertension or to monitor the response to its treatment. Indications include closed head injury, space-occupying lesions, encephalopathy and Reye's syndrome. ICP monitoring is seldom required in the conscious patient, where clinical examination and regular Glasgow Coma Scale (GCS) assessment are generally sufficient. Patients with closed head injury should have ICP monitoring in the following circumstances:

- abnormal CT scan at admission
- GCS 8 or below, or abnormal posturing
- age > 40 or hypotension at admission

Coagulopathy is a relative contraindication to ICP monitoring. Significant coagulopathy should be treated appropriately prior to the procedure. Patients with sepsis or immunosuppression should be treated with caution; intraventricular catheters should be avoided if possible owing to their greater risk of nosocomial infection.

There are four basic types of intracranial monitor. Extradural monitors are pressure transducers placed via burr hole. They can be difficult to place and inaccurate, and do not allow drainage of CSF, but have a low risk of infection. Subarachnoid bolts are simpler to place and more accurate but have a higher rate of infection; CSF drainage may be possible. Intraparenchymal monitors are pressure transducers placed via burr hole into the white matter of the cortex; they are accurate and simple to place but cannot be used to drain CSF. Intraventricular catheters are the most accurate devices and also allow therapeutic drainage of CSF and administration of drugs (e.g. antibiotics), but they are invasive, may be difficult to place and have the highest rate of infection.

Smith M. Monitoring intracranial pressure in traumatic brain injury. *Anesth Analg* 2008; 106: 240–8.

Question B40: Acute respiratory distress syndrome – causes

The following are recognised direct causes of acute respiratory distress syndrome (ARDS):

A. Trauma
B. Fat embolism
C. Pancreatitis
D. Smoke inhalation
E. Sepsis

Answer: TTFTF

Short explanation

Causes of ARDS may be classified as direct and indirect. Direct causes of ARDS, involving primary pathology of or damage to the lung, include pneumonia, smoke inhalation, gastric aspiration, thoracic trauma and fat embolism. Indirect causes, with no initial lung pathology, include sepsis (the most common cause), shock, pancreatitis and blood transfusion.

Long explanation

Acute respiratory distress syndrome (ARDS) is a condition of acute severe hypoxaemia with bilateral chest opacities, not fully explained by cardiac failure or fluid overload. It affects up to 75 per 100,000 population and has an estimated mortality of 25–30%. The pathological features include alveolar infiltration by neutrophils with haemorrhage and proteinaceous pulmonary oedema. Inflammation leads to epithelial damage, reduced surfactant (causing atelectasis) and, later, fibrosis.

Causes of ARDS may be classified as direct or indirect. Direct causes involve primary pathology of, or damage to the lung. Common direct causes of ARDS include pneumonia, aspiration, drowning, smoke inhalation, thoracic trauma and fat or amniotic fluid embolism. Indirect causes of ARDS include sepsis, shock, pancreatitis, blood transfusion and burns. Outcomes are similar for direct and indirect causes of ARDS when severity of illness is taken into account.

Ranieri VM, Rubenfeld GD, Thompson BT, *et al.* Acute respiratory distress syndrome: the Berlin definition. *JAMA* 2012; 307: 2526–33.
Wheeler AP, Bernard GR. Acute lung injury and the acute respiratory distress syndrome: a clinical review. *Lancet* 2007; 369: 1553–64.

Question B41: Equipment decontamination

According to the Spaulding classification:

A. A blood pressure cuff is a non-critical item and should be cleaned at the bedside
B. Surgical instruments should be sterilised
C. Endoscopes are critical items and should be sterilised

D. Laryngoscopes are non-critical items and should be disinfected
E. Semi-critical items should be disinfected to remove spores

Answer: TTFFF

Short explanation

Critical items, which include surgical instruments, should be sterilised. Semi-critical items such as laryngoscopes and endoscopes should be free from bacteria but not necessarily spores, so they should be disinfected.

Long explanation

The Spaulding classification was devised in 1968 to classify medical equipment according to need for decontamination. The categories are based on the risk of infection being transmitted to a patient by the object.

Critical items include surgical instruments, implants, catheters, syringes and needles. They enter tissue or the vascular system and therefore pose a high infection risk. They should be sterile.

Semi-critical items come into contact with mucous membranes and skin but not normally the blood. These surfaces are resistant to spores but not bacteria, viruses or fungi, so the equipment should undergo at least high-level disinfection prior to use. Examples include laryngoscopes, endoscopes and thermometers.

Non-critical items such as blood pressure cuffs and pulse oximeters may be cleaned at the bedside as they come into contact with intact skin only and therefore pose a low risk of infection.

Decontamination is the process of removing matter such that is unable to reach a site in sufficient quantities to initiate infection or inflammation. It starts with cleaning and is followed by disinfection or sterilisation as appropriate to the equipment.

Cleaning is the physical removal of foreign material from an object, reducing bioburden but not necessarily destroying all infectious agents. It may include detergents, enzyme solutions and automated washers.

Disinfection is the reduction of all pathogenic material on an object but not complete removal of e.g. spores.

Sterilisation is the removal of all viable microorganisms and infectious agents from an object. This may exclude prions.

Sabir N, Ramachandra V. Decontamination of anaesthetic equipment. *Contin Educ Anaesth Crit Care Pain* 2004; 4: 103–6.

Al-Shaikh B, Stacey S. *Essentials of Anaesthetic Equipment*, 3rd edn. London: Elsevier Churchill Livingstone, 2007; pp. 237–8.

Question B42: Cardiac output estimation – Fick method

The Fick method for estimating cardiac output:

A. Can use oxygen or CO_2 levels
B. Requires measurement of oxygen consumption (VO_2) or CO_2 production
C. Gives the most accurate results when based on oxygen content in the pulmonary artery and vein
D. Estimates cardiac output by dividing VO_2 by the area under the concentration/time curve
E. Commonly assumes no intracardiac shunt

Answer: TFTFT

Short explanation

The original, and most accurate, Fick method used measured VO_2 and blood samples from pulmonary artery and vein. Modifications to make the test easier and/or less invasive involve assuming a value of VO_2, and assuming no intracardiac shunt (using peripheral arterial blood instead of pulmonary vein). The NICO monitor uses end-tidal CO_2 levels during normal ventilation and periods of partial CO_2 rebreathing. The area under the concentration/time curve is not used by the Fick method.

Long explanation

Cardiac output (CO) estimation was first described in 1870 by Adolph Fick. The Fick principle as applied to CO states that the total amount of a substance produced or taken up by the body is equal to CO multiplied by the arteriovenous concentration difference:

$$VO_2 = CO \times (C_a - C_v)$$

If the amount of substance and the arterial and venous concentrations are known, then CO can be calculated. The initial method involved measurement of oxygen consumption with a closed-loop spirometer and the oxygen concentration of blood in the pulmonary artery and pulmonary vein:

$$CO = VO_2 \;/\; (C_a - C_v)$$

In modern practice, blood is sampled from a peripheral artery instead of a pulmonary vein (assuming there is no intracardiac shunt), and oxygen consumption is assumed to be 125 ml/min/m^2 body surface area. The oxygen content of blood is calculated from the amount bound to haemoglobin and the amount dissolved in blood:

$$\text{Oxygen content} = (Hb \times SpO_2 \times 1.34) + (PO_2 \times 0.003)$$

The Fick principle is used by the non-invasive cardiac output (NICO) monitor, which compares end-tidal CO_2 measured during normal ventilation and during periods of partial CO_2 rebreathing.

Marik PE. Noninvasive cardiac output monitors: a state-of-the-art review. *J Cardiothorac Vasc Anaesth* 2013; 27: 121–34.

Question B43: Community-acquired pneumonia and CURB65

Which of the following are associated with increased disease severity in adults with community-acquired pneumonia (CAP), according to CURB65?

A. Age > 60
B. Urea > 7 mmol/l
C. Mini-mental test score ≤ 8/10
D. Respiratory rate > 25 breaths/minute
E. Heart rate > 110 bpm

Answer: FTTFF

Short explanation

The CURB65 score is a validated severity of illness score for patients with CAP, with one point awarded for each of five findings. Higher scores are associated with higher mortality, and patients with a score of > 3 should be urgently assessed for admission to critical care. Age ≥ 65 years and respiratory rate ≥ 30 breaths/minute each score one point. Heart rate does not feature in CURB65.

Long explanation

The CURB65 score is a simple bedside severity of illness scoring system for use in patients presenting with community-acquired pneumonia (CAP). It has been validated by multiple studies totalling over 12,000 patients. It is based on information readily available at hospital presentation and is simple to perform at the bedside. As such, its use is recommended by the British Thoracic Society to assess the risk of mortality and to guide locus of care (home, hospital, critical care).

One point is awarded for each of the following findings:

- confusion, not long-standing (mini-mental test score ≤ 8/10)
- urea > 7 mmol/l
- respiratory rate ≥ 30 breaths/minute
- blood pressure < 90 mmHg (systolic) or ≤ 60 mmHg (diastolic)
- age ≥ 65 years

An integer score between 0 and 5 is the result, which has the following associated predicted mortality:

- score 0: mortality 0.7%
- score 1: mortality 2.1%
- score 2: mortality 9.2%
- score 3–5: mortality 15–40%

Patients with scores of 0–1 may be appropriately cared for in the community. Patients with scores ≥ 2 should be considered for hospital admission. Patients with scores of ≥ 3 should be reviewed by a senior physician and those with scores ≥ 4 should be urgently considered for critical care admission. As with all severity of illness scores, clinical judgement should also be applied to decide locus of treatment, particularly in patients with other medical comorbidities (e.g. COPD, heart disease), other markers of disease severity (e.g. respiratory rate > 40, septic shock) or poor social circumstances.

Lim W, Baudouin S, George R. BTS guidelines for the management of community acquired pneumonia in adults: update 2009. *Thorax* 2009; 64: ii1–55.

Question B44: Subarachnoid haemorrhage

Concerning acute subarachnoid haemorrhage (SAH):

A. Grading of severity is based solely on the Glasgow Coma Scale
B. Patients with suspected SAH should have a lumbar puncture
C. Control of the bleeding aneurysm should be undertaken at the earliest feasible opportunity
D. Systolic blood pressure should be kept low (< 140 mmHg) to prevent rebleeding
E. Corticosteroids should be administered to reduce cerebral oedema

Answer: TFTFF

Short explanation

All patients with suspected SAH should have CT (including CT angiography) or MRI imaging. Patients with suspected SAH but equivocal CT/MRI should undergo lumbar puncture if not contraindicated. Control of the aneurysm (surgical or radiological) should be undertaken at the earliest feasible opportunity. Blood pressure should be kept below 180 mmHg until aneurysmal control is achieved. Corticosteroids are not recommended in acute SAH.

Long explanation

Subarachnoid haemorrhage (SAH) has an incidence of 9 per 100,000, accounting for 3% of strokes but with a 60% 6-month mortality. The majority of cases of SAH are caused by ruptured intracranial aneurysms; other causes include trauma and coagulopathy. Grade of SAH is based on the Glasgow Coma Scale at presentation.

Initial diagnosis of SAH relies on clinical suspicion and neuroimaging. Typical features of SAH include 'thunderclap' headache, neck stiffness, reduced conscious level and vomiting. CT is the initial investigation of choice, as nearly all SAH will be detected on fine-cut CT within 24 hours. CT angiography or MRI may also be used, particularly if the initial CT is equivocal or there has been a delay in presentation (CT becomes less sensitive with time). Cerebral angiography is the gold-standard investigation but not always available. Lumbar puncture should be performed in patients with suspected SAH but equivocal imaging, in the absence of contraindications. Clear CSF without xanthrochromia effectively excludes recent SAH.

Control of bleeding aneurysms to prevent rebleeding is desirable and should take place at the earliest feasible opportunity, and certainly within 72 hours. Open or surgical clipping of aneurysms is becoming less common as more aneurysms are treated by endovascular coiling. Some lesions are more amenable to one technique or the other, but if either is equally feasible, then coiling should be performed.

Blood pressure (BP) should be maintained at a high-normal level and only reduced if systolic BP exceeds 180 mmHg. BP control should not reduce the mean arterial pressure to below 90 mmHg. While a lower BP will reduce the risk of rebleed, this will lead to a reduction in cerebral perfusion pressure, thus increasing the likelihood of secondary brain injury. Other supportive management includes airway, respiratory and cardiovascular support, control of fever, seizures and hyperglycaemia (> 10 mmol/l) and mechanical thromboprophylaxis. Corticosteroids are not recommended in the management of acute SAH.

Steiner T, Juvela S, Unterberg A, *et al.* European Stroke Organization guidelines for the management of intracranial aneurysms and subarachnoid haemorrhage. *Cerebrovasc Dis* 2013; 35: 93–112.

Diringer MN, Bleck TP, Claude Hemphill J, *et al.* Critical care management of patients following aneurysmal subarachnoid hemorrhage: recommendations from the Neurocritical Care Society's Multidisciplinary Consensus Conference. *Neurocrit Care* 2011; 15: 211–40.

Question B45: Acute kidney injury

The definitions of acute kidney injury (AKI) and its severity include:

A. Urine volume < 0.5 ml/kg/h for 6 hours
B. Increase in serum creatinine by > 26.5 μmol/l within 48 hours
C. Increase in serum creatinine to > 1.5 times baseline in 7 days
D. Stage 3 AKI: eGFR < 35 ml/min per 1.73 m^2 in patients aged 18 years or over
E. Stage 3 AKI: anuria for > 12 hours

Answer: TTTFT

Short explanation

In small children, where a low muscle mass may prevent large rises in creatinine, eGFR can be used to stage AKI. In adults a combination of urine output and serum creatinine is preferred, as eGFR is estimated and only validated in a steady-state situation.

Long explanation

Acute kidney injury (AKI) is a clinical syndrome with a spectrum of severity and multiple underlying aetiologies. Clinically, AKI is characterised by a rapid reduction in kidney function resulting in a failure to maintain fluid, electrolyte and acid–base homoeostasis.

Consensus definitions have been produced by Kidney Disease: Improving Global Outcomes (KDIGO), incorporating previous definitions and guidelines from the Acute Dialysis Quality Initiative (ADQI) (RIFLE definition and staging system) and the Acute Kidney Injury Network (AKIN).

AKI is defined as any of the following:

- Increase in serum creatinine by > 26.5 μmol/l within 48 hours
- Increase in serum creatinine to > 1.5 times baseline in 7 days
- Urine volume < 0.5 ml/kg/h for 6 hours

AKI is staged as follows:

Stage 1: serum creatinine 1.5–1.9 times baseline or increase by > 26.5 μmol/l within 48 hours, or urine output < 0.5 ml/kg/h for 6–12 hours

Stage 2: serum creatinine 2.0–2.9 times baseline, or urine output < 0.5 ml/kg/h for > 12 hours

Stage 3: serum creatinine 3.0 times baseline or increase to > 353.6 μmol/l, initiation of renal replacement therapy, or anuria for > 12 hours

Serum creatinine is preferred as a marker to eGFR (estimated glomerular filtration rate), because eGFR is only accurate in the steady state; while serum creatinine is increasing it will overestimate kidney function, and vice versa. In small children where a low muscle mass may prevent large rises in creatinine, eGFR may be used to stage AKI.

KDIGO clinical practice guideline for acute kidney injury. *Kidney International Supplements* 2012; 2 (1): 8–27.

Waldmann C, Soni N, Rhodes A. *Oxford Desk Reference: Critical Care*. Oxford: Oxford University Press, 2008; pp. 312–15.

Question B46: Surviving Sepsis guidelines

The following therapies are recommended for patients with severe sepsis, according to the Surviving Sepsis guidelines (2012):

A. Antimicrobial therapy must not start until two sets of blood cultures have been taken
B. Effective intravenous antimicrobials within 1 hour of recognition of severe sepsis
C. Surgical intervention for source control within 12 hours
D. The use of albumin in patients requiring large volumes of crystalloid resuscitation
E. Continuous infusion of hydrocortisone in vasopressor-refractory septic shock

Answer: FTTTT

Short explanation

At least two sets of blood cultures should be taken. This should be prior to, but must not delay, starting antimicrobial therapy (which should be intravenous, effective and started within 1 hour).

Long explanation

The third edition of the Surviving Sepsis guidelines was issued in 2012. The guidelines are a part of a wider Surviving Sepsis Campaign (SSC) to reduce deaths from sepsis across the globe. Strategies include increasing awareness, improving diagnosis and the introduction of bundles of care to improve management. Guidance covers initial resuscitation, early management of infection, cardiovascular support, ventilator management and adjuvant therapies.

Following recognition of severe sepsis or septic shock, initial resuscitation should commence along with various measures aimed at effectively treating the underlying infection. Blood cultures (at least two sets) should be taken within 45 minutes, prior to starting antimicrobial therapy, which should be started within 60 minutes. If the taking of blood cultures is likely to delay this, then the administration of antimicrobials takes precedence. Antimicrobials should be intravenous, broad-spectrum and effective against any possible causative organisms. Surgical source control (e.g. drainage of abscesses) should be as minimally invasive as possible, and should occur within 12 hours of presentation.

Initial fluid resuscitation should be with crystalloids, but albumin is recommended for patients requiring large volumes of fluid. Hydroxyethyl starches are not recommended in sepsis. Vasopressor support should be started to achieve a mean arterial pressure (MAP) of ≥ 65 mmHg. Norepinephrine is recommended as first-line, with epinephrine and/or vasopressin reserved for second-line therapy. Patients with refractory hypotension despite high-dose vasopressors should receive hydrocortisone 200 mg/day, which should be administered as a 24-hour infusion.

Dellinger RP, Levy MM, Rhodes A, *et al.* Surviving Sepsis Campaign. International guidelines for management of severe sepsis and septic shock: 2012. *Crit Care Med* 2013; 41: 580–637.

Question B47: Refeeding syndrome

Regarding refeeding syndrome:

A. Thiamine deficiency is the most clinically significant vitamin deficiency seen
B. Feed should be introduced at a rate to meet the patient's full nutritional requirements
C. Refeeding syndrome causes hyperglycaemia
D. Potassium deficiency is the most common finding
E. Refeeding syndrome is more common in patients on diuretics

Answer: TFTTT

Short explanation

Feed should be introduced at a rate below that of the patient's full nutritional requirements, and increased gradually if there are no adverse signs.

Long explanation

Refeeding syndrome refers to shifts in fluids and electrolytes in patients receiving artificial feeding (enteral or parenteral) after a period of starvation.

Metabolic changes in starvation result in fat and protein being used instead of carbohydrate as the principal source of energy, which reduces the basal metabolic rate by 20–25%. In prolonged starvation, hormone changes to reduce protein and muscle breakdown are activated with ketogenesis and reduced gluconeogenesis. Body stores of minerals and salts may be depleted although serum concentrations are normal.

Once feeding is recommenced there is increased production of insulin to stimulate glycogen, fat and protein synthesis. This process requires phosphate and magnesium as well as cofactors such as thiamine. Phosphate, potassium and magnesium are all taken up by cells, and the plasma concentration may fall precipitously due to total body depletion of these minerals. Hypophosphataemia is the commonest biochemical feature of refeeding syndrome. Sodium and water excretion is reduced with carbohydrate intake, and urine output will fall. Fluid resuscitation in this situation may lead to fluid overload and pulmonary oedema.

Hyperglycaemia occurs due to a chronic reduction in insulin secretion, and if severe may cause an osmotic diuresis, dehydration, and a metabolic acidosis with ketone production. Lipogenesis with excess glucose may cause respiratory failure due to increased carbon dioxide production. Thiamine is the most important vitamin deficiency in refeeding syndrome, as it is an essential coenzyme for carbohydrate metabolism. Thiamine deficiency results in Wernicke's encephalopathy (ocular abnormalities, ataxia, confusion, hypothermia, coma) or Korsakoff's syndrome (retrograde and anterograde amnesia with confabulation).

Any patient who has been without food for more than 5 days is at risk of refeeding syndrome. Specific risk factors include eating disorders, chronic alcohol use, oncology patients, postoperative patients and the elderly. Those on diuretics are more at risk due to pre-existing electrolyte deficiencies.

NICE guidelines recommend a thorough nutritional assessment before starting feed, with regular measurements of plasma electrolytes (especially phosphate, sodium, potassium and magnesium) and glucose and prompt replacement of deficiencies. In high-risk patients feed should be initiated at a lower rate and built up gradually if refeeding syndrome is not identified. Vitamin replacement should start immediately.

Mehanna HM, Moledina J, Travis J. Refeeding syndrome: what it is, and how to prevent and treat it. *BMJ* 2008; 336: 1495–8.

National Institute for Health and Care Excellence. *CG32: Nutrition Support in Adults*. London: NICE, 2006. http://www.nice.org.uk/cg32 (accessed June 2014).

Question B48: Invasive candidiasis

Risk factors for invasive candidiasis include:

A. Renal replacement therapy
B. Oral fluconazole
C. Oesophageal surgery
D. Perforated duodenal ulcer
E. Proton-pump inhibitors

Answer: TTTTT

Short explanation

All of the above constitute risk factors for invasive candidiasis.

Long explanation

Invasive fungal infection is becoming more common on the intensive care unit, and positive blood cultures should prompt investigation for underlying fungaemia. Risk factors for invasive candidiasis include:

- central venous catheters
- total parenteral nutrition

- broad-spectrum antibiotics
- high APACHE scores (indicating comorbidities and severity of illness)
- acute kidney injury, particularly if requiring renal replacement therapy
- surgery, particularly intra-abdominal
- gastrointestinal tract perforations and anastomotic leaks
- increased gastric pH (proton-pump inhibitor use)

The most significant risk factors for invasive candidaemia are colonisation by *Candida* followed by disruption of host defences (surgery and indwelling devices). The gastrointestinal and urogenital tracts and the skin are the main portals of entry for *Candida* infections.

Candida albicans remains the most common species isolated, followed by *C. glabrata*, *C. parapsilosis*, *C. krusei* and *C. tropicalis*. Fluconazole is inactive against *C. glabrata* and *C. krusei*. Risk factors for non-albicans candidaemia include prior fluconazole exposure and central venous catheters.

The most common *Candida* infections in ICU patients are bloodstream infections, catheter-related infections, intra-abdominal infections and urinary tract infections.

Invasive candidaemia has been shown to increase morbidity and mortality in intensive care patients with an attributable mortality rate of 20–40%. Candidaemia is also associated with increased ventilator days and length of unit and hospital stay.

Kauffman CA. Epidemiology and pathogenesis of candidaemia in adults. *UpToDate* 2012. http://www.uptodate.com (accessed June 2014).

Méan M, Marchetti O, Calandra T. Bench-to-bedside review: *Candida* infections in the intensive care unit. *Crit Care* 2008; 12: 204.

Question B49: Pleural effusions

Light's criteria for the diagnosis of pleural effusions state that:

A. Pleural fluid protein divided by serum protein > 0.5 suggests an exudate
B. Pleural fluid lactate dehydrogenase (LDH) divided by serum LDH < 0.6 suggests an transudate
C. Pleural fluid glucose < 2/3 of plasma glucose suggests an exudate
D. Pleural fluid pH < 7.2 suggests empyema
E. Pleural fluid LDH > 2/3 the upper limit of the laboratory normal value for serum LDH suggests a transudate

Answer: TTFFF

Short explanation

According to Light's criteria, pleural fluid is an exudate if pleural fluid LDH is > 2/3 the upper limit of the laboratory normal value for serum LDH. Pleural fluid glucose and pH do not form part of Light's criteria.

Long explanation

Pleural effusions should be investigated with a standardised history, examination and investigation approach. The history may elucidate a cause, while examination serves to establish any other clinical features of relevance. Routine blood tests and a posteroanterior (PA) chest x-ray should be performed in the first instance. Aspirating a bilateral transudate in the absence of suspicious features is not recommended. It is strongly recommended that pleural aspiration should be performed with ultrasound guidance to improve accuracy and reduce the risk of organ damage.

Any fluid removed for testing should be sent for protein, lactate dehydrogenase (LDH), glucose, Gram stain, cytology and culture. A fluid pH of < 7.2 is helpful in confirming the diagnosis of an empyema. Causes of a lymphocyte-predominant pleural effusion include pleural malignancy, cardiac failure and tuberculosis. Further investigations may include CT scan, thoracoscopy, bronchoscopy and biopsy.

Light's criteria help to determine whether a pleural effusion is a transudate or exudate. They state that pleural fluid is an exudate if one or more of the following criteria are met:

- Pleural fluid protein divided by serum protein is > 0.5
- Pleural fluid LDH divided by serum LDH is > 0.6
- Pleural fluid LDH is > 2/3 the upper limit of the laboratory normal value for serum LDH.

British Thoracic Society Pleural Disease Guideline Group. BTS pleural disease guideline. *Thorax* 2010; 65 (Suppl 2).

Question B50: Central venous catheter-related bloodstream infection

Central venous catheter-related bloodstream infection (CRBSI):

A. Is an opportunistic infection if the pathogen is methicillin-resistant *Staphylococcus aureus* (MRSA)
B. Is an opportunistic infection if the pathogen is a coagulase-negative *Staphylococcus*
C. Occurs in up to 25% of patients with central venous catheters
D. Is a greater risk with pulmonary artery catheters than with dialysis catheters
E. Occurs less frequently with subclavian vein cannulation than with cannulation of the femoral or internal jugular vein

Answer: TTFFT

Short explanation

CRBSI occurs in up to 16% of patients with central venous catheters. Dialysis catheters are associated with a higher risk of infection than pulmonary artery catheters.

Long explanation

An opportunistic infection is one caused by a microorganism that does not usually cause disease in a patient with a fully functioning immune system. Such infections are therefore most common in immunocompromised patients or those with chronic disease. The pathogen may be part of normal human flora (e.g. coagulase-negative *Staphylococcus*) or found in the environment. Disease caused by normal human flora may be described as endogenous infection, as the patient was colonised by the microorganism prior to developing an infection. Infection from an environmental pathogen is described as exogenous infection. Exogenous bacteria such as methicillin-resistant *Staphylococcus aureus* (MRSA) may colonise the patient in intensive care and predispose to opportunistic infection.

Risk factors for opportunistic infections are common in critically unwell patients. Surgery predisposes to deep infection, while invasive catheters and endotracheal tubes may act as ports of entry for organisms. Devices such as humidifiers may allow bacterial replication. Patients with a critical illness are often immunocompromised, and close contact between staff and patients acts as a route of cross-contamination.

CRBSI is the presence of a bacteraemia caused by an intravenous catheter. The incidence is up to 16% of catheterisations, although a better measure is the episodes per 1000 catheter days. CRBSI is rare from peripheral or arterial cannulae, highest in dialysis catheters and roughly equal in central venous catheters and pulmonary artery catheters. The site of placement also impacts on the likelihood of infection, with femoral placement carrying the highest risk, followed by internal jugular then subclavian vein cannulation. A central venous catheter care bundle incorporating all aspects from insertion to after care and removal has been shown to reduce CRBSI and should be employed in all patients with central venous access devices.

Loveday HP, Wilson JA, Pratt RJ, *et al*. epic3: national evidence based guidelines for preventing healthcare-associated infections in NHS hospitals in England. *J Hosp Infect* 2014; 86 (Suppl 1): S1–70.

Fletcher S. Catheter-related bloodstream infection. *Contin Educ Anaesth Crit Care Pain* 2005; 5: 49–51.

Question B51: ICU delirium

Regarding ICU delirium, which of the following are correct?

A. Morbidity and mortality is increased in patients with ICU delirium
B. Persisting cognitive impairment is common in patients with ICU delirium
C. Patients with ICU delirium cost more to treat
D. Hypoactive delirium is common in patients on ICU
E. Patients with hyperactive delirium are at a higher risk of long-term memory problems

Answer: TTTTF

Short explanation

The development of delirium is a strong predictor of mortality for up to 12 months following an episode. Cognitive impairment is found in many patients for months to years following an episode of delirium on ICU. This can increase healthcare costs considerably. Mixed and hypoactive delirium are commoner than hyperactive delirium. There is no published evidence showing a significant difference in long-term memory problems between the different delirium types.

Long explanation

Delirium is a serious condition with an incidence of up to 85% among the ICU patient population. The development of delirium is associated with a doubling of the risk of death in the next 12 months. Following an ICU admission, many patients experience significant cognitive deficits for months to years afterwards, and these deficits are commoner and more pronounced in those patients who have experienced delirium. The length of delirium is also relevant, as patients who experience more days of delirium score worse on cognitive tests at 1 year. If patients have significant cognitive deficits this leads to increased requirement for health and living care and so increases the cost for healthcare providers. Patients with delirium are more likely to self-extubate and remove invasive medical devices. Delirium increases hospital stay significantly, with some studies showing it to be increased by a median of 10 days.

The classification of delirium has been simplified into hypoactive, hyperactive and mixed. Patients with hypoactive delirium may appear subdued and withdrawn and will not necessarily interact with healthcare providers, family and friends. Hypoactive delirium accounts for up to 45% of cases of delirium. Patients with hyperactive delirium may be agitated and aggressive, and have hallucinations. This affects 10% of patients with delirium. Patients with mixed delirium will fluctuate between hypo- and hyperactive delirium.

Alce T, Page V, Vizcaychipi M. Delirium uncovered. *J Intensive Care Soc* 2013; 14: 53–9.

Girard T, Jackson J, Pandharipande P, *et al*. Delirium as a predictor of long-term cognitive impairment in survivors of critical illness. *Crit Care Med* 2010; 38: 1513–20.

Ouimet S, Kavanagh B, Gottfried S, Skrobik Y. Incidence, risk factors and consequences of ICU delirium. *Intensive Care Med* 2007; 33: 66–73.

Van Rompaey B, Elseviers M, Schuurmans M, *et al*. Risk factors for delirium in intensive care patients: a prospective cohort study. *Crit Care* 2009; 13: R77.

Question B52: *Clostridium difficile*

Regarding *Clostridium difficile*-associated diarrhoea:

A. Prior use of penicillins or macrolides is not a risk factor
B. Probiotics have been shown to reduce mortality from *C. difficile* in critical care
C. Meticulous use of alcohol-based hand gels reduces *C. difficile* transmission
D. Surgical resection of infected colon may be required
E. A toxin produced by the bacillus is responsible for the disease

Answer: FFFTT

Short explanation

Use of broad-spectrum antibiotics of all classes is a risk factor for *Clostridium difficile*-associated diarrhoea, but quinolones and cephalosporins are particularly associated. Probiotics may reduce rates of *C. difficile*-positive samples, but no mortality benefit has yet been shown. Alcohol-based hand gels are ineffective against *C. difficile*; soap and water should be used. Toxic megacolon may develop, which requires resection. *C. difficile* produces a toxin that causes inflammation, dilatation and necrosis of the bowel.

Long explanation

Clostridium difficile is an anaerobic Gram-positive bacillus which is the commonest cause of infective diarrhoea in critical care. It produces a toxin, which leads to bowel mucosal inflammation, dilatation and necrosis. Disease ranges from mild, which may require no treatment, to severe colitis and toxic megacolon, which often requires surgical resection. Mortality of *C. difficile* colitis in critical care approaches 20%.

In order for *C. difficile* to grow, the normal ecosystem of bowel flora must be disturbed. Risk factors include prolonged ICU stay, use of proton-pump inhibitors, enteral feeding and the current or recent use of antibacterial agents. All broad-spectrum antibacterial agents may increase the risk of *C. difficile* overgrowth and diarrhoea, but the quinolones and cephalosporins are particularly strongly associated.

Treatment is with antibacterial agents. Metronidazole (enteral or intravenous) is first-line therapy, with resistant cases treated with enteral vancomycin. Other effective agents include teicoplanin and fidaxomicin. As many as 20% of cases may require multiple courses of antibacterials.

Prevention of the disease is important. Limitation of the use of proton-pump inhibitors, careful stewardship of antibacterials and rigorous infection control procedures are key to disease control. Alcohol-based hand gels are ineffective against *C. difficile*, so soap and water should be used. Probiotics such as lactobacilli and bifidobacteria have been found to reduce rates of *C. difficile*-positive faecal samples, but no mortality or length-of-stay benefit has yet been shown.

Wiesen P, Van Gossum A, Preiser JC. Diarrhoea in the critically ill. *Curr Opin Crit Care* 2006; 12: 149–54.

Question B53: Pathophysiology of burns

With regards to the pathophysiology of burns, which of the following are correct?

A. The depth of the burn is related only to the temperature to which the skin is exposed
B. Scalds are an unusual cause of burns in children
C. Flame burns are often deep or full-thickness burns
D. The severity of electrical burns is mainly related to the voltage applied
E. Coagulative necrosis occurs at the site of burn injury

Answer: FFTTT

Short explanation

The depth of burn is related to the temperature to which the skin is exposed, the specific heat of the causative agent and the duration of exposure. Scalds are common in children, as they are prone to spilling hot liquids. The elderly are also vulnerable to scalds.

Long explanation

Burns are a major cause of injury, morbidity and mortality worldwide. The pathophysiology involves local skin changes related directly to the thermal injury in addition to systemic effects. At the site of a burn injury there is coagulative necrosis of the epidermis and underlying tissues. Burns can be caused by flame, hot liquids, hot objects, chemicals or electricity. Burns caused by flame, hot liquids or hot objects induce cellular damage by transfer of energy leading to coagulative necrosis. Chemical burns and electricity cause direct injury to cellular membranes in addition to the transfer of heat.

The area of cutaneous or superficial injury is commonly divided into three zones. The zone of coagulation, the zone of stasis and the zone of hyperaemia.

The zone of coagulation is the necrotic area where the cells have been disrupted. The area directly next to this has had a moderate amount of tissue injury with decreased tissue perfusion. This area can progress to coagulative necrosis if the wound environment is poor.

The zone of stasis is associated with vascular damage and vessel leakage. Cytokines, such as the vasoconstrictor thromboxane A_2, are involved in the processes occurring in these areas. The presence of antioxidants and bradykinin antagonists can counteract some of the problems caused by vasoconstriction.

The final zone, the zone of hyperaemia, is characterised by vasodilatation from inflammation surrounding the wound. This area contains the most viable tissue, from which the healing process begins, and is not usually at risk from further necrosis.

Hettiaratchy S, Dziewulski P. Pathophysiology and types of burns. *BMJ* 2004; 328: 1427–9.

Question B54: Cardiac tamponade

The following are signs of cardiac tamponade:

A. Enlarged cardiac silhouette on chest radiograph (CXR) with clear lung fields
B. A drop in diastolic blood pressure of > 10 mmHg during inspiration
C. Muffled heart sounds on auscultation
D. Diastolic collapse of heart chambers on echocardiography
E. Absent or reduced *x* descent on CVP trace

Answer: TFTTF

Short explanation

Beck's triad (hypotension, distended neck veins and muffled heart sounds) is classically associated with cardiac tamponade. Central venous pressure (CVP) is elevated, with absent or reduced *y* descent (diastolic). The cardiac silhouette is commonly enlarged and globular with clear lung fields on CXR. Echocardiography is usually diagnostic, with visualisation of the effusion and diastolic collapse of the atria and sometimes the right ventricle. A drop in systolic blood pressure of > 10 mmHg during inspiration is a sign of pulsus paradoxus.

Long explanation

Cardiac tamponade is a life-threatening medical emergency caused by decompensated compression of the heart by pericardial fluid and increased intrapericardial pressure. Tamponade may be 'surgical' or 'medical'. Surgical tamponade is associated with rapidly accumulating (minutes to hours) pericardial fluid, generally due to haemorrhage, and may cause precipitous deterioration in haemodynamics. Medical tamponade is associated with slower (days to weeks) accumulation of fluid, generally inflammatory in nature, which may become very large before decompensation and tamponade occur.

Beck's triad describes the classical clinical signs of tamponade: hypotension, distended neck veins and muffled or distant heart sounds. The presence of all three signs is pathognomonic of cardiac tamponade. Other clinical findings include tachycardia, dyspnoea and pulsus paradoxus. Pulsus paradoxus is defined as a drop in systolic blood pressure of > 10 mmHg in inspiration. Diastolic blood pressure tends to be maintained.

ECG may show tachycardia, reduced-amplitude QRS complexes, non-specific ST segment changes or electrical alternans; beat-to-beat alteration of QRS amplitude or axis. Chest radiography often shows an enlarged or globular cardiac silhouette with clear lung fields, with larger silhouettes in medical tamponades. The CVP is usually elevated (maybe greatly so), with a loss or diminution of the diastolic *y* descent.

Effusions are usually visualisable with echocardiography, and tamponade is suggested by evidence of impaired filling. Diastolic collapse of the atria (especially the right atrium) is seen, with collapse of the free wall of the right ventricle and/or septal displacement. Left ventricular diastolic collapse is only seen with very high intrapericardial pressures. Treatment by pericardiocentesis is indicated for large effusions (> 20 mm on echocardiography), for tamponade, or for diagnostic purposes.

Maisch B, Seferović PM, Ristić AD, *et al.* Guidelines on the diagnosis and management of pericardial diseases executive summary. *Eur Heart J* 2004; 25: 587–610.

Question B55: Anaemia

Regarding anaemia:

A. Anaemia shifts the oxyhaemoglobin dissociation curve to the left
B. Haemolysis causes a microcytic anaemia
C. There is a reduced response to erythropoietin
D. Increased hepcidin synthesis is responsible for the fall in serum iron
E. Ferritin concentrations are decreased in the critically ill

Answer: FFTTF

Short explanation

Anaemia will shift the oxyhaemoglobin dissociation curve to the right. Haemolysis causes a macrocytic anaemia. Ferritin concentrations are increased in the critically ill.

Long explanation

Anaemia is defined as a haemoglobin concentration of < 12 g/dl in women and < 13 g/dl in men. Anaemia in the critically ill patient may be pre-existing, and it may be multifactorial. Anaemia is commonly classified into microcytic, normocytic and macrocytic, and this helps narrow the list of differential diagnoses. The most common reason for anaemia on ICU is blood loss. This may be from surgery, trauma or gastrointestinal bleeding, but will be exacerbated in all patients by phlebotomy. Acute blood loss will cause a normocytic normochromic anaemia; chronic blood loss will cause a microcytic hypochromic anaemia.

Haemolysis will generally lead to a macrocytic anaemia, as increased blood production leads to a reticulocytosis. Other causes of macrocytic anaemia include hypothyroidism, and vitamin B_{12} and folate deficiency. Anaemia of chronic disease is also commonly seen in ICU patients. This generally causes a normochromic normocytic anaemia. The exact pathophysiology is unclear, but erythropoietin secretion is reduced and the marrow response blunted. Serum iron is decreased in the critically ill patient, with a fall in total iron binding capacity and a rise in ferritin (an acute-phase protein). Hepcidin reduces serum iron by binding and inactivating ferroportin, an iron-transport protein on cell membranes. This response is thought to be protective, as many bacteria require iron for metabolism.

The physiological response to anaemia is dependent on the volume status and physiological reserve of the patient, and on the chronology of the anaemia (acute vs. chronic). The TRICC study showed that patients transfused with a restrictive policy (haemoglobin > 7 g/dl) had improved outcomes over those transfused with a liberal transfusion strategy. This is now a fairly standard transfusion trigger in ICU in the absence of comorbidities that might make increased oxygen delivery desirable, e.g. ischaemic heart disease. Anaemia shifts the oxyhaemoglobin dissociation curve to the right, increasing oxygen delivery to the tissues.

Treatment of anaemia in ICU should focus on management of the underlying condition, reduction of blood loss, and optimising the patient's cardiac output. Erythropoietin and iron supplements have not been shown to make a clinically significant difference to anaemia, and blood transfusions are often required.

Hebert PC, Wells G, Blajchman MA, *et al*. A multicenter, randomized, controlled clinical trial of transfusion requirements in critical care. Transfusion Requirements in Critical Care Investigators, Canadian Critical Care Trials Group. *N Engl J Med* 1999; 340: 409–17.

Lelubre C, Vincent JL. Red blood cell transfusion in the critically ill patient. *Ann Intensive Care* 2011; 1: 43.

Retter A, Hunt BJ. Anaemia in critical care. In Waldmann C, Soni N, Rhodes A. *Oxford Desk Reference: Critical Care*. Oxford: Oxford University Press, 2008; pp. 392–3.

Question B56: APRV

Regarding airway pressure-release ventilation (APRV)

A. Peak pressures are higher than with BIPAP for a given tidal volume
B. T_{high} is usually a minimum of 4 seconds
C. Neuromuscular blockade is often required to prevent patient/ventilator asynchrony
D. Hypercapnia is a contraindication to its use
E. Spontaneous breathing is sensed by the ventilator and mandatory breaths synchronised

Answer: FTFFF

Short explanation

APRV is a ventilator mode using a prolonged high pressure with intermittent release of pressure for tidal ventilation and carbon dioxide clearance. For a given tidal volume peak airway pressure is lower than for a BIPAP ventilatory mode. If hypercapnia becomes a problem then the T_{high} may need to be shortened. A reduction in neuromuscular blockade use should be seen, as spontaneous breathing can occur throughout the ventilatory cycle.

Long explanation

APRV is a variation on bilevel pressure ventilation (BIPAP) or continuous positive airway pressure (CPAP). it is time-triggered, pressure-limited, and time-cycled. The high 'inspiratory' pressure (P_{high}) is maintained for a longer period of time than is traditional (T_{high}, usually a minimum of 4 seconds), with spontaneous breathing maintained throughout the respiratory cycle. Brief 'releases' of this higher pressure allow carbon dioxide removal (P_{low}) and tidal ventilation. If hypercapnia causing acidosis ensues the T_{high} may be shortened, but hypercapnia is otherwise tolerated.

The main indication for APRV is hypoxia from acute lung injury (ALI) or acute respiratory distress syndrome (ARDS), as the higher mean airway pressure improves oxygenation, aids recruitment and reduces atelectasis. The lower respiratory rate reduces low-volume re-expansion injury and continued spontaneous breathing may improve V/Q mismatch. Spontaneous breaths can occur at any point in the ventilator cycle and do not need require the ventilator to synchronise breaths. The higher mean airway pressure and increased alveolar recruitment ensures that spontaneous breaths occur on a more favourable part of the compliance curve, thereby reducing the work of breathing.

Advantages of APRV include a significantly lower peak airway pressure for a given tidal volume but with a higher mean airway pressure to aid oxygenation. It allows spontaneous breathing throughout the ventilatory cycle, improving lung mechanics and avoiding the use of neuromuscular blockers and deep sedation.

Disadvantages of APRV currently include a lack of familiarity amongst clinicians and limited availability of the technology (most portable ventilators are not set up for this mode). As with other pressure-controlled ventilator modes, lung compliance significantly affects pressures required, tidal volumes and carbon dioxide clearance.

Frawley PM, Habashi NM. Airway pressure release ventilation: theory and practice. *AACN Clinical Issues*. 2001; 12: 234–46.

Gould T, de Beer JMA. Principles of artificial ventilation. *Anaesth Intensive Care Med* 2007; 8: 91–101.
Waldmann C, Soni N, Rhodes A. *Oxford Desk Reference: Critical Care*. Oxford: Oxford University Press, 2008; pp. 10–11.

Question B57: P-POSSUM

The P-POSSUM system

A. Is a modification of POSSUM with reductions in predicted mortality
B. Only applies to patients undergoing surgery
C. Uses categorised clinical and observational data
D. Relies on the results of blood tests
E. Can be used to predict preoperative risk of surgery

Answer: TTTTF

Short explanation

P-POSSUM applies to patients undergoing surgery. It uses 12 physiological findings (age, observations, investigations and clinical examination findings) and 6 surgical parameters (complexity, urgency and operative findings). This means that P-POSSUM can only be calculated at the end of surgery, and cannot be used to predict surgical risk beforehand.

Long explanation

The Physiological and Operative Severity Score for the enUmeration of Mortality and morbidity (POSSUM) is a tool for assessing the risk of surgery. It was introduced in 1991 and modified in 1998 in response to criticism that mortality was overestimated, especially for lower-risk procedures. This formed the P-POSSUM, which uses the same variables but a modified equation to calculate the outcome figures.

There are two groups of variables recorded: 12 physiological parameters, including clinical findings, observations and investigation results; and 6 operative parameters, including complexity, urgency and findings at surgery.

Physiological	Age Observations (systolic BP, heart rate, GCS) Investigations (ECG, Hb, WBC, urea, Na^+, K^+) Examination findings (signs of cardiac and respiratory failure)
Surgical	Operation type (complexity, number of procedures, urgency) Findings (blood loss, peritoneal contamination, malignancy)

The reliance of the model on findings from the operating theatre means that the P-POSSUM can only be calculated at the end of surgery, and so cannot be used to predict the preoperative risk of surgery. Of course, it is possible to predict these findings, perhaps to give a 'worst-case-scenario' estimate of morbidity and mortality prior to surgery.

The primary use is to assess performance in a standardised way, thereby allowing meaningful comparison of different surgeons and hospitals. No scoring system is perfect, however, and some specialties have developed their own modifications of POSSUM to give closer predictive value for their cohorts of patients. Examples include V-POSSUM for vascular surgery and CR-POSSUM for colorectal surgery.

Copeland GP, Jones D, Walters M. POSSUM: a scoring system for surgical audit. *Br J Surg* 1991; 78: 355–60.

Palazzo M. Severity of illness and likely outcome from critical illness. In Bersten AD, Soni N. *Oh's Intensive Care Manual*, 6th edn. Edinburgh: Butterworth-Heinemann, 2009, pp. 17–30.

Question B58: Acute heart failure

The following are recognised causes of acute heart failure (AHF):

A. Pregnancy
B. Aortic stenosis
C. Sickle cell disease
D. Atrial fibrillation
E. Ventricular septal defect (VSD)

Answer: TTTTT

Short explanation

The commonest cause of AHF is ischaemic heart disease, including mechanical sequelae such as VSD or papillary muscle rupture. Critical aortic stenosis combined with a trigger (e.g. peripheral vasodilatation) can lead to rapid decompensation of cardiac output. Post-partum cardiomyopathy is an uncommon cause of AHF. Causes of high-output AHF include severe anaemia, sepsis and thyrotoxic storm.

Long explanation

Acute heart failure (AHF) is rapid onset or worsening of heart failure symptoms and signs. It is a medical emergency requiring urgent assessment and treatment. A classification of six subtypes of AHF was published in 2008 by the European Society of Intensive Care Medicine (ESICM) and the European Society of Cardiology (ESC):

- Acute decompensated heart failure (no signs of shock or pulmonary oedema)
- Pulmonary oedema (with respiratory distress)
- Hypertensive AHF (with signs of congestion)
- Cardiogenic shock (tissue hypoperfusion despite adequate preload)
- High-output failure
- Right heart failure

The commonest cause of AHF is decompensated chronic heart failure, which itself is strongly associated with ischaemic heart disease, hypertension and diabetes mellitus. Acute cardiac syndromes can trigger AHF secondary to reduced myocardial function or ischaemic sequelae such as papillary muscle rupture or VSD.

Arrhythmias, particularly ventricular arrhythmias such as VT, compromise cardiac function. Atrial arrhythmias such as fibrillation or flutter are unlikely to cause AHF alone, but may cause significant decompensation in patients with pre-existing valvular disease or cardiac failure. Valvular lesions may cause AHF if acute (such as chordae tendinae rupture or endocarditis) or in combination with a trigger (e.g. systemic vasodilatation in severe aortic stenosis).

High-output cardiac failure is characterised by increased cardiac output but symptoms and signs of AHF. Aetiologies include shunts (A-V malformations, haemangiomata), vasodilatation (pregnancy, sepsis), anaemia (e.g. caused by sickle cell disease), hyperthyroidism and beriberi.

Dickstein K, Cohen-Solal A, Filippatos G, *et al.* ESC Guidelines for the diagnosis and treatment of acute and chronic heart failure 2008: the Task Force for the Diagnosis and Treatment of Acute and Chronic Heart Failure 2008 of the European Society of Cardiology. *Eur Heart J* 2008; 29: 2388–442.

McMurray JJV, Adamopoulos S, Anker SD, *et al*. ESC guidelines for the diagnosis and treatment of acute and chronic heart failure 2012. The Task Force for the Diagnosis and Treatment of Acute and Chronic Heart Failure 2012 of the European Society of Cardiology. *Eur Heart J* 2012; 33: 1787–847.

Question B59: Paraquat poisoning

With regards to paraquat poisoning, which of the following are correct?

A. It is commoner in the developing world
B. A patient who has ingested 10 mg paraquat ion per kg body weight is likely to make a full recovery
C. Oesophageal perforation has a mortality rate of around 100%
D. Paraquat is mostly metabolised to toxic metabolites that are excreted by the kidney
E. Concentrations are lowest in the lung due to reduced uptake into cells

Answer: TTTFF

Short explanation

Paraquat is not actively metabolised, and is mostly excreted unchanged via the kidneys. Paraquat concentration is up to 20 times higher in the lungs, because of active energy-dependent uptake by alveolar epithelial type 1 and type 2 cells via the polyamine uptake pathway.

Long explanation

Paraquat is a herbicide used all over the world in agricultural industries. It is fast-acting and kills green plant tissue on contact. Its use is illegal in the European Union and highly restricted in the United States, where individuals must be licensed to use it. In the developing world it is used widely. Paraquat is highly toxic in relatively small doses and so is a major suicide agent in many countries worldwide.

Exposure on the skin can lead to systemic toxicity, although inhalation of sprayed solution rarely causes systemic problems. Less than 20% is absorbed through the gastrointestinal tract, from where it is distributed to highly perfused organs. In the lung the active uptake of paraquat by type 1 and type 2 epithelial cells leads to much higher levels than in the rest of the body. Paraquat radicals and hydroxyl free radicals are formed, which damage cells and inhibit essential enzymes.

Paraquat is highly irritant to eyes and mucosa. Oesophageal ulceration and eventually perforation can occur, leading to severe mediastinitis and death. Diffuse alveolar damage occurs, leading to respiratory failure. Severe poisoning (20–40 mg paraquat ion per kg body weight) and fulminant poisoning (> 40 mg paraquat ion per kg body weight) will almost invariably lead to death.

The urine dithionite test can confirm the diagnosis, which may not be clear in children and people with suicidal intent. Blood level results are subject to significant delays and are of negligible clinical utility, although a plasma level of > 1.6 μg/ml 12 hours after ingestion is almost invariably fatal.

Initial management should include prevention of further absorption using activated charcoal. Supportive measures such as renal replacement therapy and fluid, electrolyte and pain control are the mainstay of treatment. Oxygen can worsen lung injury. No specific antidote or treatment exists, although lung transplantation has been reported.

Benditt J. Teaching case of the month: paraquat poisoning. *Resp Care* 2005; 50: 383–5.

Question B60: Critical illness neuromyopathy

Concerning critical illness neuromyopathy (CINM):

A. CINM affects up to 30% of all ventilated patients on ICU
B. It is diagnosed by clinical examination
C. The risk is increased by hyperglycaemia
D. Development of CINM is an independent risk factor for ICU mortality
E. Steroid use is an independent risk factor for the development of CINM

Answer: FFTTT

Short explanation

CINM affects up to 80% of ICU patients. It is difficult to diagnose clinically and may be easily missed. Risk factors include sepsis, multi-organ failure, immobility, hyperglycaemia, and use of corticosteroids, muscle relaxants and aminoglycosides. CINM is an independent risk factor for ICU mortality and may lead to long-term weakness or disability, although 70% of patients recover completely.

Long explanation

Critical illness neuromyopathy (CINM) is a term used to describe two overlapping conditions which manifest in similar ways and often co-exist. Critical illness myopathy (CIM) is an acute primary myopathy causing muscle fibre damage and necrosis in severe cases. Critical illness polyneuropathy (CIP) affects sensory and motor nerves as systemic inflammation and hypotension cause neuronal dysfunction and damage.

CINM often remains undiagnosed. Electrophysiological and histological studies suggest that as many as 60–80% of critically ill patients develop elements of CINM at some point in their stay, although the majority recover before discharge. Risk factors include:

- sepsis
- multi-organ dysfunction or failure
- corticosteroid use
- hyperglycaemia
- neuromuscular blocking agents and electrolyte abnormalities (CIM)
- prolonged ICU stay and immobility

CINM is often manifested as a failure to wean from mechanical ventilation or prolonged weakness. Motor deficit usually affects all four limbs equally, with reduced or absent reflexes and loss of sensory function in up to half of patients. Clinical diagnosis is difficult, as patients are often sedated, delirious or uncooperative. Electrophysiological tests include nerve conduction studies (CIP), electromyography (CIM) or direct muscle stimulation, which is possible in uncooperative patients. Other investigations such as MRI, lumbar puncture and serum electrolytes may be required to exclude other diagnoses. Differential diagnoses include CNS lesions (tumours, haemorrhage, infarction), Guillian–Barré syndrome, multiple sclerosis and myasthenia gravis.

Treatment of CINM is supportive, and the focus is instead on prevention of its development by limiting the time a patient is immobile, aggressively managing sepsis and multi-organ failure, controlling blood glucose and limiting the use of drugs such as corticosteroids and neuromuscular blocking agents. CINM is an independent predictor for ICU mortality, and while the majority of patients make a full functional recovery, there may be mild features present for up to 5 years after ICU discharge.

Latronico N, Peli E, Botteri M. Critical illness myopathy and neuropathy. *Curr Opin Crit Care* 2005; 11: 126–32.

Question B61: Diagnosis of brain death

Brainstem reflex tests for diagnosis of neurological death include:

A. Tests of cranial nerves II to X inclusive
B. Doll's eye movements
C. Response to central and peripheral painful stimuli
D. Carinal stimulation
E. Consensual pupillary reaction to light

Answer: TFTTT

Short explanation

Doll's eye movements are not tested in the diagnosis of neurological death.

Long explanation

Brainstem reflexes are tested as part of the process of diagnosing death by neurological criteria. Prior to brainstem testing, the patient must meet essential preconditions (irreversible brain damage of known aetiology causing apnoeic coma requiring mechanical ventilation) and have other causes of apnoea or coma excluded (drugs, metabolic disturbance, haemodynamic instability).

There are six brainstem reflex tests, which test all cranial nerves (CNs) except for I (olfactory), XI (accessory) and XII (hypoglossal). The brainstem nuclei tested range from the midbrain to the medulla oblongata. Most tests involve multiple cranial nerves (different efferent and afferent pathways). The tests are outlined below.

Pupillary response to light

- A bright light is shone into each eye, looking for direct and consensual reactions.
- CN II (optic) → midbrain → CN III (oculomotor)

Corneal reflex

- Light touch to cornea should elicit blinking
- CN V (facial) → pons → CN VII (trigeminal)

Response to pain

- Painful stimulus to head (e.g. supra-orbital) and limbs should elicit a response (e.g. grimace)
- CN V (facial) → pons → CN VII (trigeminal)

Oculovestibular reflex

- 50 ml of cold saline into the external auditory meatus should elicit eye movement
- CN VIII (vestibulocochlear) → pons → CNs III, IV, VI (oculomotor, trochlear, abducens)

Gag reflex

- Pharyngeal stimulation should elicit a gag response
- CN IX (glossopharyngeal) → medulla → CN X (vagus)

Cough reflex

- Carinal stimulation (e.g. suction catheter) should elicit a cough response
- CN X (vagus) → medulla → CN X (vagus)

The doll's eyes reflex is elicited by turning the head of an unconscious subject. The eyes will normally move as if the patient is fixating on a stationary object. If the reflex is 'negative' then the eyes remain stationary with respect to the head. A negative reflex suggests a lesion in one or more of the following: the vestibular nerve and labyrinth, the neck proprioceptors, cranial nerves III and VI and/or the external ocular muscles. Doll's eye movements are not part of brainstem reflex testing.

If no brainstem reflexes are elicited, then apnoea testing should be performed. In some conditions, these tests are not possible (e.g. massive craniofacial trauma), in which case ancillary tests are required to diagnose death by neurological criteria, such as four-vessel cranial angiography or EEG.

Oram J, Murphy P. Diagnosis of death. *Contin Educ Anaesth Crit Care Pain* 2011; 11: 77–81.

Question B62: Hypermagnesaemia

Regarding hypermagnesaemia, which of the following are correct?

A. Diuretics are a common cause
B. Magnesium crosses the placenta
C. Levels over 5 mmol/l lead to cardiac arrest
D. Higher doses of non-depolarising muscle relaxants are required
E. Hypermagnesaemia leads to loss of deep tendon reflexes

Answer: FTFFT

Short explanation

Diuretics usually cause hypomagnesaemia. The commonest cause of hypermagnesaemia is excess administration. Levels over 25 mmol/l will invariably cause cardiac arrest. Non-depolarising muscle relaxants are potentiated, and lower doses are required. Onset time is also reduced.

Long explanation

Magnesium is used in clinical practice for a variety of conditions. Common uses are in the treatment of pre-eclampsia and eclampsia and acute severe asthma. Supplemental administration of magnesium is often required in patients with malabsorption. Symptomatic hypermagnesaemia is rare other than in patients who are receiving supplemental magnesium. This can occur due to excessive doses or due to renal failure, where excretion is impaired.

The normal plasma value for magnesium is 0.7–1.0 mmol/l. Therapeutic levels in patients with eclampsia are 4–8 mmol/l. Toxicity usually becomes apparent when blood levels increase beyond this. Brisk deep tendon reflexes are lost at levels beyond 10 mmol/l. At a blood level of 15 mmol/l respiratory muscle paralysis becomes evident and blockade of the sinoatrial and atrioventricular nodes occurs. Cardiac arrest is inevitable at blood levels of 25 mmol/l. Magnesium crosses the placenta, so high levels in the mother can be transferred to the fetus, which can then be apnoeic and hypotonic at birth.

Parikh M, Webb S. Cations: potassium, calcium and magnesium. *Contin Educ Anaesth Crit Care Pain* 2012; 12: 195–8.

Question B63: Acute pancreatitis

The following are recognised causes of acute pancreatitis:

A. Choledocholithiasis
B. Protozoal infection
C. Hypocalcaemia
D. Hypothermia
E. Corticosteroids

Answer: TFFTT

Short explanation

The commonest causes of acute pancreatitis are alcohol and choledocholithiasis. Other causes include trauma, surgery (including ERCP), hypothermia, hypercalcaemia, hyperlipidaemia, drugs (e.g. corticosteroids, diuretics, antiretrovirals) and mumps. Rare causes include scorpion venom, extreme exercise and helminthal infections.

Long explanation

Acute pancreatitis has an annual incidence of 2–90 per 100,000 population, which is rising steadily with time. It has an estimated mortality of 2–14%. Males are affected more than females.

The commonest causes of acute pancreatitis worldwide are alcohol and choledocholithiasis, which together account for over 80% of cases. Surgical causes include endoscopic retrograde cholangiopancreatography (ERCP), gastric and hepatobiliary surgery. Other important causes include trauma, hypothermia, ulcers, malignancy and viral infection (e.g. mumps, Coxsackie virus).

Metabolic conditions which can lead to acute pancreatitis include hypercalcaemia, hyperlipidaemia and malnutrition. People with familial hyperlipidaemias are at a higher risk. Some cases are due to drugs, such as corticosteroids, diuretics, antiretroviral agents and some antibiotics (tetracyclines and sulphonamides). Rarer causes include scorpion venom, extreme exercise and helminthal infections.

Bank S, Indaram A. Causes of acute and recurrent pancreatitis: clinical considerations and clues to diagnosis. *Gastroenterol Clin North Am* 1999; 28: 571–89.

Banks PA, Bollen TL, Dervenis C, *et al*. Classification of acute pancreatitis – 2012: revision of the Atlanta classification and definitions by international consensus. *Gut* 2013; 62: 102–11.

Question B64: Blood products

Concerning blood products:

A. Human albumin solution contains some clotting factors
B. Fresh frozen plasma (FFP) should be ABO-compatible with the recipient
C. AB-negative patients are universal recipients

D. Fresh frozen plasma (FFP) should be rhesus-compatible with the recipient
E. Fresh frozen plasma (FFP) should be stored at −18 °C

Answer: FTFFF

Short explanation

Human albumin solution (HAS) contains no clotting factors. AB-positive patients are universal recipients. FFP is unlikely to cause RhD sensitisation. FFP should be stored at −30 °C

Long explanation

Once donated, whole blood is processed in a number of different ways in order to produce the individual components in clinical use. Human albumin solution (HAS) is processed from blood that has not been snap frozen to preserve clotting factors and therefore has no procoagulant activity. Fresh frozen plasma (FFP) is separated from whole blood and quickly frozen to −30 °C. It contains all the coagulation factors in concentrations similar to that of blood and has a shelf life of up to a year. FFP does not need to be cross-matched but should be ABO-compatible. Group O FFP should only be transfused to group O recipients. If the patient's blood group is not available, FFP of a different ABO group is acceptable, provided it does not have high titres of anti-A or anti-B activity. FFP does not need to be RhD-compatible, as it is unlikely to cause RhD sensitisation.

British Committee for Standards in Haematology, Blood Transfusion Task Force. Guidelines for the use of fresh-frozen plasma, cryoprecipitate and cryosupernatant. *Br J Haematol* 2004; 126: 11–28.

Power I, Kam P. Physiology of blood. In *Priniciples of Physiology for the Anaesthetist*, 2nd edn. London: Hodder Arnold; pp. 291–2.

Question B65: Survival after cardiac arrest

Which of the following treatments have been shown to improve survival after cardiac arrest?

A. Amiodarone 300 mg after the third shock for ventricular fibrillation
B. Epinephrine 1 mg IV
C. Untrained bystander CPR
D. Bipolar defibrillation
E. Airway maintenance with a laryngeal mask airway or endotracheal tube

Answer: FFTTF

Short explanation

Early effective bystander CPR, uninterrupted high-quality chest compressions and early defibrillation are the only interventions that have been definitively shown to improve survival after cardiac arrest. No drugs or advanced airway techniques have been shown to increase survival to hospital discharge.

Long explanation

The only interventions that have been definitively shown to improve survival after cardiac arrest, regardless of whether it occurs in or out of hospital, are early effective bystander CPR, uninterrupted high-quality chest compressions and early defibrillation. Epinephrine has been shown to increase the return of spontaneous circulation, but no drugs or advanced airway techniques have been shown to increase survival to hospital discharge.

This evidence is reflected in the 2010 resuscitation guidelines. The rescuer should check that it is safe to approach and check for signs of life. If none are present, he or she should summon help before immediately starting chest compressions at a ratio of 30:2 breaths. Chest compressions should cease only for a rhythm check (10 seconds) and for defibrillation. Chest compressions should continue while the defibrillator is charging. After defibrillation the chest compressions should continue immediately, without a pulse check, as the chance of feeling a pulse is small, and chest compressions will not provoke arrhythmias if a perfusing rhythm is present. Chest compressions will increase the amplitude and frequency of ventricular fibrillation, thereby increasing the chance for successful defibrillation. They may also usefully induce VF from asystole.

Resuscitation Council (UK). Advanced life support algorithm. In *Advanced Life Support*, 6th edn. London: Resuscitation Council, 2011; Chapter 6.

Waldmann C, Soni N, Rhodes A. *Oxford Desk Reference: Critical Care*. Oxford: Oxford University Press, 2008; pp. 240–1.

Question B66: Colonic pseudo-obstruction

With regards to acute colonic pseudo-obstruction, which of the following are correct?

A. There must be clinical and radiological evidence of large bowel obstruction for diagnosis
B. It is also known as Ogilvie's syndrome
C. Ischaemia and perforation rarely occur
D. Oral neostigmine has been shown to be effective in up to 80% of patients
E. Endoscopic decompression can be performed as an alternative to surgery

Answer: TTFFT

Short explanation

Ischaemia and perforation are complications that occur in up to 15% of patients. Perforation is more likely when the caecal diameter is large, and in elderly patients. Oral neostigmine is not recommended, because absorption can be very variable in patients with pseudo-obstruction. Intravenous administration is the preferred route.

Long explanation

Critically ill patients are at risk from a number of gastrointestinal pathologies with little relation to their underlying illness. These include gastrointestinal ulceration and haemorrhage, diarrhoea, vomiting, feed intolerance, paralytic ileus and acute colonic pseudo-obstruction. In acute colonic pseudo-obstruction there is clinical and radiological evidence of large bowel obstruction in the absence of mechanical obstruction. Patients will probably fail to pass stool or flatus, they are likely to have abdominal pain and distension, and they may vomit. Clinical features are similar to those of mechanical bowel obstruction (e.g. secondary to malignancy or hernia), which should be excluded.

A plain abdominal x-ray will show dilated colon, usually the caecum and proximal colon. The diameter of the dilated bowel is important, as the risk of perforation increases with increasing dilatation. Free air suggests perforation. Water-soluble contrast-enhanced CT or radiograph demonstrates dilated large bowel in the absence of mechanical obstruction and should be performed in all patients. CT is the preferred investigation, since it gives more information regarding the viability of the bowel and may show if there is ischaemia or inflammation present.

The underlying pathophysiology of pseudo-obstruction is unknown but may involve dysfunction of the autonomic plexuses in the gut wall. Treatment includes supportive care and meticulous attention to fluid balance, electrolyte levels and haemodynamics. Neostigmine is the most widely used pharmacological agent; it should be administered intravenously with close cardiac monitoring. Invasive treatments include endoscopic decompression, radiologically guided percutaneous caecostomy and surgery. Surgery should only be attempted in patients with imminent or confirmed perforation, as mortality is high. Usual procedures are either a caecostomy or a colostomy, but both carry a risk of recurrence of pseudo-obstruction.

De Giorgio R, Knowles C. Acute colonic pseudo-obstruction. *Br J Surg* 2009; 96: 229–39.

Question B67: Tetanus

Regarding tetanus:

A. The clinical effects are due to the endotoxin tetanospasmin
B. Tetanus spores are eradicated by autoclaving
C. The neurotoxin enters the nervous system via synapses
D. Diagnosis is confirmed by culture of *Clostridium tetani*
E. *Clostridium tetani* is an aerobic Gram-positive coccus

Answer: FTFFF

Short explanation

Clostridium tetani is an anaerobic Gram-positive bacillus. Tetanospasmin is an exotoxin that enters the nervous system via the neuromuscular junction. Diagnosis is clinical, as the organism is difficult to culture.

Long explanation

Clostridium tetani is a spore-forming obligate anaerobic Gram-positive coccus. Spores are ubiquitous in the environment and can survive in extreme conditions for prolonged periods. They usually enter the body after contamination of a wound. The incubation period of the disease is 3–21 days (average 7 days). The clinical effects are due to tetanospasmin, an exotoxin which spreads into the nervous system by binding to the neuromuscular junction. Once bound, it is transported in a retrograde manner to the cell body and across synapses to adjacent motor and autonomic nerves. Tetanospasmin exerts its effect by cleaving synaptobrevin, a vesicle-associated membrane protein which is essential for the release of neurotransmitters.

Tetanus primarily affects inhibitory pathways, causing increased muscle tone, rigidity and sudden extreme muscle spasms. These initially affect the face, then spread to the rest of the body, and may be of sufficient severity to cause tendon, muscle or bony injury. Involvement of sympathetic neurons results in loss of autonomic control, sympathetic overactivity and increased catecholamine levels. Neuronal binding of the toxin is irreversible, and therefore recovery requires the growth of new nerve terminals, taking 4–6 weeks.

Tetanus is a clinical diagnosis. Early symptoms of tetanus include neck stiffness, sore throat, dysphagia and trismus. Patients with respiratory distress should be mechanically ventilated. Sudden death occurs from laryngospasm, diaphragmatic paralysis and cardiovascular instability.

Management of tetanus includes wound debridement to reduce the bacterial and toxin load, treatment with metronidazole to eradicate the tetanus bacterium and supportive care. Free circulating toxin should be neutralised with human tetanus immunoglobulin (HTIG). Infection with tetanus does not result in immunity, so the patient will require vaccination after recovery.

Muscle spasms and rigidity are treated by sedation. Dantrolene and intrathecal baclofen have also been used. Refractory muscle spasms require the use of neuromuscular blocking agents. Autonomic instability is also improved by sedation and opiate analgesia. Magnesium is increasingly being used as it blocks catecholamine release from nerves and the adrenal medulla, reduces receptor responsiveness to released catecholamines and is an antispasmodic.

Taylor AM. Tetanus. *Contin Educ Anaesth Crit Care Pain* 2006; 6: 101–4.

Question B68: Treatment of acute liver failure

Patients with severe acute liver failure (ALF) should receive:

A. *N*-acetyl-cysteine (NAC) regardless of paracetamol level
B. Hypertonic saline for cerebral oedema
C. Correction of coagulopathy with fresh frozen plasma (FFP) if INR > 4.0
D. Ornithine aspartate to reduce ammonia levels
E. Prophylactic parenteral antibiotics

Answer: TTFFF

Short explanation

NAC has been shown to be of benefit in ALF of all aetiologies, not just in paracetamol overdose. Cerebral oedema should be prevented and treated with mannitol or hypertonic saline. FFP improves coagulopathy transiently and should be used only in active bleeding or prior to invasive procedures. Ornithine aspartate has no benefit in ALF. Prophylactic antibiotics have not been shown to be of benefit, but any infection in ALF should be treated aggressively.

Long explanation

Acute liver failure (ALF) is rare (1–6 cases per million population per year) but has high morbidity and mortality. The commonest cause worldwide is viral infection; in the developed world it is paracetamol (acetaminophen). The most effective treatment is hepatic transplantation, but with donor numbers falling, supportive and medical management is increasingly important.

N-acetyl-cysteine (NAC) has been used in paracetamol-induced ALF for many years with good evidence of benefit. More recently, however, it has emerged that NAC is of benefit in ALF of all causes, possibly by improving circulatory dysfunction and oxygen delivery.

Cerebral oedema in ALF is common but poorly understood. It is thought to be related to inflammation, increased ammonia levels, hypo-osmolality and impaired cerebral autoregulation. Ornithine aspartate has been shown to reduce ammonia levels in chronic liver failure but has not been found to be effective in ALF and is not available in the UK. The use of hypertonic saline or mannitol has been found to reduce intracranial hypertension in ALF.

Coagulopathy and thrombocytopenia are common in ALF, but should only be corrected in cases of active bleeding or prior to invasive procedures. The routine use of fresh frozen plasma (FFP) to correct raised INR is short-lived, carries a risk associated with transfusion, and has not been shown to improve outcomes.

The routine use of prophylactic parenteral antibiotics in ALF has been shown to reduce the incidence of infection, but has not been found to improve outcomes. Concerns about side effects and increasing bacterial resistance to antibiotics mean that routine antibiotic prophylaxis is not recommended. However, prevention strategies (e.g. ventilator care bundles, hand washing), constant vigilance for signs of infection, and prompt, appropriate instigation of antimicrobial therapy are the keys to reducing significant infective complications.

Bernal W, Auzinger G, Dhawan A, Wendon J. Acute liver failure. *Lancet*, 2010; 376: 190–201.

Trotter JF. Practical management of acute liver failure in the intensive care unit. *Curr Opin Crit Care* 2009; 15: 163–7.

Question B69: Donation after circulatory death

Concerning donation after circulatory death (DCD):

A. DCD should not be considered if life-sustaining care is to be withdrawn
B. DCD does not apply to patients diagnosed as brainstem dead
C. DCD can be considered and organised after the death of a patient
D. The time between withdrawal and death can determine which organs are retrieved
E. DCD is only possible for liver, kidneys and pancreas

Answer: FFTTF

Short explanation

DCD should be considered in all patients who are expected to die in ICU; it can occur in brainstem-dead patients who die before a planned donation after brain death (DBD). Uncontrolled DCD is organ retrieval that has been organised after the death of a patient. If patients survive for a long time following withdrawal, warm ischaemic time may be too long for viable organs. DCD applies to liver, kidneys, lungs, pancreas and corneas.

Long explanation

Demand for transplanted organs continues to outstrip supply from donation after brain death (DBD). Improvements in transplantation medicine and the increasing age of the population have led to increased demand for organs. At the same time, improvements in road safety and treatment of intracerebral haemorrhage and traumatic brain injury have reduced the number of organs available for transplant from DBD. Donation from living donors has increased in an attempt to fill this gap, but has obvious limitations in the organs available for transplant. As a result of these pressures, donation after circulatory death (DCD) is becoming increasingly common.

DCD should be considered for all patients who have no hope of recovery, for whom withdrawal of life-sustaining therapy is under consideration, but who do not meet the criteria for DBD. The decision to withdraw life-sustaining treatment must be entirely divorced from the consideration of DCD. If familial assent is obtained, then the withdrawal of treatment should occur at a time when the organ-retrieval team is available. After confirmation of death, family members are usually allowed a short time (a few minutes) with the deceased patient before the deceased is transferred to theatre for organ retrieval. This process is a type of controlled DCD, along with organ retrieval following cardiac arrest in a patient awaiting DBD.

Uncontrolled DCD is a term describing organ retrieval organised after the death of a patient, following unsuccessful resuscitation in the community or in hospital.

Uncontrolled DCD is rare, as organ-retrieval teams need to mobilised within the warm-ischaemic time (WIT) of the organs to be retrieved. WIT is the period of time for which organs are at body temperature with inadequate oxygen delivery, defined as systolic BP < 50 mmHg, SpO_2 < 70%, or both. WITs are organ-specific, as follows:

- liver: 30 minutes
- pancreas: 30 minutes
- lung: 60 minutes
- kidneys: 2 hours

Manara AR, Murphy PG, O'Callaghan G. Donation after circulatory death. *Br J Anaesth* 2012; 108 (Suppl): i108–21.

Question B70: Acute spinal cord injury

In the management of a patient with acute spinal cord injury, which of the following are correct?

A. Pharmacological thromboprophylaxis should be commenced as early as possible following the injury
B. Intravenous methylprednisolone should be commenced as soon as possible
C. Stabilisation of unstable vertebral injuries should be performed within 24 hours
D. Patients with unstable vertebral injuries and spinal cord damage should be immobilised on a hard spinal board until definitive surgery
E. Rapid sequence induction and intubation is commonly indicated for patients with high cervical spine injuries within the first 72 hours

Answer: TFTFT

Short explanation

There has been a lot of controversy regarding the use of steroids in spinal cord injuries, and current UK guidelines from the British Association of Spinal Cord Injury Specialists do not recommend them, because of concerns about rates of sepsis and mortality. Spinal boards are for safe transport of patients only and should be removed as soon as the patient is in hospital.

Long explanation

Spinal cord injuries account for significant morbidity and mortality throughout the world. Those affected are commonly of working age, and young men are at highest risk. Road traffic accidents are the commonest cause in the UK, but other causes include sporting injuries and penetrating trauma from gunshot or stab injuries.

As with the management of all major trauma patients, a dedicated team should follow a protocolised initial assessment routine to identify and treat life-threatening injuries in the first instance. Spinal immobilisation should be maintained during transfer and assessment in all patients with suspected or potential spinal injuries. A hard collar, blocks, tape and log rolling should be part of this process. Hard spinal boards should be removed as soon as possible after arrival in hospital, as they are only suitable for transport. There is a very high risk of significant pressure injuries occurring even in a short time if the board is not removed.

Whole-spine CT should be performed at the earliest opportunity, ideally as part of the initial trauma imaging in a major trauma centre. A spinal surgeon should be consulted early, and unstable injuries should be reduced and stabilised within the first 24 hours once the patient is stable. Intravenous methylprednisolone has been shown to improve neurological outcome in patients with spinal cord injury but at increased risk of sepsis and mortality. This has meant that administration is not recommended as routine in UK hospitals.

Particular attention should be paid to maintaining haemodynamic stability in the first few days following injury. Some would advocate maintaining a mean arterial pressure of at least 85 mmHg to optimise blood flow to the spinal cord, which can become ischaemic due to oedema and disrupted blood flow, thereby worsening the primary injury. This is referred to as secondary injury. Patients with cervical cord injuries often require ventilation, particularly if the injury is above C5, as the innervation of the diaphragm becomes affected. Suxamethonium is safe to use in the first 48 hours, and rapid sequence induction is recommended because of reduced gastric emptying.

Patients with spinal injuries are at a high risk of venous thromboembolism, which accounts for a significant number of early deaths. After discussion with surgeons and consideration of other injuries, pharmacological thromboprophylaxis with low-molecular-weight heparin should begin, ideally within 72 hours. Mechanical thromboprophylaxis with foot pumps should also be undertaken.

Bonner S, Smith C. Initial management of acute spinal cord injury. *Contin Educ Anaesth Crit Care Pain* 2013; 13: 224–31.

Question B71: Thyroid storm

Which of the following apply to thyroid storm?

A. The commonest precipitant is infection
B. Iodine should be administered before antithyroid treatment is given
C. Administration of steroids is recommended
D. Thyroid surgery is a common cause of thyroid storm
E. Atrial fibrillation is the commonest arrhythmia seen

Answer: TFTFT

Short explanation

Antithyroid treatment such as propylthiouracil should be commenced at least 1 hour before the administration of iodine, to prevent stimulation of the thyroid gland and worsening of the clinical picture. Thyroid surgery is a rare cause of thyroid storm nowadays, because treatment is administered preoperatively to control hyperthyroidism. Most surgery is undertaken on patients who are relatively euthyroid, although there is still a risk.

Long explanation

Thyroid storm is an uncommon complication of hyperthyroidism. It is seen in around 1% of all patients with hyperthyroidism and tends to affect females over the age of 60. It is a life-threatening medical emergency, particularly as delayed diagnosis is common. Mortality may be as high as 30% if it is left untreated or if treatment is delayed. The correct management usually results in a favourable outcome.

There is a spectrum of disease ranging from hyperthyroidism to severe thyrotoxicosis to thyroid storm, and the delineation may not always be completely clear. A scoring system devised by Burch and Wartofsky can help assess the degree of dysfunction in a number of organ systems. It would be safe to assume that any patient with symptoms of severe thyrotoxicosis has impending thyroid storm, and to treat accordingly.

Patients with true thyroid storm are very unwell. They may have cardiac failure, life-threatening arrhythmias, seizures and extremely high temperatures. Blood tests will reveal high levels of free T_3 and T_4, with low levels of TSH. These patients should be treated with a multidrug approach, with a number of aims: to prevent synthesis of new hormone, to halt release of stored hormone from the gland, to prevent conversion of T_4 to T_3 in the periphery, to control adrenergic symptoms, and to control systemic decompensation with supportive therapy. A specialist endocrinologist should be consulted as soon as possible.

The order of administration of drugs is important. Firstly, antithyroid medication such as propylthiouracil should be given, followed by iodine therapy. The time lapse between these drugs should be at least 60 minutes. The antithyroid medication stops production of further hormone and the iodine prevents release of stored hormone. β-Blockers, usually propranolol, reduce the cardiovascular effects of T_4 and should be administered unless there are contraindications. Intravenous therapy should be carefully monitored. Steroids such as dexamethasone or hydrocortisone block peripheral conversion of T_4 to T_3 and should also be given. Supportive care in a critical care department will almost certainly be required in addition to treatment of the underlying cause or precipitant. Once the hyperthyroidism is controlled, more definitive treatment, such as thyroid surgery, can be considered and planned for.

Nayak B, Burman K. Thyrotoxicosis and thyroid storm. *Endocrinol Metab Clin N Am* 2006; 35: 663–86.

Ngo S, Chew H. When the storm passes unnoticed: a case series of thyroid storm. *Resuscitation* 2007; 73, 485–90.

Question B72: SIRS

Features of systemic inflammatory response syndrome (SIRS) include:

A. Heart rate > 100 bpm
B. Respiratory rate > 20/minute
C. Temperature < 35 °C or > 38 °C
D. > 10% immature neutrophils
E. $PaCO_2$ < 32 mmHg (4.3 kPa)

Answer: FTFTT

Short explanation

A diagnosis of SIRS requires two out of four specified clinical findings related to temperature, heart rate, respiratory rate or $PaCO_2$, and white cell count. For heart rate, the criterion is > 90 bpm. For temperature, it is < 36 °C or > 38 °C.

Long explanation

The systemic inflammatory response syndrome (SIRS) was first described in 1983, with the consensus statement of definition and diagnositic criteria published in 1992. SIRS describes an inflammatory process common to both infectious and non-infectious systemic pathologies that can lead to organ dysfunction. Causes of SIRS include systemic infection, burns, ischaemia, trauma, haemorrhagic shock, pancreatitis and autoimmune conditions.

A diagnosis of SIRS requires two of the following four clinical findings:

- temperature < 36 °C or > 38 °C
- heart rate > 90 bpm
- respiratory rate > 20/minute or $PaCO_2$ < 32 mmHg (4.3 kPa)
- white cell count < 4 × 10^9/l or > 12 × 10^9/l, or > 10% immature neutrophils ('bands') on blood film

In children, the diagnostic criteria are modified as follows:

- temperature < 36 °C or > 38.5 °C. This must be present for a diagnosis of SIRS
- heart rate > 2 standard deviations above normal for age (or less than 10th percentile for age in infants)
- respiratory rate > 2 standard deviations above normal for age
- white cell count elevated or depressed, or > 10% immature neutrophils

In combination with the detection of an infective process, a diagnosis of sepsis – an inflammatory process in response to infection – can be made. Severe SIRS is defined as SIRS without evidence of infection, but with evidence of acute organ dysfunction.

American College of Chest Physicians/Society of Critical Care Medicine Consensus Conference: definitions for sepsis and organ failure and guidelines for the use of innovative therapies in sepsis. *Crit Care Med* 1992; 20: 864–74.

Question B73: Management of raised intracranial pressure

Which of the following are methods used to reduce raised intracranial pressure (ICP)?

A. Hypertonic saline
B. Suxamethonium
C. Hypothermia
D. Vecuronium
E. Hypoventilation

Answer: TFTTF

Short explanation

Suxamethonium is used for rapid sequence induction, and its effects on ICP are disputed. There may be a momentary increase in ICP following administration. It is not routinely administered to reduce ICP. Hypoventilation would result in hypercapnia, which increases ICP.

Long explanation

The management of raised intracranial pressure (ICP) is one of the key skills required in neurointensive care. Patients with traumatic brain injury are the commonest group for whom raised ICP is a problem. ICP monitoring is commonly undertaken in these patients to guide treatment. The absolute values for an acceptable ICP are disputed, but some evidence suggests that ICP > 25 mmHg predicts a poorer outcome. A reduction in ICP, which can be achieved by a number of measures, has the aim of increasing cerebral perfusion pressure and therefore cerebral oxygen delivery.

Medical management includes a number of measures. Ventilatory control of $PaCO_2$ is crucial, as cerebral blood flow is directly linked to $PaCO_2$. A high $PaCO_2$ results in increased cerebral blood flow and hence blood volume, increasing ICP. Hyperventilation to reduce the $PaCO_2$ to normal limits will result in cerebral vasoconstriction and reduced total cerebral blood volume. It is important not to over-ventilate to a low $PaCO_2$, because cerebral blood flow may be reduced to such an extent that regional ischaemia occurs. This is particularly important in areas of damaged brain, where normal autoregulatory mechanisms are interrupted. Hyperventilation to a low $PaCO_2$ can lead to secondary brain injuries and should be avoided.

Hyperosmolar therapy aims to draw water out of the brain cells, resulting in reduced brain volume and reduced ICP. Mannitol was previously the most commonly used osmotic agent, with added activity as an osmotic diuretic. This helps treat cerebral oedema, but causes a number of side effects including intravascular hypovolaemia and hypotension if repeated doses are given. It is also thought that mannitol may cross a damaged blood–brain barrier, drawing water into the brain and worsening cerebral oedema. More recently hypertonic saline has become popular. It has similar effects to mannitol in that it results in diffusion of water out of the brain and reduction in brain tissue volume but without the side effects seen with mannitol. Its use may be combined with loop diuretics (e.g. furosemide) to prevent volume overload.

Raised central venous pressure such as during straining or coughing can also cause acute rises in ICP, and patients should therefore be adequately sedated and paralysed as necessary. Hyperthermia is known to be harmful to the brain, but the effects of hypothermia in traumatic brain injuries are not entirely known. In patients with acute rises in ICP a period of hypothermia can be induced to help reduce the ICP. Simple measures such as nursing the patient with the bed head at 45 degrees upwards and avoiding tight endotracheal ties can also make a difference to the ICP by reducing the venous pressure.

Helmy A, Vizcaychipi M, Gupta A. Traumatic brain injury: intensive care management. *Br J Anaesth* 2007; 99: 32–42.

Question B74: Metabolic acidosis

Causes of a high anion gap acidosis include:

A. Short gut syndrome
B. Chronic paracetamol (acetaminophen) ingestion
C. Resuscitation with 0.9% sodium chloride
D. Urine reabsorption from ileal conduit
E. Acetazolamide

Answer: TTFFF

Short explanation

Urine reabsorption from an ileal conduit, acetazolamide and 0.9% sodium chloride cause a normal anion gap or hyperchloraemic metabolic acidosis.

Long explanation

A metabolic acidosis is defined as a serum pH < 7.35 due to excess hydrogen ions or bicarbonate loss. The anion gap is the difference between the measured cation and anion concentrations in the plasma. The sum of the sodium and potassium concentrations exceeds that of chloride and bicarbonate by 4–11 mmol/l, depending on the laboratory assays used. The difference is due to anionic proteins, phosphate and sulphate ions.

$$\text{Anion gap} = [\text{NA}^+ + \text{K}^+] - [\text{Cl}^- + \text{HCO}_3^-]$$

Causes of a high anion gap acidosis include lactic acidosis, ketoacidosis, acute or chronic kidney disease, alcohol poisoning, salicylate poisoning and staggered paracetamol overdose. This is seen with chronic ingestion of a normal dose in thin malnourished patients and is thought to be due to glutathione deficiency. The accumulating acid is pyroglutamic acid. D-lactic acidosis is caused by bacterial fermentation of carbohydrates in the gut with excessive absorption of D-lactic acid from the gut lumen. It is usually seen in patients with jejunoileal bypasses or short bowel syndrome.

Normal anion gap metabolic acidosis is seen with loss of bicarbonate or gain of chloride and therefore is synonymous with the term 'hyperchloraemic acidosis'. Causes of a normal anion gap metabolic acidosis are diarrhoea, proximal (type 2) renal tubular acidosis and ileal conduits. Excessive administration of chloride-containing fluids may also lead to a normal anion gap acidosis. A hyperchloraemic metabolic acidosis is encountered in patients with ileal or colonic urinary reconstruction (following cystectomy), as sodium is exchanged for hydrogen and bicarbonate for chloride in the bowel wall. Ammonia, ammonium, hydrogen ions and chloride may be reabsorbed as well.

Acetazolamide is a reversible, non-competitive carbonic anhydrase inhibitor in the proximal convoluted tubule. Carbonic anhydrase catalyses the conversion of bicarbonate and hydrogen ions into carbonic acid then carbon dioxide and water. When the availability of hydrogen ions in the distal tubule (where they are usually exchanged for sodium ions) is decreased, there is a loss of sodium and bicarbonate ions with a resultant hyperchloraemic metabolic acidosis.

The picture may be mixed, e.g. severe diarrhoea with hypovolaemia and resultant lactic acidosis.

Emmett M. Approach to the adult with metabolic acidosis. *UpToDate* 2013. http://www.uptodate.com (accessed June 2014).

Power I, Kam P. Acid–base physiology. In *Priniciples of Physiology for the Anaesthetist*, 2nd edn. London: Hodder Arnold; pp. 251–68.

Question B75: Drowning

With regards to the presentation and management of patients with a history of submersion in water or drowning, which of the following are correct?

A. Pulmonary complications are unlikely if the PaO_2 is normal 1 hour after the episode
B. 'Secondary drowning' occurs with aspiration of salt water into the alveoli, but not with fresh water
C. Cervical spine immobilisation should be considered in all patients
D. Exogenous surfactant can improve outcome in patients with progressive respiratory distress
E. Immersion in cold water results in hyperventilation and reduced breath-hold time

Answer: FFTFT

Short explanation

Pulmonary complications such as pulmonary oedema can occur up to 12 hours after submersion in water. Patients should be observed for at least 6 hours. Extravasation of fluid into the alveoli, also known as 'secondary drowning', occurs with both salt and fresh water. There is no good evidence base to support exogenous surfactant administration to these patients.

Long explanation

Drowning is a major cause of death worldwide, particularly among children. The incidence is much higher in the developing world than in developed nations. Drowning is defined by the WHO as 'the process of experiencing respiratory impairment from submersion/immersion in liquid'. This definition encompasses immediate death and late death from respiratory complications, previously known as 'near-drowning'. This term should now be avoided; the terms 'non-fatal drowning' and 'fatal drowning' should be used, depending on outcome.

There are a number of physiological changes that occur when a person is suddenly submerged in water, particularly if it is cold. Respiratory drive is increased in water

< 25 °C. Initial gasping is followed by uncontrollable hyperventilation and a reduced breath-hold time. This means that many people, even if they are good swimmers, will be unable to swim to safety in open water. If the water is choppy, then significant aspiration of water can occur. The intense peripheral vasoconstriction due to the sudden drop in temperature can put significant strain on the heart. In patients with cardiovascular comorbidities this can be quite significant and lead to cardiac arrest.

Aspiration of water into the alveoli causes a disruption to normal surfactant function. The presence of salt water in the alveoli leads to fluid accumulation in the alveoli due to altered osmotic gradients. The opposite is true of fresh water. This movement of water disrupts the delicate alveolar membrane and leads to increased permeability, allowing protein and fluid to accumulate in the alveoli. Some alveoli will collapse due to altered osmotic gradients. This can occur over a number of hours and leads to significant hypoxaemia due to pulmonary shunting. A normal chest x-ray and normal oxygen saturations at first presentation may not exclude later deterioration, as fulminant pulmonary oedema has been seen up to 12 hours following injury. Loss of surfactant will also reduce normal lung compliance, leading to difficulty with mechanical ventilation and increased work of breathing in self-ventilating patients.

Artificial surfactant, inhaled nitric oxide and liquid ventilation with perfluorocarbons have been studied in these patients, but there is little or no evidence to support their routine use in victims of drowning. It is important to take note of the history of the drowning incident, as the vast majority will be trauma-related and therefore normal trauma assessment protocols should be applied. This is particularly important when considering the cervical spine and the possibility of internal injuries. Cervical spine immobilisation should be instigated if there is any doubt.

Golden F, Tipton M, Scott R. Immersion, near-drowning and drowning. *Br J Anaesth* 1997; 79: 214–25.

Szpilman D, Bierens J, Handley A, Orlowski J. Drowning. *N Engl J Med* 2012; 366: 2102–10.

Question B76: Intercostal chest drains

Regarding intercostal chest drains (ICDs):

A. Wide-bore ICDs are more likely to cause pleural infection than Seldinger ICDs
B. Trocars should only be used under direct vision, to prevent complications
C. Seldinger ICDs should not be used in acute haemothorax
D. Chest-drain tubing should be clamped prior to transfer
E. ICDs should be secured with 'purse-string' sutures, gauze and tape

Answer: FFTFF

Short explanation

Infection rates are similar with all types of ICD. Trocars should never be used; blunt dissection is the recommended technique for wide-bore ICD insertion. Wide-bore ICDs are recommended in acute haemothorax, to allow monitoring of blood loss. Bubbling chest drains should never be clamped. Otherwise, drains may be clamped under the supervision of a respiratory physician or thoracic surgeon. 'Purse-string' sutures are painful and leave disfiguring scars. Dressings should be transparent.

Long explanation

Intercostal chest drains are used in the treatment of pneumothorax, haemothorax, pleural effusions and following intrathoracic or upper gastrointestinal surgery. They should be sited in the 'triangle of safety' above the level of the nipple and below the axilla, between the lateral border of pectoralis major and the anterior border of latissimus dorsi.

Large-bore ICDs are inserted by blunt dissection through an initial lateral skin incision at the upper border of the rib. They are packaged with a trocar, but this should not be used under any circumstances because of the risk of catastrophic damage to intrathoracic structures. Small-bore drains are inserted using the Seldinger technique and are preferred in most cases as they are more comfortable for patients.

There is no evidence that either type of ICD is clinically superior, although air leaks around very small (9F) drains may lead to inadequate treatment of pneumothorax. Even thick fluid associated with empyema or malignant effusions may be adequately drained by small-bore drains. Acute haemothoraces should be treated using large-bore drains, however, to allow regular monitoring of ongoing haemorrhage.

A bubbling chest drain should never be clamped, but post-pneumonectomy patients or cases of large pleural effusions may need intermittent clamping to prevent mediastinal shifts and re-expansion pulmonary oedema, respectively. ICD clamping should be done under the supervision of a respiratory physician or thoracic surgeon, and in a specialist area. Patients with clamped drains should be closely monitored, and the drain should be unclamped if they show signs of deterioration.

ICDs should be carefully secured to the patient using sutures and tape. Linear sutures using a thick, strong material such as 1 silk are recommended. 'Purse-string' sutures create circular holes which are painful, slow to heal and leave disfiguring scars. They are therefore not recommended.

Laws D, Neville E, Duffy J. BTS guidelines for the insertion of a chest drain. *Thorax* 2003; 58 (Suppl 2): ii53–9.

Question B77: Lithium toxicity

With regards to the management of patients with lithium toxicity, which of the following are correct?

A. The presence of a goitre suggests acute intoxication
B. Oral bioavailability of lithium is poor
C. ACE inhibitors promote the excretion of lithium from the kidneys
D. A plasma lithium concentration above 3.5 mEq/l is classed as severe toxicity
E. Lithium is the most dialysable common toxin known

Answer: FFFTT

Short explanation

The presence of a goitre in a euthyroid patient is evidence of chronic lithium toxicity. Acute overdose will not cause this. Lithium is almost 100% absorbed via the gastrointestinal tract. ACE inhibitors and other diuretics increase the reabsorption of lithium in the proximal tubule and reduce excretion, which can lead to toxicity.

Long explanation

Lithium therapy is central to the management of a variety of psychiatric conditions. In particular it is administered for the treatment of bipolar disorder, mania and depression. Long-term lithium therapy can lead to chronic accumulation of the drug and a number of side effects. These include goitre, leukocytosis and nephrogenic diabetes insipidus. Increased thirst usually prevents electrolyte abnormalities in the last of these.

Acute intoxication can lead to serious or even fatal consequences. Lithium has a narrow therapeutic index above which toxicity is commonly seen. The recommended therapeutic plasma levels are between 0.6 and 1.5 mEq/l, depending upon the condition being treated. It is also thought that plasma levels below 0.6 mEq/l may still be effective. Blood levels should be taken 12 hours after dose administration. Gastrointestinal absorption is rapid and complete after oral administration. Lithium is distributed throughout body water, and toxicity will be more likely in circumstances where total body water levels are reduced. Such conditions include renal impairment, dehydration, drug administration (such as ACE inhibitors or NSAIDs) and in the elderly.

As plasma lithium levels rise above 1.5 mEq/l up to 3.5 mEq/l the mild symptoms of lithium toxicity become more severe. Symptoms include neuromuscular irritation, coarse tremors, muscle weakness, ataxia, delirium, sinus bradycardia and hypotension. Seizures and coma occur late and can lead to death or permanent neurological sequelae such as dementia.

Treatment of lithium toxicity involves repletion of effective circulating volume and supportive treatment. Activated charcoal does not inhibit absorption of charged particles such as lithium and so is ineffective. Haemodialysis should be considered in patients with very high plasma levels (> 4 mEq/l, regardless of symptoms), or in patients with renal impairment and levels above 2.5 mEq/l, There are some concerns about a rebound increase in plasma levels of lithium after cessation of haemodialysis as cellular levels of lithium equilibrate. Some people advocate at least 8–12 hours of dialysis and to repeat if levels rise above 1 mEq/l.

Waring WS. Management of lithium toxicity. *Toxicol Rev* 2006; 25: 221–30.

Question B78: Hyperbaric oxygen therapy

Which of the following statements correctly describe the uses of hyperbaric oxygen therapy?

A. It can be useful in the management of patients with ARDS following chest trauma
B. It is usually administered at 8–10 times atmospheric pressure at sea level
C. Charles's law governs the increase in oxygen partial pressure of the blood
D. Necrotising fasciitis is an indication for the use of hyperbaric oxygen therapy
E. Seizures are common and often prolonged and may lead to permanent neurological disability

Answer: TFFTF

Short explanation

Hyperbaric oxygen therapy is usually administered at 2–3 times the atmospheric pressure at sea level. Boyle's law governs the reduction in volume of gas in a space due to the increased pressure exerted on it. This reduces the bubble size of dissolved oxygen in the blood and increases the dissolved amount of oxygen. Seizures are rare and usually self-limiting. Permanent neurological sequelae are also very rare.

Long explanation

Hyperbaric oxygen therapy is not widely available in the UK, and only a few centres have the facility. 100% oxygen is delivered at a pressure of 2–3 atmospheres at sea level. This leads to a large increase in the dissolved oxygen content of the blood and raises the arterial oxygen tension to more than 2000 mmHg. The dissolved oxygen content can be as high as 6 ml per dl, meaning that dissolved oxygen content alone will meet tissue requirements without any need for oxygen bound to haemoglobin.

It is used in a number of conditions. Decompression sickness following deep sea diving causes excess nitrogen bubbles forming in the tissues and organs. These bubbles cause pain, systemic upset and neurological dysfunction. Carbon monoxide poisoning can be fatal, as carbon monoxide binds avidly to haemoglobin and prevents oxygen delivery to tissues. Hyperbaric oxygen therapy greatly increases the oxygen content of the blood and restores tissue oxygenation. In addition, the dissociation of carbon monoxide from haemoglobin greatly increased in hyperbaric oxygen. The half-life of carboxyhaemoglobin is reduced from 4–5 hours to 20 minutes in oxygen at 2.5 atmospheres.

Tissue hypoxia leads to poor wound healing, and hyperbaric oxygen may therefore be used to help treat difficult wounds. It is also used for the treatment of infections by anaerobic organisms such as clostridia, which are killed by oxygen. Other uses include the treatment of arterial gas embolism, refractory osteomyelitis, compromised skin grafts and flaps, anaemia due to exceptional blood loss (for example in Jehovah's witnesses), thermal burns and radiation-induced tissue injury.

Hyperbaric oxygen is usually administered via endotracheal tube or tight-fitting mask, and sessions last from 90 minutes to 5 hours for some types of decompressive illnesses. The most common side effect is reversible myopia due to the effects of oxygen on the lens. Mild to moderate pain from rupture of the middle ear or the cranial fossae is rare. Seizures are rare and usually self-limiting. Reversible tracheal burning, sternal discomfort and cough can occur after repeated exposures. A patient who has been receiving high concentrations of normobaric oxygen and then has hyperbaric therapy is more prone to toxic pulmonary effects.

Tibbles PM, Edelsberg JS. Hyperbaric-oxygen therapy. *N Engl J Med* 1996; 334: 1642–8.

Question B79: Notifiable diseases

Regarding notifiable diseases in the UK, which of the following are correct?

A. Responsibility for notification lies with the patient's general practitioner
B. Acute infective hepatitis of any cause is a notifiable disease
C. Notification of certain infectious diseases first came into practice in the 1800s
D. Acute meningitis of any cause is a notifiable disease
E. Microbiological confirmation via microscopy or culture is required for official notification

Answer: FTTTF

Short explanation

Responsibility for notification lies with the attending registered medical practitioner responsible for the patient's care at the time of diagnosis. This may be a primary or secondary care clinician. Notification should be completed on diagnosis of the suspected disease and not delayed until laboratory confirmation is available.

Long explanation

At the end of the nineteenth century legislation came into force to ensure notification of diseases such as cholera, diphtheria and smallpox. Initially, responsibility lay with the head of the family or landlord to report the disease to the local 'proper office'. The aim of the notifications system is to identify and prevent outbreaks and epidemics.

Notification only requires clinical suspicion of a disease, and diagnostic accuracy can be reviewed at a later date. Doctors in England and Wales have a statutory duty to report certain diseases to the local Health Protection Unit. The certificate required for notification is available online at the Health Protection Agency (HPA) website.

The HPA collates data and produces statistics related to the incidence and prevalence of the diseases. The list of diseases now stretches to over 30. It includes a number of tropical diseases rarely seen in the UK other than in travellers and immigrants, as well as infectious diseases that are commonly seen on the intensive care unit. The list of notifiable diseases is as follows:

- Acute encephalitis
- Acute infectious hepatitis
- Acute meningitis
- Acute poliomyelitis
- Anthrax
- Botulism
- Brucellosis
- Cholera
- Diphtheria
- Enteric fever (typhoid/paratyphoid)
- Food poisoning
- Haemolytic uraemic syndrome (HUS)
- Infectious bloody diarrhoea
- Invasive group A streptococcal disease
- Legionnaires' disease
- Leprosy
- Malaria
- Measles
- Meningococcal septicaemia
- Mumps
- Plague
- Rabies
- Rubella
- SARS
- Scarlet fever
- Smallpox
- Tetanus
- Tuberculosis
- Typhus
- Viral haemorrhagic fever (VHF)
- Whooping cough
- Yellow fever

Other diseases that might present significant risk to human health may also be reported.

Public Health England. Notifications of infectious diseases (NOIDs). http://www.gov.uk/government/collections/notifications-of-infectious-diseases-noids (accessed October 2014).

Question B80: Obstetric haemorrhage

In a case of massive obstetric haemorrhage, which of the following are correct?

A. It can be defined as blood loss > 500 ml following caesarean section
B. The commonest cause of secondary post-partum haemorrhage is uterine atony
C. Administration of recombinant activated factor VII is contraindicated
D. Carboprost 250 μg boluses can be repeated up to a total of 2 mg

E. First-line medical management for post-partum haemorrhage is intramuscular ergometrine

Answer: FFFTF

Short explanation

Blood loss of 500 ml following vaginal delivery or 1000 ml following caesarean section can be considered as normal. Massive obstetric haemorrhage is sometimes defined as blood loss > 1500 ml. The commonest cause of primary post-partum haemorrhage is uterine atony. Secondary post-partum haemorrhage occurs 24 hours to 6 weeks after delivery. First-line medical management is intravenous oxytocin (syntocinon). Refractory haemorrhage has been treated with recombinant activated factor VII, although this is an unlicensed use for this product.

Long explanation

Massive obstetric haemorrhage remains a significant cause of maternal morbidity and mortality, although management has improved over the past few decades. Obstetric haemorrhage can be antepartum (defined as bleeding after 24 weeks gestation) or post-partum haemorrhage (PPH). Primary PPH occurs within 24 hours of delivery. Secondary PPH occurs from 24 hours to 6 weeks following delivery. Massive obstetric haemorrhage can be defined as > 1500 ml blood loss, a decrease in haemoglobin of > 4 g/dl, or acute transfusion requirement > 4 units.

Causes of massive antepartum haemorrhage include placental abruption, placenta praevia and uterine rupture. Massive primary PPH is caused by uterine atony, genital tract trauma, retained products of conception, clotting defects or uterine inversion. Massive secondary PPH is usually caused by infection or retained products of conception. Massive haemorrhage can occur abruptly and quickly. The uterine blood supply is up to 12% of cardiac output at term (up to 900 ml/minute). The 40% increase in circulating blood volume seen in mothers at term protects against blood loss to a certain extent but also masks the signs of haemorrhage. Tachycardia may be the only sign until 30–40% of circulating volume is lost.

General resuscitation measures should be provided in addition to specific obstetric interventions designed to stop the bleeding. Drugs to increase uterine tone include syntocinon (oxytocin analogue), ergometrine and carboprost. Surgical interventions include manual uterine massage, manual removal of the placenta, uterine packing, uterine artery ligation and hysterectomy. Some centres have interventional radiological services where selective embolisation of pelvic vessels can be performed.

Most hospitals have a massive haemorrhage policy in place to facilitate the fast availability of blood products in an emergency. Early discussion with the laboratory staff is important, and involvement of haematologists should be considered early. Refractory haemorrhage has been treated with recombinant activated factor VII, although this is an unlicensed use for this product. Following cessation of haemorrhage, patients may require admission to the intensive care unit for ongoing fluid balance management, blood component replacement and monitoring.

Banks A, Norris A. Massive haemorrhage in pregnancy. *Contin Educ Anaesth Crit Care Pain* 2005; 5: 195–8.

Neligan P, Laffey J. Clinical review. Special populations: critical illness and pregnancy. *Crit Care* 2011; 15: 227.

Question B81: Percutaneous tracheostomy

Indications for percutaneous tracheostomy insertion include:

A. A contraindication to surgical tracheostomy placement
B. Insertion by day 4 in patients expected to be ventilated for more than 14 days
C. Irreversible brain injury
D. Failure of needle cricothyroidotomy
E. Excessive respiratory secretions

Answer: FFTTT

Short explanation

Percutaneous tracheostomy should not be performed if there is a contraindication to surgical tracheostomy placement. The TracMan study showed no improvement in mortality or other end-points from early tracheostomy placement.

Long explanation

Tracheostomy is a common procedure in intensive care. Once confined to patients with upper airway obstruction or malignancy, it now has numerous indications including prolonged mechanical ventilation, weaning from ventilation, failure of airway protective reflexes, secretion management and obstructive sleep apnoea. It may also be used as a rescue technique in a 'can't intubate can't ventilate' scenario where needle cricothyroidotomy placement has failed. Surgical tracheostomy in this scenario may be quicker, but familiarity with the technique may be an advantage to the percutaneous approach.

Tracheostomies on intensive care are commonly performed percutaneously, a procedure which has a similar rate of complications to surgical tracheostomy and reduces the need for the patient to be transferred to the operating theatre. If a surgical tracheostomy is contraindicated then a percutaneous procedure should not proceed. Relative contraindications for percutaneous tracheostomy include children < 12 years old, coagulopathy, active infection in anterior neck, local malignancy, unstable cervical spine fracture, morbid obesity, anatomical distortion, previous neck surgery, radiotherapy or tracheostomy, high ventilatory requirements, haemodynamic instability and raised intracranial pressure.

Timing of tracheostomy placement in critical care patients requiring prolonged ventilation has always been a subject of debate. The TracMan trial (Young *et al.* 2013) showed that tracheostomy within 4 days of critical care admission was not associated with an improvement in 30-day mortality, and furthermore the ability of clinicians to predict which patients required extended ventilatory support was limited.

Regan K, Hunt K. Tracheostomy management. *Contin Educ Anaesth Crit Care Pain* 2008; 8: 31–5.

Young D, Harrison DA, Cuthbertson BH. Effect of early vs late tracheostomy placement on survival in patients receiving mechanical ventilation: the TracMan randomized trial. *JAMA* 2013; 309: 2121–9.

Question B82: Parenteral nutrition

Parenteral nutrition:

A. Should be started as soon as enteral nutrition is deemed unsuitable
B. Should not overlap with enteral feeding
C. Should meet at least 66% of a patient's nutritional needs
D. Is a recognised cause of lipolysis
E. Should be adjusted to take account of propofol sedation

Answer: FFFFT

Short explanation

Current guidelines on when to start parenteral nutrition (PN) vary from 3 to 7 days. It is thought that later administration may be beneficial. Cessation of PN may overlap with enteral feeding. PN should meet 33–66% of a patient's requirements; exceeding this may lead to lipogenesis.

Long explanation

Parenteral nutrition (PN) is used when enteral nutrition is contraindicated. It is expensive, associated with hyperglycaemia and infection, and has no beneficial effects on gut integrity. Current guidelines vary in when they recommend starting PN; however, a recent study has shown better outcomes in patients commencing PN later (day 8).

Prescribing PN is a complex process requiring many assumptions, as calorimetric measurements on ICU are rarely practicable. The Schofield equation calculates basal metabolic rate based on age, sex and weight and uses adjustments for illness states. This gives an estimate of the kcal/kg/day requirement. Metabolic requirements are high in critically ill patients but they receive supplemental nutrients from catabolic tissue breakdown, so supplying full nutritional requirements as feed may lead to overfeeding. Generally outcomes are best in patients receiving 33–66% of their estimated nutritional needs. Calorie requirements are generally 20–35 kcal/kg/day (NICE and ESPEN).

The formulation of PN varies. In general, carbohydrate is supplied as glucose, which may cause hyperglycaemia and often requires insulin to stabilise blood sugars. Oversupply of glucose results in lipogenesis with an increase in carbon dioxide production and hence implications for respiratory function. Lipids in the form of fatty acids are essential but are associated with fatty liver, immune dysfunction and altered pulmonary function. Propofol sedation contributes a significant lipid load and should be taken into account. Protein is used to replace nitrogen losses and reduce muscle loss, and is supplied as amino acids. NICE guidelines suggest 0.13–0.24 g/kg/day of nitrogen, including all essential amino acids and glutamine, which is conditionally essential in critical illness. Trace elements (such as copper, zinc and selenium) need to be added, as do vitamins, especially thiamine and B-vitamins.

PN should be discontinued when the patient's nutritional needs are reliably met via the enteral route. Some degree of overlap with enteral feeding is common.

Monitoring of a patient on PN includes regular assessment of fluid status, electrolyte and liver function measurements daily, and regular triglyceride levels in longer-term PN.

Casaer MP, Mesotten D, Hermans G, *et al.* Early versus late parenteral nutrition in critically ill adults. *N Engl J Med* 2011; 365: 506–17.

Macdonald K, Page K, Brown L, Bryden D. Parenteral nutrition in critical care. *Contin Educ Anaesth Crit Care Pain* 2013; 13: 1–5.

National Institute for Health and Care Excellence. *CG32: Nutrition Support in Adults.* London: NICE, 2006. http://www.nice.org.uk/cg32 (accessed June 2014).

Question B83: Sengstaken–Blakemore tubes

Sengstaken–Blakemore tubes:

A. Have three lumens – gastric balloon, oesophageal balloon and oesophageal aspiration port
B. Control around 90% of cases of variceal bleeding
C. When correctly sited, should be attached to 5 kg of traction

D. Usually have the oesophageal balloon inflated before the gastric balloon
E. Should only be left in for 12 hours

Answer: FTFFF

Short explanation

Sengstaken–Blakemore tubes have three lumens – gastric balloon, oesophageal balloon and gastric aspiration port. Bleeding control occurs in around 90% of cases of variceal bleeding. Traction should not be applied, owing to the risk of necrosis of the gastro-oesophageal junction and nose. The gastric balloon is inflated first; the oesophageal balloon is rarely required. Balloons should be deflated after 12 hours (much sooner if the oesophageal balloon is inflated) but may stay in for 36–48 hours.

Long explanation

Sengstaken–Blakemore tubes are used in cases of bleeding oesophagogastric varices. Their use should be considered in cases where endoscopic therapy has failed to control bleeding, or in cases where endoscopic therapy is not available in a clinically appropriate timeframe. Bleeding is controlled in up to 90% of cases, at least for the duration of the insertion of the tube. Bleeding recurs in half of cases on deflation, and so definitive therapy is usually required (e.g. further endoscopy, transjugular intrahepatic portosystemic shunt (TIPS), partial gastrectomy).

Sengstaken–Blakemore tubes have three lumens – gastric balloon, oesophageal balloon and gastric aspiration port. They are usually inserted via the nose in the same manner as a nasogastric tube. Once past the gastro-oesophageal junction (> 55–60 cm), the gastric balloon should be partially inflated with air or water. A chest radiograph should be performed to check correct placement (water-soluble contrast may aid location). Once the location is confirmed, the balloon should be fully inflated (to 300 ml) and gentle traction applied to bring the balloon to the gastro-oesophageal junction. Taping the tube to the nose is generally sufficient traction. Weighted tubes increase the risk of necrosis of the gastro-oesophageal junction and nose.

The gastric lumen should be regularly aspirated or placed on continuous low-pressure suction. The balloon should be deflated every 12 hours, but may be reinflated if bleeding recurs. Sengstaken–Blakemore tubes should not stay in longer than 48 hours. The oesophageal balloon is rarely required. If used for cases of intractable bleeding, the balloon pressure should be kept below 40 mmHg and deflated every 1–4 hours to reduce the risk of oesophageal necrosis.

National Institute for Health and Care Excellence. *CG141: Acute Upper Gastrointestinal Bleeding: Management*. London: NICE, 2012. http://www.nice.org.uk/cg141 (accessed June 2014).

Question B84: Norepinephrine

Norepinephrine:

A. Is a weak base
B. Stimulates β-adrenergic receptors to cause coronary vasodilatation
C. Must not be infused into a peripheral vein
D. Should be used with caution in patients taking linezolid, amitriptyline or atenolol
E. Increases platelet aggregation and GI tract relaxation

Answer: TTFTT

Short explanation

Norepinephrine is an endogenous catecholamine. It is a potent agonist at α_1- and α_2-adrenergic receptors, causing peripheral vasoconstriction, gastrointestinal tract relaxation, bronchoconstriction and platelet aggregation. It has also has significant β_1 activity, causing inotropy and coronary vasodilatation. Peripheral infusion should be avoided if possible owing to the risks of extravasation. Linezolid, tricyclic antidepressants and β-blockers exaggerate hypertensive effects, and norepinephrine should be used with caution.

Long explanation

Norepinephrine is an endogenous catecholamine that is in widespread use in critical care. It is an important neurotransmitter both centrally (e.g. in the locus coeruleus) and peripherally (postganglionic sympathetic neurons). It is also released from the adrenal medulla as part of the stress response. Norepinephrine is a weak base with a pKa of 8.58.

Norepinephrine has activity at all classes of adrenergic receptor. It is a very potent α_1 agonist, causing arterial and venous vasoconstriction in all but coronary and cerebral vascular beds. Its α_2 activity causes inhibition of endogenous norepinephrine release, gastrointestinal relaxation and platelet aggregation. In addition, norepinephrine has significant β_1 activity, leading to increased myocardial contractility and coronary and peripheral vasodilatation.

Norepinephrine is usually diluted in 5% dextrose and administered as an infusion via a central venous catheter. Peripheral administration is sometimes necessary but should be avoided if possible owing to the risk of extravasation, which causes tissue necrosis.

Important drug interactions with norepinephrine include tricyclic antidepressants and monoamine oxidase (MAO) inhibitors, both of which block the metabolism of norepinephrine and increase its hypertensive effects. Linezolid is an antibiotic with MAO inhibitory properties, so should also prompt caution if co-administered with norepinephrine. The concomitant use of norepinephrine with β-blockers leads to an inhibition of the vasodilatory β_1 effects of norepinephrine and can lead to extreme hypertension and coronary vasoconstriction.

DrugBank. Norepinephrine. http://www.drugbank.ca/drugs/DB00368 (accessed June 2014).

Joint Formulary Committee. *British National Formulary*, 65th edition. London: British Medical Association and Royal Pharmaceutical Society of Great Britain, 2013.

Rang HP, Dale M, Henderson G, Ritter JM, Flower RJ. *Rang and Dale's Pharmacology*, 7th edn. Edinburgh: Elsevier Churchill Livingstone, 2012.

Question B85: Immunoglobulin therapy

With regards to the use of intravenous immunoglobulin use in critically ill adult patients, which of the following are correct?

A. The most widely practised use of immunoglobulin is for group B streptococcal toxic shock syndrome
B. The recommended dose for severe sepsis is 1 mg/kg/day for 2 days
C. The Surviving Sepsis Campaign guidelines recommend its use in patients with septic shock who fail to respond to initial resuscitation measures
D. Intravenous immunoglobulin is a pooled blood product from over 1000 donors
E. IgM-enriched immunoglobulin is not routinely used in clinical practice

Answer: FFFTT

Short explanation

The most widely practised use of immunoglobulin is for group A streptococcal toxic shock syndrome. The usual dose for an adult with severe sepsis would be 1 g/kg/day for 2 days. However, the most recent Surviving Sepsis Campaign guidelines do not support its use in patients with sepsis.

Long explanation

The search for an agent that significantly improves the outcome of the most severely ill patients on the critical care unit has centred on immunomodulatory agents, including recombinant activated protein C (APC) and intravenous immunoglobulin. Unfortunately none of these agents have proven to be 'wonder drugs', and their use is not recommended in routine clinical practice.

Studies looking at the benefits of intravenous immunoglobulin are relatively small and heterogeneous. This means that even meta-analyses are not sufficient to elucidate which patients will benefit most from this expensive treatment. The most widely accepted use for intravenous immunoglobulin is for patients with group A streptococcal toxic shock syndrome. The evidence for this use is of poor quality, although many still continue to administer intravenous immunoglobulin in this situation.

Immunoglobulin is a pooled blood product from over 1000 donors (and sometimes up to 10,000 donors). Most intravenous immunoglobulin is the IgG isomer. There is currently one company which produces IgM-enriched product, and there is some evidence to suggest that this is more effective. It is usually administered in a 5% solution at a dose of 1g per kg body weight per day. This results in a large volume of fluid, which can have implications in patients with pulmonary oedema. Other complications include anaphylaxis, thromboembolic events and renal dysfunction.

Dellinger RP, Levy MM, Rhodes A, *et al*. Surviving Sepsis Campaign. International guidelines for management of severe sepsis and septic shock: 2012. *Crit Care Med* 2013; 41: 580–637.

Shankar-Hari M, Spencer J, Sewell W, Rowan K, Singer M. Bench-to-bedside review: immunoglobulin therapy for sepsis – biological plausibility from a critical care perspective. *Crit Care* 2011; 16: 206.

Question B86: Management of multiple injuries

Regarding the early management of the multiply injured patient:

A. If a serious head injury is suspected the patient should be cooled to a temperature of < 35 °C
B. Diaphragmatic rupture in blunt trauma is typically on the right
C. Laboratory clotting studies are helpful in guiding blood product administration to the multiply injured patient with ongoing blood loss
D. Around 10% of patients with cervical spine injury have another non-contiguous vertebral fracture
E. Chest wall subcutaneous emphysema is a worrying sign in a patient with normal chest x-ray

Answer: FFFTT

Short explanation

Normothermia should be maintained if at all possible, given the deliterious effects of hypothermia on coagulation. There is no conclusive evidence of neuroprotection with cooling in the traumatically injured brain. Diaphragmatic rupture in blunt trauma is typically on the left, because the right side is 'protected' by the liver. Laboratory investigations of clotting are often too slow, and soon become obsolete when a shocked patient is actively bleeding.

Long explanation

Management of the multiply injured patient should always be coordinated by a well-trained trauma team. The recent introduction of regional trauma centres in the UK is an attempt to ensure that trauma patients receive the most appropriate care from the moment they reach the emergency department. The traditional ATLS-style assessment (primary and secondary survey) is a good starting point. This ensures that life-threatening injuries are identified and dealt with in a timely fashion. Ongoing volume resuscitation, respiratory support and cardiovascular support should be managed by critical care physicians with experience in the trauma setting.

Diaphragmatic rupture in blunt trauma is typically on the left, as the right side is 'protected' by the liver.

A particular area of interest is blood product administration. Military experience during recent conflicts has helped change hospital practice. Red cell transfusion, correction of coagulopathy and near-patient testing have all become central to the first few hours following the injuries. There is evidence to suggest that coagulopathy which is present at admission to intensive care indicates a worse 30-day mortality. It is important to avoid over-transfusion and to identify the difference between surgical bleeding and bleeding due to coagulopathy. Near-patient testing such as TEG (thromboelastography) or rotational thromboelastometry (ROTEM) should be available, because discrete laboratory values such as PT or APTT are a poor reflection of the haemostasis picture in vivo. Markedly deranged values indicate significant coagulopathy, but attempts to normalise the values may result in over-transfusion of coagulation products and volume overload.

Hypothermia should be avoided, particularly because of its effects on the coagulation system. In the hours and days following admission to critical care, attention should be paid to identifying and managing hyperglycaemia, adrenal insufficiency, transfusion-associated complications, abdominal compartment syndrome, rhabdomyolysis, hyperkalaemia, hypocalcaemia, acute lung injury and acute respiratory distress syndrome (ARDS). These are commonly seen in the multiply injured patient and can lead to serious consequences if left untreated.

Shere-Wolfe RF, Galvagno SM, Grissom TE. Critical care considerations in the management of the trauma patient following initial resuscitation. *Scand J Trauma Resusc Emerg Med* 2012; 20: 68.

Question B87: Renal transplant

In renal transplant patients:

A. ARDS frequently occurs early in the post-transplant period
B. The mortality rate on ICU is higher than in other patients
C. The incidence of critical care admission is higher than among liver transplant patients
D. The most common reason for ICU admission is the requirement for renal replacement therapy
E. Immunosuppression is a significant factor in the need for intensive care

Answer: FTFFT

Short explanation

ARDS is not common in renal transplant patients, although it does occur more often than in other patients. It usually occurs late in the post-transplant period due to immunosuppression or graft failure. Sepsis, in particular pulmonary infections, is the commonest reason for ICU admission. Liver transplant patients are much more likely to require critical care admission than renal transplant patients.

Long explanation

The number of patients receiving transplanted organs, particularly kidney and liver transplants, is increasing annually in the UK. This is partly due to the hugely successful recent initiative to encourage and increase organ donation rates. In addition, the long-term survival of these patients continues to increase. Immunosuppressive techniques are continually advancing, and post-transplant care is improving all the time.

Despite the success of the organ donation programmes, some of these patients will require critical care services at some time around their transplant. Liver transplant patients tend to require critical care during the perioperative period, particularly those with acute liver failure. Renal transplant patients, in contrast, do not routinely require formal critical care admission.

In the medium to long term following transplantation, patients may require critical care. Commonly this is due to infective causes. The lifelong significant immunosuppression predisposes these patients to serious and unusual infections. For this reason, it is important to involve the relevant specialists early in the admission. This would include the relevant transplant team and local microbiologists. Decisions that need to be carefully considered include choice of antibiotic, monitoring of immunosuppressive medication, and use of steroids.

Klouche K, Amigues L, Massanet P, *et al*. Outcome of renal transplant recipients admitted to an intensive care unit: a 10-year cohort study. *Transplantation* 2009; 87: 889–95.

Shorr A, Abbott, K, Agadoa L. Acute respiratory distress syndrome after kidney transplantation: Epidemiology, risk factors, and outcomes. *Crit Care Med* 2003; 31: 1325–30.

Question B88: Metabolic acidaemia

With regards to the management of patients with metabolic acidaemia, which of the following are correct?

A. Rapidity of correction of severe acidaemia on admission to ICU is inversely proportional to mortality
B. The administration of bicarbonate to patients with severe metabolic acidosis has been shown to improve prognosis
C. Bicarbonate administration can result in reduced ionised calcium levels and therefore arrhythmias
D. Bicarbonate administration to patients with chronic kidney disease is widely practised
E. It is recommended that bicarbonate be administered to patients with diabetic ketoacidosis if the pH is < 7.2

Answer: TFTTF

Short explanation

There are no large randomised controlled trials studying the effects of bicarbonate administration to patients with acidaemia. No mortality benefits have been demonstrated in the small prospective studies published. Some texts recommend bicarbonate be administered to patients with pH < 7.0. In the case of diabetic ketoacidosis, however, this is not usually necessary unless the patient has severe or chronic renal impairment, where excess bicarbonate losses occur.

Long explanation

The administration of intravenous bicarbonate to patients with metabolic acidosis has long been a controversial intervention among critical care and renal physicians. Patients who have chronic kidney disease in whom bicarbonate losses are excessive (e.g. renal tubular acidosis) routinely take oral bicarbonate supplements as part of their ongoing treatment. Improvement of the pH has been reported to improve cardiovascular stability when patients are haemodynamically compromised and requiring vasopressors. Unfortunately this has not been demonstrated by the limited studies available. In addition, no mortality benefit has been shown.

Some conditions, such as diabetic ketoacidosis, result in a reduction in the plasma bicarbonate levels as it is converted to another anionic base, such as acetoacetate and β-hydroxybutyrate. Once the underlying cause is treated, these anionic bases are converted back to bicarbonate, resulting in a normalising pH. The body has not in effect lost bicarbonate, so administration of exogenous bicarbonate is not the answer. Some conditions that result in loss of bicarbonate from the body, such as diarrhoea, may be more appropriately managed with exogenous bicarbonate administration. If bicarbonate is to be administered to patients with acidaemia, then some recommendations state that this should only occur when the plasma pH is < 7.0, and only enough to return the pH to 7.2 should be given.

Jung B, Rimmele T, Le Goff C, *et al*. Severe metabolic or mixed acidemia on intensive care unit admission: incidence, prognosis and administration of buffer therapy. a prospective, multiple-center study. *Crit Care* 2011; 15: R238.

Mathieu D, Neviere R, Billard V, Fleyfel M, Wattel F. Effects of bicarbonate therapy on hemodynamics and tissue oxygenation in patients with lactic acidosis: a prospective, controlled clinical study. *Crit Care Med* 1991; 19: 1352–6.

Sabatini S, Kurtzman N. Bicarbonate therapy in severe metabolic acidosis. *J Am Soc Nephrol* 2009; 20: 692–5.

Question B89: Snake bites

In the treatment of patients with bites from venomous snakes, which of the following are correct?

A. Children and adults are affected similarly by adder bites
B. A tourniquet should be applied to the affected limb to prevent systemic spread of venom
C. Secondary cellulitis develops quickly, and prophylactic antibiotics should be commenced early
D. Antivenom is widely available, and the standard dose is the same for all patients
E. Blood transfusion may be required, but heparin should be avoided

Answer: FFFTT

Short explanation

Children are more vulnerable to the toxic effects of adder bites, and mortality is higher. Application of tourniquets or bandages to the affected limb should be avoided, and the skin wound should not be interfered with if at all possible. The limb should be immobilised with bandages or splints. Secondary cellulitis does occur, but erythema around the wound is common and does not usually signify infection. Prophylactic antibiotics are not recommended.

Long explanation

In the UK the only indigenous venomous snake is the adder, *Vipera berus*. Hundreds of adults and children are bitten annually. Other venomous snake bites occur from snakes kept in zoos and as pets. The National Poisons Information Service can advise physicians on how best to identify and treat the bites. Mortality from adder bites is low, the last death in the UK occurring in 1976. However, mortality is more common in children, and the morbidity in adults can be significant.

Local envenoming (venom injection into the skin and subcutaneous tissues only) results in pain, erythema and tender enlargement of local lymph nodes. If the venom reaches the bloodstream (also known as systemic envenoming), the symptoms include sweating, fever, rash, vomiting, tachycardia, angioedema and bronchospasm. These can develop hours after the bite. Hypotension is a worrying sign and should prompt critical care review. Bleeding can occur due to thrombocytopenia and mild coagulopathy, although disseminated intravascular coagulation (DIC) is rare. A range of arrhythmias can occur, and myocardial infarction has also been described.

The limb should be immobilised with bandages or splints. Tourniquets or bandages should be avoided, as the increased concentration of venom either to the affected area or just prior to tourniquet release may be more hazardous, and the skin wound should not be interfered with if at all possible.

Antivenom is a specific antidote, and it is widely available, although it is underused in the UK. Indications are hypotension, signs of systemic envenoming (such as ECG changes, neutrophilia, elevated serum creatinine kinase or metabolic acidosis), or extensive or rapidly spreading swelling. Two ampoules are given to all patients, including children. 10% may develop a non-allergic anaphylactic ('anaphylactoid') type reaction, and so epinephrine should be available. The dose should be repeated after 1 hour if there is no improvement. Other treatment should include prevention of contractures in the immobilised limb, fluid resuscitation and blood transfusion if required. Recovery is usually complete by 1 month in children but can take longer in adults (up to 9 months). The affected limb may continue to be achy and swollen during the recovery period.

Warrell D. Treatment of bites by adders and exotic venomous snakes. *BMJ* 2005; 331: 1244.

Question B90: Hyperkalaemia – ECG changes

In a case of hyperkalaemia, which of the following ECG changes are seen?

A. The QRS complex is often narrowed
B. A prolonged PR interval is the first ECG change to be seen
C. The P wave is often absent
D. U waves are a late ECG sign
E. A normal ECG is incompatible with severe hyperkalaemia

Answer: FFTFF

Short explanation

Although the ECG may be entirely normal in severe hyperkalaemia, it is typically associated with a number of characteristic ECG changes. The QRS complex widens in hyperkalaemia; it is narrowed in hypokalaemia. Tented T waves are seen first on the ECG in hyperkalaemia, followed by a prolonged PR interval and then flattened or absent P waves. U waves are a feature of hypokalaemia.

Long explanation

Hyperkalaemia is a common electrolyte disturbance in critically ill patients. There are a number of causes including renal failure, rhabdomyolysis, administration of potassium-containing fluids and diuretic therapy. The ECG changes of potassium can help decide on the severity of hyperkalaemia and guide the urgency of treatment. It is important to remember that even in cases of severe hyperkalaemia the ECG can appear entirely normal. The speed of onset of hyperkalaemia probably affects the changes seen on an ECG.

Patients with chronic kidney disease appear relatively resistant to the effects of hyperkalaemia, and potassium levels can rise much higher than in other patients before clinical deterioration occurs. As the serum potassium starts to rise, cardiac cell membranes become depolarised, ventricular contraction is slowed and the duration of the action potential is decreased.

The first sign on the ECG is the presence of tented T waves, usually seen at serum levels of between 5.5 and 6.5 mmol/l. At serum levels above 6.5 mmol/l, the PR interval gradually increases and the P waves become flattened and eventually absent. The QRS complex widens at levels between 7.0 and 8.0 mmol/l. Eventually, the QRS complex merges with the T wave, forming a sine wave pattern. Worsening hyperkalaemia greatly increases the risk of cardiac arrest due to ventricular fibrillation, although other arrhythmias, such as ventricular tachycardia or bradycardia, may be seen.

Webster A, Brady W, Morris F. Recognising signs of danger: ECG changes resulting from an abnormal serum potassium concentration. *Emerg Med J* 2002; 19: 74–7.

Weisberg L. Management of severe hyperkalaemia. *Crit Care Med* 2008; 36: 3246–51.

Exam C: Questions

Question C1

Regarding catecholamines:

A. Phenylephrine acts mainly on α_2 receptors
B. Epinephrine acts predominantly on β receptors at low doses, and α receptors at higher doses
C. Dobutamine is a synthetic inodilator drug acting chiefly on β_1 receptors
D. Salbutamol causes tachycardia owing to its β_1 receptor activity
E. All non-synthetic catecholamines are derived from dopamine

Question C2

With regards to the basal energy requirements for an adult, which of the following are true?

A. The greatest elevations in resting energy expenditure are seen in patients with polytrauma
B. Normal resting energy expenditure is generally accepted as around 20 kcal/kg/day actual body weight
C. Fever does not increase resting energy expenditure
D. Profound sedation and muscle relaxation are likely to reduce resting energy expenditure
E. The Faisy equation can be used to calculate basal energy expenditure in ventilated critically ill patients

Question C3

Needle pericardiocentesis:

A. Is indicated for effusions > 20 mm in patients without haemodynamic compromise
B. Requires direct ECG monitoring on the puncturing needle to reduce the risk of cardiac perforation
C. Is most safely performed via the subxiphoid approach
D. Should never be undertaken without imaging (fluoroscopy or echocardiography)
E. Should not be performed in the presence of aortic dissection

Question C4

According to the Surviving Sepsis guidelines (2012), the following are goals of initial resuscitation for patients with sepsis-induced tissue hypoperfusion:

A. Central venous pressure (CVP) > 15 mmHg
B. Mean arterial pressure (MAP) ≥ 65 mmHg
C. Urine output ≥ 0.5 ml/kg
D. Central venous (SVC) saturations of 75%
E. Haematocrit ≥ 30%

Question C5

Ventilator-associated pneumonia (VAP)

A. Is underdiagnosed by bronchoalveolar lavage
B. After 4 days of ventilation is commonly due to *Streptococcus pneumoniae*
C. Is reduced by the use of proton-pump inhibitors
D. Is reduced by the use of high-volume, low-pressure cuffs on endotracheal tubes
E. Is increased by non-invasive ventilation (NIV)

Question C6

The antecubital (cubital) fossa:

A. Is a quadrilateral area on the anterior surface of the forearm
B. Contains the brachial, radial and ulnar arteries
C. Contains the median, radial and ulnar nerves
D. Contains the cephalic vein, which runs through the medial part of the fossa
E. Is the site where the median cubital vein links the cephalic and basilic vein under the bicipital aponeurosis

Question C7

Diagnosis of death by neurological criteria (brain death):

A. Requires a diagnosis of irreversible brain damage of known aetiology
B. Can only be made in a patient with a normal pH
C. Requires a wait of 3 half-lives of any sedative drugs to ensure clearance
D. Includes blood glucose analysis
E. Cannot be made in cases of high cervical spine injury

Question C8

The Multiple Organ Dysfunction Score (MODS):

A. Evaluates dysfunction of six organ systems
B. Includes the gastrointestinal and central nervous systems
C. Is calculated daily
D. Can be used to predict mortality
E. Requires the platelet count, bilirubin and creatinine levels

Question C9

Which of the following are appropriate treatments for airway obstruction?

A. CPAP
B. Abdominal thrusts
C. Sevoflurane
D. Intramuscular epinephrine
E. 21% oxygen and 79% helium

Question C10

Which of these statements about the transfer of antibiotic resistance between organisms are correct?

A. Naked DNA from killed bacteria is a common way for resistance to be transferred between organisms on the ICU
B. Plasmids are an unusual route for transfer of genetic information between bacteria on the ICU
C. Conjugation is the process through which resistance is transferred between bacteria via bacteriophages
D. Transposons can be independently mobile
E. Bacteria have a variable susceptibility to infection with bacteriophages

Question C11

In the initial assessment of a patient who appears acutely confused:

A. Capillary blood glucose level should be measured early in the assessment
B. Hyponatraemia should be urgently corrected if the patient is acutely agitated
C. If meningitis is strongly suspected, CT head is not required before lumbar puncture
D. Consent should be sought from relatives for invasive procedures
E. Benzodiazepines are the first-line drugs for the management of an agitated patient

Question C12

Regarding microbiological surveillance in critical care:

A. Its aim is to guide prophylactic antibiotic use
B. Its aim is to identify pre-existing infections
C. Its aim is to identify bacterial colonisation of patients
D. Its aim is to collate national data on healthcare-associated infections (HCAIs)
E. Its aim is to guide antimicrobial treatment protocols

Question C13

Regarding status epilepticus (SE):

A. It is defined as generalised tonic–clonic seizure activity for > 30 minutes, continuously or without intervening periods of consciousness
B. It has a hospital mortality rate > 10%
C. Neurological damage is unlikely to occur until seizure activity has lasted 30 minutes

D. First-line therapy is phenytoin 20 mg/kg
E. Buccal administration of benzodiazepine is likely to prove ineffective

Question C14

With regards to the causes and recognition of hypoxaemia, which of the following are correct?

A. Anaemic patients will appear cyanosed at an earlier stage of hypoxaemia than patients with a normal haemoglobin concentration
B. The alveolar–arterial gradient is high in patients with pulmonary embolism
C. Lobar collapse is a common cause of shunt
D. Administration of supplemental oxygen will not be beneficial in shunt
E. Hypoxaemia due to large pulmonary embolus is usually accompanied by a normal or low $PaCO_2$

Question C15

With regards to the use of the intraosseous (IO) route of access in adults, which of the following are correct?

A. The EZ-IO access device is battery-powered
B. The Big Injection Gun (BIG) device is designed for sternal access
C. Intravenous infusion pumps are a useful way of administering fluid via the IO route
D. The humerus provides a reliable, well-protected IO access site
E. The FAST 1 access device is manually powered

Question C16

The physiological effects of positive-pressure ventilation include:

A. Increased portal venous pressure
B. A reduction in renal sodium and water excretion
C. Decreased intracerebral pressure
D. Increased ventilation in the non-dependent areas of the lung
E. A reduction in left ventricular end-diastolic volume

Question C17

When considering a T-piece trial to wean a patient from mechanical ventilation, the following physiological parameters may predict successful weaning:

A. Frequency/tidal volume ratio of < 100 seconds/litre
B. PaO_2/FiO_2 > 27.5 kPa
C. Maximum inspiratory pressure of −15 cmH_2O
D. Vital capacity > 8 ml/kg
E. Static lung compliance with inspiratory pressure of 30 cmH_2O giving a tidal volume of > 10 ml/kg

Question C18

Regarding the measurement of base excess:

A. Base excess refers to the amount of acid or base (in mmol) required to restore 1 litre of blood to normal pH at 21 °C
B. It is inaccurate in the presence of a respiratory acidosis
C. Normal base excess is −2 to +2 mmol/l
D. It is an in-vivo test
E. The base excess is calculated with an assumed $PaCO_2$ of 5.3 kPa

Question C19

In the treatment of shockable rhythms the 'defibrillation threshold' is the amount of current required to produce defibrillation. Factors affecting the defibrillation threshold include:

A. Acidosis
B. Positive end-expiratory pressure (PEEP)
C. Amiodarone
D. Electrode polarity with a biphasic defibrillator, but not with a monophasic defibrillator
E. QRS width

Question C20

Cardiac output (CO) monitoring using oesophageal Doppler monitoring (ODM):

A. Uses frequency shifts in reflected sound waves to estimate flow velocity
B. Will overestimate values of stroke volume (SV) and CO if the probe is poorly positioned
C. Can be used in children
D. Does not measure blood flow to the head or arms
E. Requires measurement or estimation of aortic cross-sectional area

Question C21

Vancomycin-resistant enterococci (VREs):

A. Are associated with increased mortality in critically ill patients
B. Have a higher virulence than sensitive enterococci
C. Most commonly present in intensive care as a urinary tract infection
D. Are associated with central venous catheters
E. Are more likely to be *Enterococcus faecium* than *Enterococcus faecalis*

Question C22

With regards to the use of therapeutic hypothermia in patients who have had a cardiac arrest, which of the following are correct?

A. Current recommendations advise cooling patients to 30–32 °C for 24 hours following an out-of-hospital cardiac arrest due to ventricular fibrillation
B. The risk of sepsis is increased following therapeutic hypothermia
C. There is good evidence for beneficial effects from therapeutic hypothermia following in-hospital PEA cardiac arrest
D. Patients should be rewarmed to normothermia over a period of at least 12 hours
E. The number needed to treat to prevent unfavourable neurological outcome at 6 months after cardiac arrest is 6

Question C23

Coagulopathy following blood transfusion:

A. May be dilutional in nature
B. Is avoided by the use of whole blood
C. Requires the use of cryoprecipitate if the fibrinogen level is < 2 g/l
D. Should be treated on the basis of laboratory coagulation tests
E. Has become more common since the introduction of leucodepletion

Question C24

Pharmacological strategies to reduce the risk of acute kidney injury in critically ill patients include:

A. *N*-acetyl-cysteine
B. Fenoldopam
C. Low-dose dopamine infusion
D. Vasopressin in preference to norepinephrine
E. Furosemide

Question C25

Regarding 12-lead ECG monitoring:

A. Each lead combines the electrical signals from two or more electrodes
B. The leads display electrical signals in different directions across the heart
C. Leads I, II and III compare the arms and the left leg with a fourth reference electrode
D. The chest leads use a combined reference electrode from leads aVR, aVL and aVF
E. Leads aVR, aVL and aVF correspond to the signals from the limb electrodes

Question C26

Concerning the Advanced Trauma Life Support (ATLS) style of assessment and management of a patient with multiple injuries, which of the following are correct?

A. The primary survey should be completed within the first 24 hours of admission to hospital
B. A brief history of the patient's allergies, medical history, medications, last meal and events surrounding the incident should be sought
C. Large-volume external haemorrhage should be dealt with before assessing the airway and cervical spine
D. Life-threatening chest injuries should be assessed and excluded or managed in the primary survey
E. If the patient is combative, the cervical collar and stabilisation can be removed safely

Question C27

Regarding the risk of electrocution, which of the following are correct?

A. A current of 5 mA will cause ventricular fibrillation if applied directly to the myocardium
B. Direct current is less likely to cause ventricular fibrillation than alternating current
C. The muscles present the highest impedance to current flow when current is applied to the patient
D. As current frequency increases above 50 Hz the risk of ventricular fibrillation increases linearly
E. Microshock can occur when external ECG leads are applied to the chest

Question C28

Regarding hand hygiene:

A. Alcohol gel is effective against *Clostridium difficile* spores
B. Alcohol gels are not virucidal
C. The palms and thumbs are often missed areas when hand washing
D. Up to 40% of healthcare-associated infections (HCAIs) are prevented by adequate hand hygiene
E. Some alcohol gels are ineffective after repeated applications

Question C29

Causes of hyponatraemia include:

A. Citalopram
B. Small-cell lung cancer
C. Conn's syndrome
D. Bacterial meningitis
E. Hyperthyroidism

Question C30

The following are direct measures of peripheral tissue perfusion:

A. Serum lactate levels
B. Central venous oxygen saturations ($ScvO_2$)
C. Capillary refill time (CRT)
D. Forearm-to-finger skin temperature gradient
E. Near-infrared spectroscopy (NIRS)

Question C31

With regards to the use of echocardiography on the intensive care unit, which of the following are correct?

A. Transducers are often made of PZT-5 crystals
B. Transoesophageal echocardiography uses higher-frequency transducers than transthoracic
C. A pericardial collection with a diameter > 1 cm is likely to be significant if cardiac tamponade is suspected
D. Transthoracic echocardiography is the investigation of choice for suspected endocarditis
E. Transthoracic echocardiography gives the best results in a ventilated patient

Question C32

In the absence of intravenous access, these drugs should be administered tracheally, in the doses specified:

A. Epinephrine 3 mg
B. Atropine 3 mg
C. Bicarbonate 50 ml 8.4%
D. Amiodarone 300 mg
E. Naloxone 800 μg

Question C33

Regarding intra-abdominal pressure monitoring, which of the following are correct?

A. The standard way of monitoring intra-abdominal pressure is via an intravesical catheter
B. An intra-abdominal pressure of < 20 mmHg is normal
C. Intra-abdominal compartment syndrome rarely requires surgical intervention
D. Following laparotomy, primary closure of the wound should always be attempted
E. Increased functional residual capacity leads to gas trapping in abdominal compartment syndrome

Question C34

The following are ECG changes associated with hyperkalaemia:

A. Peaked P waves
B. Shortened PR interval
C. Widened QRS complexes
D. Peaked, inverted T waves
E. U waves

Question C35

Regarding the aminoglycoside antibiotics:

A. Peak levels correlate with toxicity
B. Trough levels correlate with toxicity
C. They are bacteriostatic
D. They exhibit good streptococcal cover
E. They exhibit no anaerobic activity

Question C36

With regards to the calculation of the surface area of skin which is burnt, which of the following are correct?

A. The rule of nines is as useful in children as in adults
B. Calculations made on the first assessment are usually the most accurate
C. The area of a child's palm including the adducted fingers approximates 1% of body surface area

D. It is important to calculate the burnt area accurately
E. The whole of the anterior of the trunk in an adult approximates 9% of body surface area

Question C37

Regarding trauma scoring systems:

A. The Trauma Injury Severity Score (TRISS) is used for triage in the field
B. The Injury Severity Score (ISS) is a purely anatomical injury score
C. The Revised Trauma Score (RTS) uses GCS, respiratory rate and systolic BP only
D. An Abbreviated Injury Score (AIS) of 6 is unsurvivable
E. Major trauma is defined as ISS > 15

Question C38

The following are sources of inaccuracy in invasive arterial blood pressure measurement:

A. Flexible connection tubing
B. Transducer height not at the level of the patient's heart
C. Peripheral site of arterial cannulation
D. Long arterial cannulae
E. Small air bubbles in fluid column within the giving set

Question C39

With regards to the management of patients with delirium, which of the following are correct?

A. Patients who remain unsedated while intubated have been shown to have a lower incidence of delirium
B. There is strong evidence for the use of atypical antipsychotics in the treatment of delirium
C. Haloperidol is useful as a first-line treatment for delirium
D. Benzodiazepines should be avoided in the treatment of delirium
E. Sedation breaks should be attempted regularly

Question C40

Regarding hypertensive emergencies:

A. Around 10% of people with hypertension will develop a hypertensive crisis during their lifetime
B. During treatment of hypertensive emergencies the goal of pharmacological therapy is a normal blood pressure
C. Renal disease is the commonest cause of secondary malignant hypertension
D. Patients of Afro-Caribbean origin are at a higher risk of hypertensive crises than Caucasian patients
E. Short-acting intravenous antihypertensive agents should be used for patients with hypertensive crises and evidence of end-organ damage

Question C41

Regarding cervical spine injuries in the unconscious trauma patient:

A. All patients should have cervical spine immobilisation until radiological clearance is complete
B. Good-quality three-view plain radiographs (lateral, anterior–posterior and open-mouth views) will exclude cervical spine injuries
C. Magnetic resonance imaging is required to exclude ligamentous injuries
D. In the absence of distracting injuries, clinical examination and passive movement is sufficient to clear the cervical spine
E. Multi-plane helical CT scans reviewed by a consultant radiologist are sufficient to exclude all significant cervical spine injuries

Question C42

On the Glasgow Coma Scale (GCS) in traumatic brain injury:

A. Abnormal flexion to pain scores 3 on the motor scale
B. Unintelligible sounds scores 2 on the verbal scale
C. Localising to painful stimulus scores 5 on the motor scale
D. Spontaneous eye opening scores 5 on the eye-response scale
E. Abnormal extension to pain scores more than abnormal flexion on the motor scale

Question C43

With regards to the assessment and management of severe hypercalcaemia, which of the following are correct?

A. Hypercalcaemic crisis is most commonly caused by primary hyperparathyroidism
B. Digoxin is the drug of choice for arrhythmias associated with hypercalcaemia
C. Malignant hypercalcaemia does not develop into a hypercalcaemic crisis
D. Acute kidney injury and anuria occur when calcium levels are > 4 mmol/l
E. Renal replacement therapy may be required if intravenous fluid resuscitation is unsuccessful

Question C44

In adult epiglottitis, which of the following are correct?

A. A small proportion of patients require admission to intensive care
B. MEWS score is a poor predictor of clinical outcome
C. Lateral neck x-ray can be helpful in diagnosis
D. The presence of stridor is the strongest predictor of the need for airway intervention
E. Positive blood cultures for *Haemophilus influenzae* type B are usually obtained

Question C45

A 35-year-old man with no significant medical history is diagnosed with community-acquired pneumonia (CAP). The following are likely causative organisms:

A. *Klebsiella pneumoniae*
B. *Streptococcus pneumoniae*
C. Methicillin-resistant *Staphylococcus aureus* (MRSA)
D. *Pseudomonas aeruginosa*
E. *Escherichia coli*

Question C46

According to the Advanced Life Support guidelines, the precordial thump:

A. Should be used only if the cardiac arrest is both witnessed and monitored
B. Is more effective for VF than for VT
C. Has been shown to induce sinus rhythm from asystole
D. Has been shown to induce VF from sinus rhythm
E. Should not be used post cardiac surgery

Question C47

Regarding spontaneous primary pneumothorax:

A. A posteroanterior (PA) chest x-ray in expiration is the diagnostic test of choice
B. A large pneumothorax is defined as one with an interpleural distance of > 2 cm at any point
C. Small pneumothoraces are managed conservatively
D. The prognosis is better than for secondary spontaneous pneumothoraces
E. Needle decompression is as effective as large-bore chest-drain insertion

Question C48

Regarding seasonal and pandemic influenza:

A. Influenza B is responsible for most pandemic cases of flu
B. Influenza A is less virulent than influenza B
C. Oral amantadine is the second-line treatment for pandemic flu
D. Oral oseltamivir is the first-line treatment for seasonal flu
E. Viral shedding occurs as soon as the patient is symptomatic

Question C49

In patients who have ingested strong acid or alkali solutions:

A. Gastric damage is greater with acidic solutions than with alkali
B. A nasogastric tube should be used to remove residual chemical
C. The risk of squamous cell cancer of the oesophagus is increased
D. Late stricture formation will be reduced by steroid administration
E. Upper gastrointestinal endoscopy should not be performed within the first 24 hours

Question C50

The following are appropriate initial management steps for patients with acute stroke:

A. CT brain for all patients with suspected acute stroke within 1 hour
B. Thrombolysis with alteplase if haemorrhage is excluded
C. Aspirin 300 mg unless the patient has a history of dyspepsia with aspirin
D. Glucose control to between 4 and 11 mmol/l
E. Urgent control of blood pressure if > 185/110

Question C51

Regarding a patient with suspected amniotic fluid embolus, which of the following are correct?

A. It only occurs during labour and delivery in the third trimester
B. Mortality is higher than 50%
C. Bronchospasm is the commonest cause of hypoxia
D. Inotropic support should not be delayed because of concerns over fetal toxicity or uterine hypoperfusion
E. Disseminated intravascular coagulation (DIC) and thrombocytopenia are hallmark signs of amniotic fluid embolism

Question C52

The following are recognised complications of pulmonary artery (PA) catheters:

A. Air embolism
B. Complete heart block
C. Pulmonary infarction
D. Pneumothorax
E. Neuropathy

Question C53

With regards to the risk factors for delirium in patients on the intensive care unit, which of the following are correct?

A. Chronic alcohol dependence is not a risk factor for delirium
B. Use of benzodiazepines is associated with a reduced risk of delirium
C. Hearing impairment increases the risk of delirium
D. Anaemia increases the risk of delirium
E. Hypotension increases the risk of delirium

Question C54

Regarding herpes simplex encephalitis:

A. It is most commonly caused by HSV-1
B. Treatment of choice is intravenous ganciclovir
C. It usually affects the frontal lobes
D. Untreated, mortality is up to 25%
E. It is characterised by a very high CSF protein level

Question C55

Indications for renal replacement therapy on the intensive care unit include:

A. Serum potassium > 6.0 mmol/l in an anuric patient
B. Oliguria
C. Anuria
D. pH < 7.2 due to hypovolaemic shock
E. Urea > 20 mmol/l

Question C56

Regarding disseminated intravascular coagulation (DIC):

A. Fibrin degradation products (FDPs) have a high diagnostic sensitivity
B. Gram-negative bacterial sepsis is more likely to induce DIC than Gram-positive bacterial sepsis
C. Fibrin degradation products (FDPs) have a high diagnostic specificity
D. Platelet count should be maintained > 100 × 10^9/l in a bleeding patient with DIC
E. Coagulation factor concentrates are an alternative to fresh frozen plasma in the treatment of DIC

Question C57

In hypokalaemia:

A. Peaked T waves are seen on the ECG
B. U waves are seen after the T waves on the ECG
C. The duration of the action potential and refractory period are reduced
D. Ventricular arrhythmias are more likely following myocardial infarction
E. Patients taking digoxin are relatively resistant to the effects of hypokalaemia

Question C58

With regards to the measurement of jugular venous bulb oxygen saturation, which of the following are correct?

A. The jugular bulb is a dilatation of the internal jugular bulb just inside the skull
B. Jugular saturation is normally lower than central venous saturation
C. Continuous jugular bulb oxygen saturation monitoring accurately reflects tissue oxygenation in the injured brain
D. The internal jugular vein is cannulated in a retrograde manner to place the catheter
E. It should be considered for all patients with traumatic brain injury on the ICU

Question C59

Which of these statements correctly describe the management of burn injury?

A. Fluid resuscitation should be commenced as early as possible even in the absence of shock
B. Prophylactic antibiotics should be administered to prevent ventilator-associated pneumonia
C. Early institution of enteral nutrition is recommended in major burns
D. Escharotomy is not usually required in full-thickness burns, because swelling is rarely a problem
E. Referral to a regional burns centre is advised for adults with 8% burns and inhalational injury

Question C60

Concerning the management of carbon monoxide poisoning, which of the following are correct?

A. Carbon monoxide in the blood is made up of endogenously produced and exogenously inhaled carbon monoxide
B. Carboxyhaemoglobin levels > 10% are invariably fatal
C. Patients with chronic obstructive pulmonary disease are protected from the toxic effects of carbon monoxide
D. Carbon monoxide binds less avidly to cardiac myoglobin than to haemoglobin
E. The relationship between inspired levels of carbon monoxide and arterial carboxyhaemoglobin levels is linear

Question C61

The following are absolute contraindications to thrombolysis in STEMI:

A. Significant closed head injury 5 months ago
B. Ischaemic stroke 6 weeks ago
C. 6 cm abdominal aortic aneurysm diagnosed 2 weeks ago
D. Cardiopulmonary resuscitation 3 hours ago
E. Intracranial meningioma

Question C62

Regarding the investigation and management of Guillain–Barré syndrome (GBS):

A. Patients with a vital capacity < 15 ml/kg are likely to need intubation
B. Gastroparesis in GBS means that intubation using a rapid sequence induction (RSI) with suxamethonium is required
C. Intravenous immunoglobulin is more effective than plasma exchange
D. Corticosteroids are a useful early treatment
E. Miller–Fisher syndrome is a subtype of GBS characterised by autonomic instability

Question C63

With regards to the prevention and management of venous thromboembolism in critical care patients, which of the following are correct?

A. Mechanical thromboprophylaxis has benefits similar to those obtained with pharmacological methods in preventing PE
B. Factor Xa levels need not be routinely monitored in patients receiving low-molecular-weight heparin (LMWH)
C. Aspirin therapy should be considered in high-risk patients with contraindications to heparin therapy
D. Fondaparinux can be used as an alternative to LMWH in patients with a previous history of heparin-induced thrombocytopenia (HIT)
E. Patients recovering from major trauma are at the highest risk of venous thromboembolism

Question C64

Methicillin-resistant *Staphylococcus aureus* (MRSA) can be successfully treated with the following antibiotics:

A. Intravenous ceftazidime
B. Oral vancomycin
C. Intravenous teicoplanin
D. Intravenous linezolid
E. Intravenous rifampicin

Question C65

Regarding massive blood transfusion:

A. It is defined as the replacement of the circulating volume in 4 hours
B. Hypothermia shifts the oxyhaemoglobin dissociation curve to the right
C. Blood giving sets should have 50-micron filters in situ
D. Platelets may be given through a blood giving set
E. Transfusion aims to keep haemoglobin > 10 g/dl with ongoing bleeding

Question C66

Regarding the management of severe acute pancreatitis (SAP):

A. Patients with a Glasgow score of 3 or more should be managed in a critical care unit
B. Enteral feeding should be avoided for the first 7 days
C. Empirical antibiotics should be prescribed
D. Endoscopic retrograde cholangiopancreatography (ERCP) should be considered in patients with SAP and jaundice
E. Necrotic pancreatic tissue should be surgically debrided as soon as possible

Question C67

In cases of abdominal trauma, which of the following are correct?

A. Bleeding patients with coagulopathy at presentation have a higher mortality than those without coagulopathy
B. Patients with isolated abdominal trauma and evidence of significant haemorrhage should undergo CT scanning as the first-line radiological intervention
C. Aortic cross-clamping is of use in the exanguinating patient
D. Tranexamic acid should be administered in the bleeding trauma patient
E. Definitive repairs of bleeding organs should be undertaken as soon as possible after injury

Question C68

Concerning the femoral triangle:

A. The roof is formed by the fascia iliaca
B. The femoral artery enters the triangle between the medial and middle thirds of the inguinal ligament

C. The femoral vein lies medial to the femoral artery throughout the femoral triangle
D. The great saphenous vein empties into the femoral vein within the femoral triangle
E. The femoral nerve lies lateral to the femoral sheath

Question C69

With respect to botulism:

A. Antibiotics should be given empirically on clinical grounds
B. Antitoxin treatment may result in anaphylaxis
C. It causes an ascending flaccid paralysis
D. It invalidates brainstem death testing
E. Sensory nerves are affected first

Question C70

In a case of paracetamol-induced acute liver failure:

A. The liver injury is due to a direct toxic effect of paracetamol on hepatocytes
B. Activated charcoal should be administered if within 4 hours of overdose
C. *N*-acetyl-cysteine is ineffective if given by the oral route
D. Patients with pH < 7.3 after fluid resuscitation should be referred for transplant
E. Intravenous *N*-acetyl-cysteine causes adverse reactions in up to 20% of patients

Question C71

With regards to the management of obtunded adult trauma patients, which of the following are correct?

A. Level 1 evidence exists to guide radiological investigations and subsequent management of potential cervical spine injury
B. Patients with low risk of cervical spine injury should undergo dynamic fluoroscopy
C. MRI is the gold-standard investigation with the highest sensitivity and specificity for bone and ligamentous injuries
D. CT scan alone has been reported to have a false-negative rate as high as 4% for cervical spine injury
E. MRI should be performed as early as possible in all patients with clinical signs of spinal cord pathology

Question C72

Regarding vasculitides:

A. They can be secondary to infective, inflammatory or malignant conditions
B. Wegener's granulomatosis (WG) affects large arteries
C. Churg–Strauss syndrome (CSS) is associated with asthma
D. Negative ANCA serology effectively excludes primary vasculitis
E. Management is purely supportive

Question C73

Which of the following statements about patient decision making are correct?

A. An advance decision to refuse treatment is legally binding in England and Wales
B. An advance decision to refuse life-sustaining procedures must be in writing, signed and witnessed
C. No-one can make medical decisions on behalf of another adult in England
D. Patients can nominate more than one lasting power of attorney
E. Patients can make advance decisions to insist upon all life-sustaining treatment

Question C74

In the management of raised intracranial pressure (ICP):

A. Glucocorticoids should be used to reduce oedema secondary to diffuse axonal injury (DAI)
B. Hypertonic saline is more effective than mannitol in treating raised ICP
C. ICP monitoring should be used in ventilated patients with open head injuries
D. Rebound intracranial hypertension is a risk with hyperventilation to a $PaCO_2$ of 4–4.5 kPa
E. Therapeutic hypothermia should be used as first-line therapy for raised ICP in sedated patients

Question C75

Causes of a metabolic alkalosis include:

A. Diuretics
B. Eating disorders
C. Corticosteroids
D. Conn's syndrome
E. Citrate haemofiltration

Question C76

Regarding ethylene glycol poisoning:

A. Activated charcoal should be given within 1 hour of ingestion
B. A normal anion gap metabolic acidosis is usually seen
C. Fomepizole should be administered intravenously because of poor oral bioavailability
D. Ethylene glycol is metabolised by alcohol dehydrogenase to non-toxic metabolites
E. Haemodialysis is a useful treatment

Question C77

In the management of a critically ill pregnant patient, which of the following are correct?

A. Sepsis is a rare cause of maternal death in the developed world
B. Antibiotics should be withheld until an organism is identified, to prevent fetal toxicity

C. Central venous oxygen saturations will be lower than in the non-pregnant patient
D. Group A *Streptococcus* infection is implicated in a large proportion of maternal deaths resulting from sepsis
E. Vasopressors should be administered to maintain acceptable systemic blood pressure following fluid resuscitation

Question C78

Complications of percutaneous tracheostomy placement:

A. Include tracheo-oesophageal fistula formation
B. Are reduced by use of standard operating procedures
C. Include erosion into subclavian veins
D. Make continuous capnography mandatory in ventilated patients
E. Are less common than with surgical tracheostomy placement

Question C79

With regards to the nutritional requirements of an adult patient, which of the following are correct?

A. Vitamin B_1 should be provided to prevent lactic acidosis
B. Vitamins A, E and C have antioxidant properties that may counteract cell damage in critically ill patients
C. Zinc deficiency results in delayed wound healing
D. Selenium supplementation in parenteral nutrition is not recommended
E. Copper deficiency can lead to arrhythmias and altered immunity

Question C80

Concerning the insertion of a nasogastric (NG) feeding tube:

A. Prior to insertion, the tube length required should be estimated using the NEX measurement
B. When using a chest radiograph to confirm correct placement, the feeding tube should always be seen below the diaphragm
C. If no aspirate is obtainable then the tube should be flushed
D. A pH of aspirated contents of > 4 is a contraindication to feeding
E. On a chest radiograph a correctly placed NG tube should bisect the carina

Question C81

With regards to stress ulceration prophylaxis in the critically ill patient, which of the following are correct?

A. There is strong evidence that stress ulcer prophylaxis reduces mortality in septic patients
B. Histamine H_2 receptor antagonists (H_2RAs) are superior to proton-pump inhibitors (PPIs) in preventing gastrointestinal ulceration in the critically ill patient

C. Upper gastrointestinal bleeding is reduced in patients taking stress ulcer prophylaxis
D. Sucralfate is not as effective as H_2RAs in preventing stress ulceration
E. Evidence suggests that higher rates of hospital-acquired and aspiration pneumonia are seen in patients taking acid-suppressive medication

Question C82

Transfusion-related acute lung injury (TRALI):

A. Is acute lung injury occurring within 12 hours of blood transfusion
B. Is more common than haemolytic reactions, HIV and hepatitis B and C transmission
C. Is more likely with platelets than with red blood cells
D. Has no specific treatment
E. Carries a higher mortality than other causes of acute lung injury (ALI)

Question C83

Regarding the guidelines for red cell transfusion in adult critically ill patients:

A. The default target Hb range should be > 9 g/dl
B. A transfusion threshold of ≤ 7 g/dl should be the default unless specific factors are present
C. Anaemic patients with stable angina should have Hb maintained > 10 g/dl
D. In patients who are weaning from the ventilator, Hb should be maintained > 9 g/dl
E. In patients with subarachnoid haemorrhage the target Hb should be 8–10 g/dl

Question C84

With regard to chronic kidney disease (CKD):

A. The commonest cause of CKD is hypertension
B. The combined use of an angiotensin-converting enzyme (ACE) inhibitor and an angiotensin II blocking agent is recommended to slow the progression to end-stage renal failure
C. Platelet transfusion is effective as a means of improving coagulation in patients prior to surgery
D. The free drug fraction of highly protein-bound drugs is decreased with CKD
E. Maximum doses of local anaesthetics are unchanged in CKD

Question C85

Which of the following statements correctly describe the metabolism of drugs in critically ill patients?

A. Non-renal metabolism of vancomycin remains unaltered in patients with acute kidney injury (AKI)
B. Uraemic molecules present due to AKI may prevent the normal hepatic metabolism of drugs
C. Renal replacement therapy ensures that metabolism of renally excreted drugs is maintained

D. Hyper- and hypothermia can prevent drug metabolism by means of enzyme dysfunction and reduced activity
E. Patients who have thyroid dysfunction will be particularly sensitive to the effects of sedative agents

Question C86

Regarding surgical site infection:

A. Colonisation with methicillin-sensitive *Staphylococcus aureus* (MSSA) increases the risk of postoperative wound infection
B. Blood sugar should be kept at 4–6 mmol/l to reduce surgical site infection
C. Blood transfusion is associated with a higher incidence of surgical site infection
D. Oxycodone should be used in preference to morphine to reduce postoperative infection
E. Povidone–iodine is as effective as 2% chlorhexidine in preventing infections

Question C87

Regarding selective decontamination of the digestive tract (SDD):

A. It is associated with a reduction in mortality
B. It increases the likelihood of infection with resistant bacteria
C. Topical therapy alone (selective oral decontamination) reduces ventilator-associated pneumonia
D. SDD does not affect fungal infections
E. SDD is a method of controlling exogenous infections in critical care patients

Question C88

Post-traumatic stress disorder (PTSD) in patients after intensive care:

A. Is reduced in incidence by a self-help recovery package given to patients on discharge
B. Is more common in patients with delusional memories
C. Occurs in up to 1 in 10 ICU patients
D. Should be assessed using validated screening tools
E. Should prompt psychiatric referral in all patients at risk

Question C89

Concerning organ donation and transplantation:

A. Organ donation should be considered in every patient expected to die in ICU
B. Family members have no right to refuse to authorise donation if the patient is on the organ donor register (ODR)
C. Family members may authorise donation if there is no indication of the prior views of the patient
D. Donation after circulatory death (DCD) can be classified as controlled or uncontrolled
E. Organ donation coordinators may only be approached after authorisation for donation has been received

Question C90

With regards to central pontine myelinolysis (CPM), which of the following are correct?

A. It is more commonly seen in patients with alcohol dependence
B. Rapid correction of acute hyponatraemia is the main cause
C. MRI is the imaging modality of choice for diagnosis
D. Microscopically there is degeneration of axons in the pons with preservation of oligodendrocytes
E. Parkinsonism, catatonia and movement disorders suggest extrapontine myelinolysis

Exam C: Answers

Question C1: Catecholamines

Regarding catecholamines:

A. Phenylephrine acts mainly on α_2 receptors
B. Epinephrine acts predominantly on β receptors at low doses, and α receptors at higher doses
C. Dobutamine is a synthetic inodilator drug acting chiefly on β_1 receptors
D. Salbutamol causes tachycardia owing to its β_1 receptor activity
E. All non-synthetic catecholamines are derived from dopamine

Answer: FTTTT

Short explanation

Phenylephrine acts principally through α_1 receptors. Epinephrine acts on all adrenergic receptors, but β activity predominates at low doses. Salbutamol is moderately selective for β_2 receptors, but also acts on β_1 receptors to cause tachycardia. Dobutamine is a synthetic β_1 agonist. All catecholamines are synthesised from dopamine in the body.

Long explanation

Catecholamines can be naturally occurring in the body (dopamine, norepinephrine, epinephrine) or synthetic (dobutamine, dopexamine, isoprenaline). Their chemical structure consists of an aromatic ring and a tertiary amine linked by a carbon chain. The synthetic pathway starts with the amino acid tyrosine, through DOPA and dopamine, to norepinephrine and finally epinephrine. Catecholamines are rapidly broken down in the body; their half-life is 1–2 minutes and steady state can be reached by infusion within 5 minutes.

There are two main classes of adrenergic receptor, α and β. These have multiple subtypes ($\alpha_{1A\ \&\ B}$, $\alpha_{2A,\ B\ \&\ C}$, β_1, β_2, β_3) which are distributed in different tissues. Each catecholamine has differing patterns of affinity for these receptors, which means that each drug has a different spectrum of effects and side effects:

	α_1	α_2	β_1	β_2
Epinephrine	++	++	+++	+++
Norepinephrine	+++	+++	++	+
Dopamine	+	–	++	–
Dobutamine	–	–	+++	+
Salbutamol	–	–	+	+++
Isoprenaline	–	–	+++	+++
Phenylephrine	++	–	–	–
Clonidine	–	+++	–	–

+++ highly active; ++ moderately active; + some activity; – no activity.

α_1 receptors are found in blood vessels, particularly in the skin, kidney, gut and liver. α_1 stimulation causes vasoconstriction and increased SVR, at the expense of reduced perfusion to these areas. α_2 receptors can be postsynaptic (with similar activity to α_1 receptors) or presynaptic, where stimulation reduces endogenous catecholamine release and hence vasodilatation and negative inotropy.

β_1 receptors are predominantly found in the heart. Stimulation causes increased heart rate and force of contraction, with associated increased myocardial work and oxygen demand. β_2 receptors are found in smooth muscle in the bronchii, blood vessels, bladder, uterus and gut. Stimulation leads to smooth muscle relaxation.

Rang HP, Dale M, Henderson G, Ritter JM, Flower RJ. *Rang and Dale's Pharmacology*, 7th edn. Edinburgh: Elsevier Churchill Livingstone, 2012.

Question C2: Resting energy expenditure

With regards to the basal energy requirements for an adult, which of the following are true?

A. The greatest elevations in resting energy expenditure are seen in patients with polytrauma
B. Normal resting energy expenditure is generally accepted as around 20 kcal/kg/day actual body weight
C. Fever does not increase resting energy expenditure
D. Profound sedation and muscle relaxation are likely to reduce resting energy expenditure
E. The Faisy equation can be used to calculate basal energy expenditure in ventilated critically ill patients

Answer: FTFTT

Short explanation

The greatest elevations in resting energy expenditure are seen in patients with severe sepsis, ARDS and burns. It can rise by as much as 80%. Fever increases resting energy expenditure by around 10% for every 1 °C rise in body temperature.

Long explanation

Critically ill patients have different nutritional requirements to healthy adults due to the body's stress response. The stress response to injury and sepsis is mediated via a number of pathways involving cytokines and stress hormones. This ultimately results in an increased metabolic rate, increased gluconeogenesis, increased lipolysis and a net loss of lean body mass.

The normal energy requirement for an adult is generally accepted to be 20–30 kcal/kg/day, based on basal energy expenditure. This can increase significantly in critically ill patients, and different disease processes appear to have different effects on basal energy expenditure. An increase of around 10–15% is often seen in patients with severe infection or polytrauma. Increases are much more significant in patients with uncontrolled sepsis and major burns. Interestingly, patients who are sedated, who have undergone prolonged starvation, who are physically immobilised, or who have severe protein calorie malnutrition have a reduced energy expenditure, by up to 15–20%.

In addition to these factors, it is important to be aware of the alterations in energy requirements seen throughout the patient's illness. It is a dynamic process which changes as the stress response develops through the theoretical 'ebb' and 'flow' phases. This means that the situation in ICU can be complicated, and measuring or estimating energy requirements is not an exact science.

It is difficult in clinical practice to measure energy expenditure via indirect calorimetry, which is effectively limited to research only. There are some equations that can be used to estimate energy requirements. These can guide clinicians when prescribing artificial nutrition. The Harris–Benedict formulae can be used to derive the basal energy expenditure but can be inaccurate in ventilated patients. The Faisy equation is thought to be more accurate in this group of patients, as it corrects for minute ventilation and body temperature.

Singer P, Berger M, Van den Berghe G, *et al*. ESPEN guidelines on parenteral nutrition: intensive care. *Clin Nutr* 2009; 28: 387–400.

Question C3: Pericardiocentesis

Needle pericardiocentesis:

A. Is indicated for effusions > 20 mm in patients without haemodynamic compromise
B. Requires direct ECG monitoring on the puncturing needle to reduce the risk of cardiac perforation
C. Is most safely performed via the subxiphoid approach
D. Should never be undertaken without imaging (fluoroscopy or echocardiography)
E. Should not be performed in the presence of aortic dissection

Answer: TTTFT

Short explanation

Pericardiocentesis is indicated for effusions > 20 mm without haemodynamic compromise, for smaller effusions with haemodynamic compromise, or for diagnostic purposes. It should be performed under fluoroscopic or echocardiographic guidance except in extreme emergencies. The subxiphoid approach is safest, avoiding the pleura and major blood vessels. ECG monitoring of the puncturing needle should be used but is insufficient on its own to safeguard against cardiac puncture. Aortic dissection is an absolute contraindication to needle pericardiocentesis.

Long explanation

Needle pericardiocentesis can be a life-saving intervention in cardiac tamponade. It is indicated in cases of pericardial effusions causing haemodynamic compromise, for large effusions (> 20 mm measured in diastole by echocardiography) without compromise, or for diagnostic reasons. Aortic dissection is an absolute contraindication; relative contraindications include coagulopathy, posterior collections, traumatic haemopericardium and purulent pericarditis.

The safest and most common approach is subxiphoid, which avoids the pleural space and the coronary and internal mammary arteries. Other possible approaches include parasternal and apical. Pericardiocentesis should be image-guided in all but the most extreme emergencies (e.g. cardiac arrest). Fluoroscopic guidance requires the transfer of the patient to the cardiac catheterisation laboratory but has the highest success rate, particularly for small or posterior effusions. Echocardiographic guidance also greatly improves success rate and reduces complications, and can be utilised at the bedside. ECG and haemodynamic monitoring are also required. Direct ECG monitoring of the puncturing needle is not an adequate safeguard against cardiac puncture.

Cardiac complications include cardiac perforation, coronary vessel laceration, arrhythmias and haemorrhage. Other complications include pneumothorax, air embolus and damage to the peritoneum or abdominal viscera. Infective pericarditis is a late complication. Complication rates are greatly reduced by image guidance to rates of around 1.5%.

Maisch B, Seferović PM, Ristić AD, *et al*. Guidelines on the diagnosis and management of pericardial diseases executive summary. *Eur Heart J* 2004; 25: 587–610.

Question C4: Sepsis-induced tissue hypoperfusion

According to the Surviving Sepsis guidelines (2012), the following are goals of initial resuscitation for patients with sepsis-induced tissue hypoperfusion:

A. Central venous pressure (CVP) > 15 mmHg
B. Mean arterial pressure (MAP) ≥ 65 mmHg
C. Urine output ≥ 0.5 ml/kg
D. Central venous (SVC) saturations of 75%
E. Haematocrit ≥ 30%

Answer: FTFFF

Short explanation

Initial goals (within 6 hours) of resuscitation in sepsis-induced tissue hypoperfusion include CVP 8–12 mmHg, urine output ≥ 0.5 ml/kg/hour, central venous saturations 70%. Blood transfusion to increase haematocrit to ≥ 30% is recommended to improve central venous or mixed venous saturation but is not a goal in itself.

Long explanation

The third edition of the Surviving Sepsis guidelines were issued in 2012. The guidelines are a part of a wider Surviving Sepsis Campaign (SSC) to reduce deaths from sepsis across the globe. Strategies include increasing awareness, improving diagnosis, and the introduction of bundles of care to improve management. The SSC resuscitation bundle has six components:

(1) initial resuscitation (protocolised and goal-directed)
(2) screening for sepsis and performance improvement
(3) diagnosis: early blood cultures (< 45 minutes) and other tests
(4) antimicrobial therapy (within 1 hour of recognition of severe sepsis or septic shock)

(5) source control (early drainage of collections, removal of infected lines etc.)
(6) infection prevention (selective oral or digestive decontamination)

Initial resuscitation goals should be used to guide therapy in patients with sepsis-induced tissue hypoperfusion (serum lactate > 4 mmol/l or hypotension despite fluid resuscitation), as soon as it is recognised. The goals are as follows:

- central venous pressure (CVP) 8–12 mmHg
- mean arterial pressure (MAP) ≥ 65 mmHg
- urine output ≥ 0.5 ml/kg/hour
- central venous saturations of 70% or mixed venous saturations of 65%
- normalised lactate in patients with elevated lactate levels

Therapy should be targeted to improving these parameters. Initial intravenous fluid boluses should be at least 30 ml/kg, comprising crystalloids and/or albumin, to achieve CVP 8–12 mmHg and urine output ≥ 0.5 ml/kg/hour. Hypotension should be treated with norepinephrine initially, although epinephrine, vasopressin and corticosteroids may be required to achieve MAP ≥ 65 mmHg. Low central venous saturations ($ScvO_2$ < 70% or SvO_2 < 65%) should be treated initially with packed red cells to achieve a haematocrit ≥ 30%, followed by dobutamine infusion.

Dellinger RP, Levy MM, Rhodes A, *et al.* Surviving Sepsis Campaign. International guidelines for management of severe sepsis and septic shock: 2012. *Crit Care Med* 2013; 41: 580–637.

Question C5: Ventilator-associated pneumonia

Ventilator-associated pneumonia (VAP)

A. Is underdiagnosed by bronchoalveolar lavage
B. After 4 days of ventilation is commonly due to *Streptococcus pneumoniae*
C. Is reduced by the use of proton-pump inhibitors
D. Is reduced by the use of high-volume, low-pressure cuffs on endotracheal tubes
E. Is increased by non-invasive ventilation (NIV)

Answer: TFFFF

Short explanation

Early VAP (< 4 days) is commonly due to *Streptococcus pneumoniae*. It is increased by the use of proton-pump inhibitors and high-volume, low-pressure cuffs, and decreased by using NIV instead of mechanical ventilation.

Long explanation

Ventilator-associated pneumonia (VAP) occurs in patients ventilated for > 48 hours. The incidence is currently reported as 15–20% but varies greatly due to differing diagnostic criteria and microbiological surveillance practices. Classification of VAP is described by the Hospitals in Europe Link for Infection Control through Surveillance (HELICS) criteria. These combine clinical and microbiological criteria to aid diagnosis. Clinical criteria include the development of new infiltrates on chest x-ray, fever, leucocytosis, purulent tracheobronchial secretions and increasing oxygen or ventilatory requirements.

Microbiological confirmation of the diagnosis may be obtained invasively or non-invasively. Invasive sampling methods include bronchoalveolar lavage (BAL), mini-BAL and protected specimen brushing. Mini-BAL, or blind BAL, is performed using catheters that allow sampling of the distal airways without contamination from the tube or trachea. Non-invasive sampling is by analysis of routine tracheal suction specimens. The sensitivity and specificity of both non-invasive and invasive methods varies widely, and it is not yet clear which method accurately diagnoses infection as opposed to airway colonisation.

The likely pathogen in VAP depends on length of stay, prior antibiotics and comorbidities. In general, early-onset VAP (< 4 days) is due to antibiotic-sensitive bacteria such as *Haemophilus*, *Streptococcus pneumoniae* and methicillin-sensitive *Staphylococcus aureus*. Late infection is more commonly caused by multidrug-resistant pathogens, including *Pseudomonas aeruginosa*, *Acinetobacter* and MRSA. Treatment of VAP is with broad-spectrum antibiotics, which should be rationalised once the organism and sensitivities are known to reduce the emergence of resistant bacteria. The antibacterial course should be no more than 8 days in most cases.

Prevention of VAP centres around a 'ventilator care bundle', including nursing the patient in the semi-recumbant position, subglottic suctioning, sedation holds and the use of non-invasive ventilation (NIV) to reduce ventilated days. The use of proton-pump inhibitors and enteral feeding both increase the risk of VAP, but are important and are therefore still recommended. The use of chlorhexidine mouthwashes and selective digestive tract decontamination also reduces VAP. The use of silver-impregnated tubes and ultrathin cuffs may also reduce VAP, although an impact on mortality, length of stay and ventilator-free days has yet to be shown.

Hunter JD. Ventilator associated pneumonia. *BMJ* 2012; 344: e3325.

Coppadoro A, Bittner E, Berra L. Novel preventive strategies for ventilator-associated pneumonia. *Crit Care* 2012; 16: 210.

Question C6: The antecubital fossa

The antecubital (cubital) fossa:

A. Is a quadrilateral area on the anterior surface of the forearm
B. Contains the brachial, radial and ulnar arteries
C. Contains the median, radial and ulnar nerves
D. Contains the cephalic vein, which runs through the medial part of the fossa
E. Is the site where the median cubital vein links the cephalic and basilic vein under the bicipital aponeurosis

Answer: FTFFF

Short explanation

The antecubital fossa is triangular. The brachial artery divides into the radial and ulnar arteries within the fossa. The cephalic vein runs superficial to the cubital fossa along the lateral border and is linked to the basilic vein by the median cubital vein superficial to the bicipital aponeurosis. The median and radial nerves run through the antecubital fossa; the ulnar nerve runs posterior to the elbow.

Long explanation

The antecubital or cubital fossa is a triangular area on the anterior surface of the upper forearm that is a regular site for venepuncture and arterial and venous cannulation. It is bounded laterally by the brachioradialis muscle, medially by the pronator teres muscle, and superiorly by a line joining the humeral epicondyles. Its floor is formed by the supinator and brachialis muscles and its roof by deep fascia (including the bicipital aponeurosis).

The brachial artery runs inferiorly through the antecubital fossa medial to the biceps tendon, where it divides into the radial and ulnar arteries at the level of the radial head. The brachial veins accompany the brachial artery throughout its course.

Other veins lie superficial to the antecubital fossa, separated from it by the bicipital aponeurosis, which protects the brachial artery from damage during attempts at cannulation or phlebotomy. The basilic vein runs superiorly along the anteromedial aspect of the forearm and lower arm before passing deep to the deep fascia and becoming the axillary vein. The cephalic vein passes along the anterolateral aspect of the upper forearm and arm before emptying into the axillary vein at the deltopectoral triangle. The median cubital vein links the cephalic and basilic veins, running superficial to the bicipital aponeurosis anterior to the cubital fossa.

The median nerve runs alongside the brachial artery along the humerus and into the cubital fossa medial to the artery. The radial nerve descends through the lateral side of the cubital fossa, dividing into deep (motor) and superficial (sensory) branches in the fossa. The ulnar nerve runs posterior to the elbow joint, passing between the medial humeral epicondyle and the olecranon.

Moore KL, Dalley AF, Agur AMR. *Clinically Oriented Anatomy*, 7th edn. Philadelphia, PA: Lippincott, Williams & Wilkins, 2013.

Question C7: Diagnosis of brain death

Diagnosis of death by neurological criteria (brain death):

A. Requires a diagnosis of irreversible brain damage of known aetiology
B. Can only be made in a patient with a normal pH
C. Requires a wait of 3 half-lives of any sedative drugs to ensure clearance
D. Includes blood glucose analysis
E. Cannot be made in cases of high cervical spine injury

Answer: FTFTF

Short explanation

In the absence of a clear cause of irreversible brain damage, further observation and ancillary tests (e.g. four-vessel angiography) may be required. Haemodynamic and biochemical stability is required for brain death testing, including normal pH and glucose. Any drugs that may contribute to apnoeic coma should be allowed 4 half-lives to clear from the body. In high cervical spine injury, apnoea testing is not applicable, so ancillary tests are required to diagnose neurological death.

Long explanation

Diagnosis of death by neurological criteria has a UK code of practice and recently updated guidelines by the Academy of Medical Royal Colleges (AoMRC). There are three components:

(1) fulfilment of preconditions
(2) exclusion of confounding factors
(3) brainstem and apnoea testing

The essential preconditions are that the patients must be in a state of apnoeic coma and mechanically ventilated. There should be a diagnosis of irreversible brain damage of known aetiology (e.g. cerebral hypoxia, intracerebral haemorrhage, malignant intracranial hypertension). In some cases, a prolonged period of observation and/or ancillary tests (e.g. angiography) may be required in the absence of a formal diagnosis.

There should be no other cause for apnoea or coma in the patient. This includes drugs (sedatives, muscle relaxants), biochemical disturbance, hypothermia (< 34 °C) and haemodynamic instability. Drugs should be allowed a period of 4 half-lives for clearance (increased in hepatic or renal failure) and/or antidotes (e.g. naloxone) should be administered. Biochemical and haemodynamic requirements are:

- pH 7.35–7.45
- $PaCO_2$ < 6.0 kPa
- PaO_2 > 10.0 kPa
- Na^+ 115–160 mmol/l
- K^+ > 2.0 mmol/l
- Mg^{++} 0.5–3.0 mmol/l
- Phosphate 115–160 mmol/l
- Glucose 3–20 mmol/l

Brainstem testing is performed by two doctors (both registered for at least 5 years, one of whom must be a consultant) on two separate occasions. All tests involve efferent and afferent cranial nerves and different parts of the brainstem. Pupillary response, corneal reflex, oculovestibular reflex, response to pain, gag and cough reflexes are all tested.

Apnoea testing is only performed after negative brainstem tests. Patients are disconnected from the ventilator with passive oxygenation and watched for respiratory effort for 5 minutes. If there is no respiration despite a $PaCO_2$ rise of 0.5 kPa, then a diagnosis of death may be made. Time of death is taken as the time of the first episode of testing.

Oram J, Murphy P. Diagnosis of death. *Contin Educ Anaesth Crit Care Pain* 2011; 11: 77–81.

Question C8: MODS

The Multiple Organ Dysfunction Score (MODS):

A. Evaluates dysfunction of six organ systems
B. Includes the gastrointestinal and central nervous systems
C. Is calculated daily
D. Can be used to predict mortality
E. Requires the platelet count, bilirubin and creatinine levels

Answer: TFTTT

Short explanation

MODS is a weighted aggregate scoring system based on a single measure of the function of six organ systems: respiratory (PO_2/FiO_2 ratio); cardiovascular (heart rate/ABP – CVP); hepatic (bilirubin); renal (creatinine); haematological (platelet count); and CNS (GCS). Each system is scored 0–4, giving a score out of 24. Scores are calculated daily and correlate well with mortality.

Long explanation

Organ failure scores are used to describe the severity of organ dysfunction. There are many such scores in use, but one of the simplest is the Multiple Organ Dysfunction Score (MODS), first described in 1995. Six organ systems are included, each represented by a single parameter with weighted scores of 0 to 4 for each system. The score is calculated daily using the first set of parameters of the day, so the progression of the patient's clinical condition can be monitored throughout the ICU stay.

The six organ systems and parameters are:

- respiratory: PO_2:FiO_2 ratio
- cardiovascular: pressure-adjusted heart rate (heart rate/ABP – CVP)
- hepatic: serum bilirubin
- renal: serum creatinine
- haematological: platelet count
- CNS: Glasgow Coma Scale

While the original intention of the MODS was as a descriptor of organ dysfunction, scores correlate well with mortality. First-day scores correlate particularly well with outcome, with greater predictive value than many more complex severity of illness scoring systems. Mortality correlates not only with raw score, but also with the number of organ systems failing scores and the delta MODS (the difference between maximum score and score on admission), which may have even greater outcome-predictive power.

Marshall JC, Cook DJ, Christou NV, *et al.* The multiple organ dysfunction (MOD) score: a reliable descriptor of a complex clinical outcome. *Crit Care Med* 1995; 23: 1638–52.

Palazzo M. Severity of illness and likely outcome from critical illness. In Bersten AD, Soni N. *Oh's Intensive Care Manual*, 6th edn. Edinburgh: Butterworth-Heinemann, 2009, pp. 17–30.

Question C9: Airway obstruction

Which of the following are appropriate treatments for airway obstruction?

A. CPAP
B. Abdominal thrusts
C. Sevoflurane
D. Intramuscular epinephrine
E. 21% oxygen and 79% helium

Answer: TTTTT

Short explanation

All are appropriate, depending on the circumstances: CPAP for partial upper airway obstruction (e.g. sleep apnoea); abdominal thrusts (Heimlich manoeuvre) in choking; gaseous induction of anaesthesia for epiglottitis; intramuscular epinephrine for anaphylactic angioedema; heliox for upper and lower airway obstruction.

Long explanation

Airway obstruction is a medical emergency. It may occur at any point from the mouth, pharynx, larynx and trachea to the bronchi. In ventilated patients, obstruction may involve ventilator valves, tubing, HME filters, endotracheal tubes or tracheostomies (intraluminal or displaced) as well as the patient's airway. Causes are legion, but include trauma, choking, reduced level of consciousness, reduced pharyngeal muscle tone, epiglottitis, angioedema, post-surgical haematoma, burns, fibrosis, asthma and secretions.

Clinical features of upper airway obstruction include snoring, stridor, gurgling or silence, the use of expiratory muscles, tracheal tug or paradoxical 'seesaw' movements of chest and abdomen. Patients with airway obstruction are commonly in respiratory distress with tachycardia and hypertension, although reduced level of consciousness may be seen as either a cause or an effect of obstruction.

Lower airway obstruction may present with wheeze, coughing, hyperexpansion, use of accessory muscles and respiratory distress. In the ventilated patient, airway obstruction may present as reduced volumes or increased airway pressures, reduced expansion, hypercapnia, hypoxia or wheeze.

Management is divided between general supportive measures and treatments specific to underlying causes. Oxygen therapy is mandatory. Basic airway manoeuvres, airway adjuncts, supraglottic airways and tracheal intubation may all be required. Experienced help should always be sought.

Disease-specific treatments include continuous positive airway pressure (CPAP) for partial upper airway obtruction (e.g. sleep apnoea); abdominal thrusts (Heimlich manoeuvre) in choking; gaseous induction of anaesthesia for epiglottitis; intramuscular epinephrine for anaphylactic angioedema; heliox for upper and lower airway obstruction.

Resuscitation Council (UK). *Advanced Life Support*, 6th edn. London: Resuscitation Council, 2011.

Yentis SM, Hirsch NP, Smith GB. *Anaesthesia and Intensive Care A–Z*, 4th edn. London: Churchill Livingstone, 2009.

Question C10: Transfer of antibiotic resistance

Which of these statements about the transfer of antibiotic resistance between organisms are correct?

A. Naked DNA from killed bacteria is a common way for resistance to be transferred between organisms on the ICU
B. Plasmids are an unusual route for transfer of genetic information between bacteria on the ICU
C. Conjugation is the process through which resistance is transferred between bacteria via bacteriophages
D. Transposons can be independently mobile
E. Bacteria have a variable susceptibility to infection with bacteriophages

Answer: TFFTT

Short explanation

Plasmids are a very common route for transfer of resistance between bacteria on the ICU. Conjugation refers to a process by which genetic information is transferred between bacteria via plasmids. Bacteriophages can also transfer genetic information between bacteria, but this is termed transduction.

Long explanation

Evidence shows that prior to antibiotic use bacteria were 100% susceptible to appropriate antibiotics. Resistance emerged early in the history of antibiotic use and now presents one of the most important challenges to physicians in critical care. Transfer of resistance between organisms occurs frequently, by a number of means. This is also termed horizontal gene transfer (HGT).

Transformation is the process by which naked DNA from killed bacteria is transferred and incorporated into different bacteria. This is common in patients on antibiotics on the ICU, although the DNA is unstable and quickly degraded if not incorporated into a host genome. Meningococci and streptococci are two clinically relevant strains of organisms which acquire resistance by transformation.

Transduction occurs when bacteriophages infect bacteria. Bacteriophages are viruses that only infect bacteria, and their DNA can be incorporated into the host genome. Not all bacteria are susceptible to infection from bacteriophages.

Conjugation is the process by which circles of DNA, called plasmids, transfer genetic material. They cannot live independently of the bacteria but are self-replicating. Plasmid transfer is the commonest way for resistance to spread between bacteria. Transposons are small pieces of DNA and code for their own mobility, which allows them to move between plasmids or within the main genotype. Integrons are gene acquisition units present in many bacterial genomes; they propagate the transfer of genetic material, in particular resistance genes.

Davies J, Davies D. Origins and evolution of antibiotic resistance. *Microbiol Mol Biol Rev* 2010; 74: 417–33.

Varley AJ, Williams H, Fletcher S. Antibiotic resistance in the intensive care unit. *Contin Educ Anaesth Crit Care Pain* 2009; 9: 114–18.

Question C11: Acute confusion

In the initial assessment of a patient who appears acutely confused:

A. Capillary blood glucose level should be measured early in the assessment
B. Hyponatraemia should be urgently corrected if the patient is acutely agitated
C. If meningitis is strongly suspected, CT head is not required before lumbar puncture
D. Consent should be sought from relatives for invasive procedures
E. Benzodiazepines are the first-line drugs for the management of an agitated patient

Answer: TFFFF

Short explanation

Hyponatraemia should be corrected slowly, based on estimation of total body sodium. Hypertonic saline should only be used in patients with severe hyponatraemia and/or seizures. CT head should be performed before lumbar puncture in all patients. Consent cannot be given by relatives, and patients who lack capacity should be treated in line with their best interests. Benzodiazepines increase the risk of delirium.

Long explanation

The approach to the patient who presents with acute confusional state should be structured and meticulous. Hypoxia and hypercarbia can be diagnosed early in the assessment. Primary CNS pathology should be considered in the first instance. Vascular accidents and CNS infection should be actively excluded as a cause of confusion. This will require an urgent CT head, which may or may not require sedation (usually in the form of intubation and ventilation). If there is evidence to suggest meningitis or encephalitis then broad-spectrum antibiotics should be commenced immediately with the advice of the local microbiology team. Lumbar puncture may be indicated, but anticoagulation or radiological or clinical evidence of raised intracranial pressure will contraindicate this.

Sedation of confused patients is a controversial area, and the patient should only be sedated if it is in his or her best interests. Benzodiazepines should be avoided, as they are associated with increased delirium. Formal anaesthesia and ventilation is usually safer than sedation, where protection of the airway may be compromised. Plasma glucose level should also be performed early in the assessment, as hypoglycaemia can occur in patients taking insulin or those taking oral hypoglycaemic agents such as gliclazide.

Other electrolyte abnormalities which commonly cause acute confusion include hyponatraemia. The actual sodium value is less important than the clinical presentation or the rate of decrease in the sodium level. Hypertonic saline should be reserved for patients who have life-threatening hyponatraemia (< 119 mmol/l) or those who are having seizures. In addition, it should be administered based on advice of the local biochemistry team or renal team. The cause of the hyponatraemia should be actively sought and all contributing drugs withheld. The sodium should be corrected slowly over 24–48 hours, and ideally no more than 0.5 mmol/l per hour.

Girard T, Jackson J, Pandharipande P, *et al.* Delirium as a predictor of long-term cognitive impairment in survivors of critical illness. *Crit Care Med* 2010; 38: 1513–20.

Question C12: Microbiological surveillance

Regarding microbiological surveillance in critical care:

A. Its aim is to guide prophylactic antibiotic use
B. Its aim is to identify pre-existing infections
C. Its aim is to identify bacterial colonisation of patients
D. Its aim is to collate national data on healthcare-associated infections (HCAIs)
E. Its aim is to guide antimicrobial treatment protocols

Answer: FTTTT

Short explanation

Prophylactic antibiotic use is not generally recommended as routine care in critically ill patients. Microbiological surveillance is a wide-reaching audit and data collection exercise aimed at reducing risk and improving patient care.

Long explanation

Surveillance is the ongoing, systematic collection, analysis and interpretation of information related to health. Microbiological surveillance is a wide-reaching audit and data collection exercise aimed at reducing risk and improving patient care. Patients are screened for infection on admission to intensive care, and any subsequent infections are subjected to culture and sensitivity tests. This allows the identification of bacterial colonisation (e.g. MRSA) which may develop into infection in susceptible patients. It also allows a map of resistance to be built up for individual units, national healthcare systems and international public health studies.

Prophylactic antibiotic therapy is rarely recommended, but there is evidence that targeted antibiotic therapy based on the commonest organisms found in a unit and known resistance patterns improves outcomes. Identification of pre-existing infections and bacterial colonisation allows not only treatment of that patient but procedures for isolation and containment of the pathogen, where appropriate. Data on healthcare-associated infections (HCAIs) is collated by Public Health England (previously the Health Protection Agency).

Inweregbu K, Dave J, Pittard A. Nosocomial Infections. *Contin Educ Anaesth Crit Care Pain* 2005; 5: 14–17.

Loveday HP, Wilson JA, Pratt RJ, *et al*. epic3: national evidence based guidelines for preventing healthcare-associated infections in NHS hospitals in England. *J Hosp Infect* 2014; 86 (Suppl 1): S1–70.

Question C13: Status epilepticus

Regarding status epilepticus (SE):

A. It is defined as generalised tonic–clonic seizure activity for > 30 minutes, continuously or without intervening periods of consciousness
B. It has a hospital mortality rate > 10%
C. Neurological damage is unlikely to occur until seizure activity has lasted 30 minutes
D. First-line therapy is phenytoin 20 mg/kg
E. Buccal administration of benzodiazepine is likely to prove ineffective

Answer: FTFFF

Short explanation

SE is seizure activity for 30 minutes, either continuously or without intervening recovery to baseline. It may be generalised convulsive (GCSE) or non-convulsive (NCSE). Hospital mortality is 10–20% for GCSE and 18–50% for NCSE. Neuronal damage can occur with much less than 30 minutes of seizure activity. Benzodiazepines are first-line therapy for seizure control. Nasal, buccal, intramuscular and rectal routes are all effective in the absence of intravenous access (preferred route).

Long explanation

Status epilepticus (SE) is a medical emergency. It is defined as seizure activity lasting for > 30 minutes, either continuously or without intervening recovery to baseline. SE may be generalised convulsive (GCSE) with tonic–clonic activity and impaired consciousness, or non-convulsive (NCSE) with subclinical seizure activity and normal or impaired consciousness. While GCSE poses more of an immediate threat to life, its hospital mortality rate (9–20%) is significantly lower than that of NCSE (18–52%).

Traditional definitions of seizure activity lasting longer than 30 minutes were based on evidence of neuronal damage occurring within this timeframe. However, recent data suggest that neuronal damage may occur much earlier, and many advocate the reduction of the defining seizure period to 5 minutes.

Underlying causes of SE may be categorised as acute or chronic processes. Acute causes include metabolic disturbance, trauma, sepsis, stroke, drugs and hypoxia. Chronic causes include pre-existing epilepsy (worsening or following changes to therapy), alcohol use or withdrawal and CNS disease (tumours, previous trauma or stroke). Acute processes may serve as triggers in patients with pre-existing chronic causes.

There are multiple initial management aims. Airway support and control (intubation often required), intravenous access and immediate termination of the seizure are initial priorities, followed by investigation of the cause and prevention of further seizures. First-line therapy for seizure termination is a benzodiazepine, preferably intravenous lorazepam, although buccal midazolam and rectal diazepam may be equally effective and should be used if a significant delay to establishing intravenous access is anticipated. Antiepileptic medications should be administered early unless an easily remedial cause is found (e.g. hypoglycaemia). Sodium valproate, phenytoin, levetiracetam, phenobarbital and continuous midazolam infusions are all recommended for initial control.

If seizure activity continues despite first-line management, further antiepileptic agents should be added in accordance with patient-specific factors (prior antiepileptic therapy, likely aetiology, type of seizure) and local protocols. Any of the first-line antiepileptic agents may be added until control is gained. Highly resistant SE may require full sedation with midazolam, propofol or thiopental while further investigation and definitive management occurs.

Brophy GM, Bell R, Claassen J, *et al*. Guidelines for the evaluation and management of status epilepticus. *Neurocrit Care* 2012; 17: 3–23.

Question C14: Hypoxaemia

With regards to the causes and recognition of hypoxaemia, which of the following are correct?

A. Anaemic patients will appear cyanosed at an earlier stage of hypoxaemia than patients with a normal haemoglobin concentration
B. The alveolar–arterial gradient is high in patients with pulmonary embolism
C. Lobar collapse is a common cause of shunt
D. Administration of supplemental oxygen will not be beneficial in shunt
E. Hypoxaemia due to large pulmonary embolus is usually accompanied by a normal or low $PaCO_2$

Answer: FTFFT

Short explanation

Anaemic patients appear cyanosed at a later stage of hypoxaemia, because the amount of deoxyhaemoglobin is reduced. Lobar collapse will not always cause shunt, given areduction in both ventilation and perfusion. Administration of oxygen can be beneficial in small shunts, as it will increase the dissolved oxygen content in the blood.

Long explanation

Cyanosis is the blue appearance of the skin and mucous membranes caused by the presence of elevated levels of deoxyhaemoglobin. Cyanosis is usually apparent once the deoxyhaemoglobin level reaches 5 g/dl. If a patient is anaemic, then cyanosis will not usually be apparent until the oxygen content is considerably lower than in a patient with a normal or high haemoglobin.

In patients with pulmonary embolism, blood flow is obstructed to part of the lung. This leads to a ventilation/perfusion defect, or dead space. The area without blood flow continues to be ventilated but not perfused. The smaller surface area for gas exchange leads to a reduction in the PaO_2. Compensatory hyperventilation usually ensures that $PaCO_2$ is low or normal.

There are different types of shunt, including extra- and intrapulmonary shunt. Extrapulmonary shunt refers to a range of cardiac conditions such as septal defects. Intrapulmonary shunt describes a situation where an area of the lung is perfused but not ventilated. This means that some blood leaves the lung still in a deoxygenated state and will mix with oxygenated blood, resulting in hypoxaemia. Administration of oxygen may improve the oxygenation of the blood which takes part in gas exchange by a small amount by increasing the amount of oxygen dissolved in plasma (as haemoglobin will already be fully saturated). This improvement is usually negligible and will not be clinically relevant in normal clinical settings. It can be relevant if the shunt is extremely large, if there is severe anaemia, or if the patient is in a hyperbaric chamber (where dissolved oxygen content will be increased). Shunt is seen in pneumonia, drowning and pulmonary oedema. When there is lobar collapse present this does not always lead to a state of shunt, as both ventilation and perfusion are impaired. In practice, however, there is often some blood flow to the collapsed lung, leading to a variable degree of shunt.

McLellan S, Walsh T. Oxygen delivery and haemoglobin. *Contin Educ Anaesth Crit Care Pain* 2004; 4: 123–6.

Question C15: Intraosseous access in adults

With regards to the use of the intraosseous (IO) route of access in adults, which of the following are correct?

A. The EZ-IO access device is battery-powered
B. The Big Injection Gun (BIG) device is designed for sternal access
C. Intravenous infusion pumps are a useful way of administering fluid via the IO route
D. The humerus provides a reliable, well-protected IO access site
E. The FAST 1 access device is manually powered

Answer: TFFFT

Short explanation

The FAST 1 access device is the only one currently licensed for sternal access in the UK. Intravenous infusion pumps will often alarm and not work effectively, because of the high pumping pressure required for infusion via IO access devices. The humeral access point is more exposed and prone to dislodgement, particularly during resuscitation.

Long explanation

The use of intraosseous (IO) access in adults has become more common in recent years, mainly due to the introduction of specialist handheld devices designed to make gaining this access easier. Previously, IO access was mainly restricted to children, whose softer bones made it is easier to obtain. But recent resuscitation guidelines have recommended IO access in the cardiac arrest scenario in adults, as the use of the transtracheal route for drug administration is no longer recommended.

There are three main devices currently used in clinical practice. The EZ-IO needles are battery-operated, and the depth of placement is controlled by the operator. It is licensed for use at three sites: the proximal tibia, the distal tibia and the proximal humerus. The BIG device is spring-loaded and licensed for use at two sites: the proximal tibia and the proximal humerus. The depth of insertion is set prior to use, depending on the site of access being used. The FAST 1 device is licensed for use in the sternum. The manubrium is the intended site of access, and this device is also manually activated. Blood flows from the sternum directly into the central veins via the internal mammary and azygos veins. All of these devices require familiarisation and training prior to use, but they are easy and quick to operate and their use is not restricted to physicians. In the military scenario they have been invaluable in recent conflicts.

Day M. Intraosseous devices for intravascular access in adult trauma patients. *Crit Care Nurse* 2011; 31: 76–81.

Resuscitation Council (UK). Use of intraosseous (IO) access during cardiac arrest. *Advanced Life Support*, Appendix D. http://www.resus.org.uk/pages/IOaccess.pdf (accessed June 2014).

Question C16: Positive-pressure ventilation

The physiological effects of positive-pressure ventilation include:

A. Increased portal venous pressure
B. A reduction in renal sodium and water excretion
C. Decreased intracerebral pressure
D. Increased ventilation in the non-dependent areas of the lung
E. A reduction in left ventricular end-diastolic volume

Answer: TTFTT

Short explanation

Positive-pressure ventilation, especially with the use of positive end-expiratory pressure (PEEP), will increase intracranial pressure.

Long explanation

The physiological effects of positive-pressure ventilation include the following:

Respiratory system

There is increased ventilation of the non-dependent areas of the lung, which are more compliant in the supine position. Combined with an alteration in the perfusion pattern of the lungs, with increased perfusion in the dependent areas, positive-pressure ventilation can lead to a significant ventilation/perfusion mismatch.

Cardiovascular system

Increased intrathoracic pressure impedes venous return and causes a reduction in preload and therefore both right and left ventricular end-diastolic volume. Pulmonary vascular resistance increases with hypoxic pulmonary vasoconstriction and atelectasis therefore it may be reduced by appropriate ventilation strategies. However, if the capillary pressure is exceeded by the alveolar pressure (e.g. overinflation) then the blood vessels collapse and pulmonary vascular resistance will increase. With an increase in pulmonary vascular resistance the right ventricle may fail.

In patients with existing heart failure, positive-pressure ventilation may improve the heart's function by reducing the preload and therefore left ventricular end-diastolic volume, placing the heart on a more favourable part of the Starling curve. Afterload may also be reduced as the positive pressure is transmitted through the heart, effectively reducing left ventricular wall tension and thereby decreasing the work of the heart.

Hepatic

The reduction in cardiac output leads to a fall in hepatic arterial supply. The venous congestion associated with increased intrathoracic pressure causes an increase in portal venous pressure, and may impede flow if severe.

Renal

The reduction in cardiac output and mean arterial pressure is sensed by arterial baroreceptors, increasing sympathetic output and antidiuretic hormone release. The renin–angiotensin system is activated by the reduction in renal blood flow. Aldosterone secretion leads to sodium and water retention, assisted by a reduction in atrial natriuretic peptide release (reduced venous return and atrial stretch).

Central nervous system

Autoregulation normally regulates cerebral perfusion pressure to counteract the increase in intracranial pressure from the reduction in jugular venous flow due to increased intrathoracic pressures. Brain injury may disrupt this, and therefore positive-pressure ventilation must be used with caution in these patients.

Gould T, de Beer JMA. Principles of artificial ventilation. *Anaesth Intensive Care Med* 2007; 8: 91–101.

Waldmann C, Soni N, Rhodes A. *Oxford Desk Reference: Critical Care*. Oxford: Oxford University Press, 2008; pp. 8–9.

Question C17: Weaning from mechanical ventilation

When considering a T-piece trial to wean a patient from mechanical ventilation, the following physiological parameters may predict successful weaning:

A. Frequency/tidal volume ratio of < 100 seconds/litre
B. PaO_2/FiO_2 > 27.5 kPa
C. Maximum inspiratory pressure of −15 cmH_2O
D. Vital capacity > 8 ml/kg
E. Static lung compliance with inspiratory pressure of 30 cmH_2O giving a tidal volume of > 10 ml/kg

Answer: TTFFF

Short explanation

Predicting successful weaning from mechanical ventilation is very difficult, but physiological parameters associated with successful weaning include a maximum inspiratory pressure of −20 to −25 cmH_2O, a vital capacity > 10 ml/kg and a static lung compliance where an inspiratory pressure of < 30 cmH_2O gives a tidal volume of > 8 ml/kg.

Long explanation

Weaning from mechanical ventilation describes the transition between full ventilatory support and spontaneous breathing, and the removal of any artificial airway. Prolonged ventilation is problematic for both the patient, with increased morbidity and mortality, and for organisational reasons (increased length and cost of stay, consumption of resources).

Many parameters have been studied as predictors of weaning success, with the aim of identifying patients who are ready to wean and excluding those who are not. Studies looking at the incidence of unplanned extubation have shown that almost half of patients who are being weaned who self-extubate do not require reintubation. This suggests that in some cases we prolong the period of ventilation unnecessarily. Equally, there is a significant mortality associated with failure of extubation, either because this selects the highest-risk patients in whom extubation was not appropriate, or because of events associated with failure and reintubation, such as aspiration, atelectasis and pneumonia.

Generally speaking, weaning will only occur successfully when the capacity of the respiratory system exceeds the load on it. Cardiovascular and neurological diseases also play an important part in assessing the patient's capacity for unassisted ventilation. The underlying condition that necessitated ventilation in the first place should be resolved or improving.

Respiratory parameters
Respiratory parameters associated with successful weaning include:

- frequency/tidal volume ratio on trial disconnection of < 100 seconds/litre
- $FiO_2 < 0.5$
- tidal volume > 5 ml/kg
- vital capacity > 10 ml/kg
- PEEP < 8 cmH_2O
- $PaO_2/FiO_2 > 20$ kPa (150 mmHg)
- $SaO_2 > 90\%$
- static lung compliance: inspiratory pressure < 30 mmHg for a tidal volume of > 8 ml/kg
- maximum inspiratory pressure of −20 to −25 cmH_2O
- adequate cough and not excessive secretions

Of these, probably the most reliable is the frequency/tidal volume ratio, which has a sensitivity of 97% and a specificity of 65%.

Cardiovascular parameters
- heart rate < 120 bpm
- stable blood pressure (with or without inotropes and vasopressors)
- lactate not elevated

Neurological parameters
- no evidence of severe critical illness myopathy
- awake and cooperative patients
- adequate analgesia

Nutritional parameters
- adequate nutrition
- normal phosphate and potassium levels

Boles JM, Bion J, Connors A, *et al*. Weaning from mechanical ventilation. Statement of the Sixth International Consensus Conference on Intensive Care Medicine. *Eur Respir J* 2007; 29: 1033–56.
Intensive Care Society. Weaning guidelines. http://www.ics.ac.uk/ics-homepage/guidelines-standards (accessed June 2014).
Waldmann C, Soni N, Rhodes A. *Oxford Desk Reference: Critical Care*. Oxford: Oxford University Press, 2008; pp.16–17.

Question C18: Base excess

Regarding the measurement of base excess:

A. Base excess refers to the amount of acid or base (in mmol) required to restore 1 litre of blood to normal pH at 21 °C
B. It is inaccurate in the presence of a respiratory acidosis
C. Normal base excess is −2 to +2 mmol/l

D. It is an in-vivo test
E. The base excess is calculated with an assumed $PaCO_2$ of 5.3 kPa

Answer: FFTFT

Short explanation

The base excess or deficit refers to the amount of acid or base (in mmol) required to restore 1 litre of blood to normal pH at a $PaCO_2$ of 5.3 kPa (40 mmHg) at body temperature. It is unaffected by a respiratory acidosis and is an in-vitro test.

Long explanation

The base excess or deficit refers to the amount of acid or base (in mmol) required to restore 1 litre of blood to normal pH at a $PaCO_2$ of 5.3 kPa (40 mmHg) at body temperature. It is a useful measure of the severity of a metabolic acidosis or alkalosis and may be used to guide bicarbonate replacement.

It is based on the assumption that the blood behaves as a simple bicarbonate buffer system and is therefore unaffected by a respiratory acidosis, as carbon dioxide dissociates into equal amounts of hydrogen and bicarbonate ions.

The main limitation of the base excess system is that it is an in-vitro test that takes no account of non-bicarbonate intravascular buffers or the role of intracellular and extracellular fluid compartments.

Power I, Kam P. Acid–base physiology. In *Prinicples of Physiology for the Anaesthetist*, 2nd edn. London: Hodder Arnold; pp. 251–68.

Question C19: Defibrillation threshold

In the treatment of shockable rhythms the 'defibrillation threshold' is the amount of current required to produce defibrillation. Factors affecting the defibrillation threshold include:

A. Acidosis
B. Positive end-expiratory pressure (PEEP)
C. Amiodarone
D. Electrode polarity with a biphasic defibrillator, but not with a monophasic defibrillator
E. QRS width

Answer: TTTFT

Short explanation

Factors affecting the defibrillation threshold include the underlying cardiac condition and the characteristics of the rhythm; transthoracic impedence (increased with increasing lung volume and PEEP); medication, including amiodarone; and metabolic disturbance. Electrode polarity is of less significance with biphasic than with monophasic defibrillators.

Long explanation

The current required to produce myocardial defibrillation is known as the 'defibrillation threshold'. It is expressed in terms of joules, and it determines whether a delivered shock will be successful in cardioverting the abnormal rhythm. The lowest energy possible is used for shocks, as higher energy is associated with myocardial damage.

The factors affecting the defibrillation threshold include:

- Electrode position: this can increase or decrease cardiothoracic impedance by extending or reducing the pathway to the myocardium. With monophasic defibrillators the polarity of the shock may also be relevant, so the position of the paddles should be guided by the manufacturer's recommendations. For biphasic devices this is of less importance.
- Shock impedance: with the use of hands-free 'sticky' paddles, the interface between paddles and chest is of less importance unless the patient is particularly hairy or the skin is wet. Transthoracic impedance depends on lung volume and tissue thickness. Lung volume is increased by PEEP.
- Charge characteristics: biphasic defibrillators are associated with lower defibrillation thresholds and lower post-shock myocardial depression than monophasic defibrillators. The inductor in the defibrillator circuit is designed to alter the time and profile of the current for maximal effect.
- Cardiac condition: the longer the time spent in VF or VT prior to defibrillation, and the more severe the cardiac disease underlying the arrhythmia, the less the chance of successful defibrillation. The wider the QRS complex, the less likely that defibrillation will cardiovert an abnormal rhythm.
- Metabolic disturbance: defibrillation thresholds are increased by hypoxia and acidosis.
- Drugs: acutely, amiodarone will decrease defibrillation thresholds, but chronically it will increase them. Fentanyl also decreases debrillation thresholds.

Davey AJ, Diba A. *Ward's Anaesthetic Equipment*, 5th edn. Philadephia, PA: Elsevier Saunders, 2005; pp. 474–7.

Resuscitation Council (UK). Defibrillation. In *Advanced Life Support*, 6th edn. London: Resuscitation Council, 2011; Chapter 9.

Question C20: Oesophageal Doppler monitoring of cardiac output

Cardiac output (CO) monitoring using oesophageal Doppler monitoring (ODM):

A. Uses frequency shifts in reflected sound waves to estimate flow velocity
B. Will overestimate values of stroke volume (SV) and CO if the probe is poorly positioned
C. Can be used in children
D. Does not measure blood flow to the head or arms
E. Requires measurement or estimation of aortic cross-sectional area

Answer: TFTTT

Short explanation

ODM measures shifts in the frequency of reflected sound waves to estimate flow velocity in the descending thoracic aorta (and thus does not measure blood flow to the heart, head or arms). It can be used in children and adults. Poor probe position underestimates values of SV and CO. The aortic diameter is required to calculate SV. This may be measured or estimated using demographic and physical data.

Long explanation

The ODM is a device used to monitor CO in adults and children. An ultrasound transducer is placed in the oesophagus, usually in sedated patients, adjacent to the descending aorta. The transducer is set at an angle and must be rotated and moved to achieve an optimal aortic signal. Ultrasound waves are emitted from the transducer, reflected by erythrocytes in the descending aorta and detected again by the transducer. The frequency of the reflected sound waves will be altered in proportion to the velocity of the erythrocytes relative to the probe, in accordance with the Doppler effect. The frequency shift can be used to calculate the velocity of blood cells, using the following equation, where c is the speed of sound in the body and θ is the probe angle:

$$\text{Velocity} = (c \times \text{Doppler shift frequency}) / (\text{transmitted frequency} \times 2 \cos \theta)$$

The velocity of the blood cells divided by the time for each heartbeat gives the stroke distance: the distance travelled by the blood in each stroke. Multiplication of the stroke distance by the cross-sectional area of the aorta gives a value for stroke volume (SV). Some ODM probes measure the aortic area with ultrasound, while others use an estimate based on demographic and physical data. ODM has been validated in many studies and shown to have accuracy for CO measurement and change tracking at clinically acceptable levels, with similar results to other minimally invasive CO monitors.

There are sources of error in ODM. Probe positioning is crucial for accurate data, but is done blind. Poor positioning underestimates values of SV and CO. Secondly, only blood flow in the descending thoracic aorta is measured. A correction factor is applied to estimate total CO from this, but this assumes that the partition of blood between the carotid/subclavian arteries and the rest of the body remains constant. In fact, fluid resuscitation may be disproportionately redistributed to the carotid arteries.

Marik PE. Noninvasive cardiac output monitors: a state-of-the-art review. *J Cardiothorac Vasc Anaesth* 2013; 27: 121–34.

Question C21: Vancomycin-resistant enterococci

Vancomycin-resistant enterococci (VREs):

A. Are associated with increased mortality in critically ill patients
B. Have a higher virulence than sensitive enterococci
C. Most commonly present in intensive care as a urinary tract infection
D. Are associated with central venous catheters
E. Are more likely to be *Enterococcus faecium* than *Enterococcus faecalis*

Answer: FFFTT

Short explanation

VREs are not associated with increased mortality when severity of illness is accounted for. They have the same virulence as vancomycin-sensitive enterococci. They more commonly present as abdominal infections or bacteraemias in intensive care.

Long explanation

Vancomycin-resistant enterococci (VREs) were identified in 1986 in France but are now found worldwide. Enterococci are part of the normal bowel flora and generally have low virulence, only causing serious infections in the immune-compromised or chronically ill patient. Infection with enterococci is associated with increased morbidity and mortality, but the role of vancomycin resistance is less clear. VREs are no more virulent than vancomycin-sensitive enterococci, and studies so far have failed to show increased mortality or morbidity when comorbidities and illness severity have been corrected for. Infection with a VRE is, however, associated with a longer hospital and ICU stay.

Enterococcus faecalis and *E. faecium* are the most common enterococci of clinical significance. Of these, *E. faecalis* infection is more common, but *E. faecium* is more likely to be vancomycin-resistant. *Enterococcus* infection in the community commonly presents as urinary tract or peritoneal cavity infections. In intensive care bacteraemias, particularly associated with indwelling catheters, abdominal cavity infections or surgical wound infections, is the most common.

Niederman MS. Impact of antibiotic resistance on clinical outcomes and the cost of care. *Crit Care Med* 2001; 29(4) (Suppl.): N114–20.

Varley AJ, Williams H, Fletcher S. Antibiotic resistance in the intensive care unit. *Contin Educ Anaesth Crit Care Pain* 2009; 9: 114–18.

Waldmann C, Soni N, Rhodes A. *Oxford Desk Reference: Critical Care*. Oxford: Oxford University Press, 2008; pp. 228–9.

Question C22: Therapeutic hypothermia after cardiac arrest

With regards to the use of therapeutic hypothermia in patients who have had a cardiac arrest, which of the following are correct?

A. Current recommendations advise cooling patients to 30–32 °C for 24 hours following an out-of-hospital cardiac arrest due to ventricular fibrillation
B. The risk of sepsis is increased following therapeutic hypothermia
C. There is good evidence for beneficial effects from therapeutic hypothermia following in-hospital PEA cardiac arrest
D. Patients should be rewarmed to normothermia over a period of at least 12 hours
E. The number needed to treat to prevent unfavourable neurological outcome at 6 months after cardiac arrest is 6

Answer: FTFTT

Short explanation

Current recommendations advise cooling patients to 32–34 °C. Temperatures lower than this can cause cardiac arrhythmias. The evidence to support therapeutic hypothermia following PEA cardiac arrest is less strong, as the studies do not include large numbers of patients.

Long explanation

The risk of neurological morbidity following survival from cardiac arrest is a significant concern to both patients and healthcare providers. The incidence of cardiac arrest in Europe is estimated at 375,000 annually. With survival rates following out-of hospital (OOH) cardiac arrest being targeted by government campaigns, increasing availability of defibrillators in the community and standardised resuscitation protocols, it is important to ensure that any opportunity to improve the neurological outcome of survivors is maximised.

The mechanism for neurological damage following cerebral hypoxia is multifaceted. The so-called cerebral reperfusion injury is mediated by increased levels of intracellular glutamate, increased intracellular calcium and accumulation of oxygen free radicals. Altered cerebral haemodynamics probably also play a part. Many ways of reducing neurological damage in these patients have been studied, including corticosteroid administration, thiopental and nimodipine. Therapeutic hypothermia has shown the most promising and reproducible results for reducing neurological morbidity following cardiac arrest. The use of therapeutic hypothermia in patients following OOH cardiac arrest was first recommended by the Advanced Life Support (ALS) Task Force of the International Liaison Committee on Resuscitation (ILCOR) in 2003:

> Unconscious adult patients with spontaneous circulation after out-of-hospital cardiac arrest should be cooled to 32 °C to 34 °C for 12 to 24 hours when the initial rhythm was ventricular fibrillation (VF).

The most recent Cochrane meta-analysis included three studies, giving a total of 481 patients, and concluded that the quality of the studies was good and overall results were in agreement with the individual studies: that mild hypothermia improves neurological recovery and reduces mortality following cardiac arrest, with no statistically significant increased risk of adverse events. The evidence is predominantly for OOH cardiac arrest with either VF or VT as the primary rhythm disturbance. The numbers for other types of cardiac arrest were deemed too small to be commented upon.

Arrich J, Holzer M, Havel C, Müllner M, Herkner H. Hypothermia for neuroprotection in adults after cardiopulmonary resuscitation. *Cochrane Database Syst Rev* 2012; (9): CD004128.

Nolan JP, Morley PT, Vanden Hoek TL, *et al.* Therapeutic hypothermia after cardiac arrest: an advisory statement by the Advanced Life Support Task Force of the International Liaison Committee on Resuscitation. *Circulation* 2003; 108: 118–21.

Question C23: Coagulopathy after transfusion

Coagulopathy following blood transfusion:

A. May be dilutional in nature
B. Is avoided by the use of whole blood
C. Requires the use of cryoprecipitate if the fibrinogen level is < 2 g/l
D. Should be treated on the basis of laboratory coagulation tests
E. Has become more common since the introduction of leucodepletion

Answer: TTFFF

Short explanation

A fibrinogen level of < 1 g/l should be treated with cryoprecipitate. Laboratory tests of coagulation are non-specific and time-consuming, and therefore clinical expertise and bedside testing should guide management in the acute stage. Coagulopathy due to transfusion reactions is less common since the advent of leucodepletion.

Long explanation

Coagulopathy usually occurs with massive transfusions and may be due to a number of factors. Dilutional coagulopathy occurs because packed red cells have little plasma present, so that there are few clotting factors present to replace those lost to haemorrhage. Coagulopathy may also be due to disseminated intravascular coagulation (DIC). DIC may develop as a direct result of massive haemorrhage or, rarely, as a result of a transfusion reaction. It is therefore not necessarily related to the amount of blood transfused. Leucodepletion of blood in the UK has resulted in fewer transfusion reactions, and the same process removes the microaggregates postulated to activate the haemostatic system with resulting DIC. Whole blood contains plasma and coagulation factors in normal quantities, so it will not cause a dilutional coagulopathy. However, it is not routinely used in the UK.

Cryoprecipitate is prepared from plasma that has been snap-frozen and then defrosted. It contains factors VIII and XIII, fibrinogen, von Willebrand factor and fibronectin. It is generally used to treat hypofibrinogenaemia. A fibrinogen level of < 1 g/l should be treated in the context of massive transfusion or ongoing haemorrhage.

Laboratory tests of coagulation are generally the prothrombin time (PT) and the activated partial thromboplastin time (APTT). These are crude and time-consuming assessments, and the results will be abnormal at a late stage of a coagulopathic process. The modern treatment of massive transfusion therefore centres around a more protocolised approach or the use of near-patient testing, e.g. thromboelastometry. The exact ratio of fresh frozen plasma (FFP) and platelet units to red cell units transfused is an ongoing area of research, but there is good evidence to start coagulation factor replacement as soon as massive haemorrhage is suspected. Any coagulopathy after blood transfusion will be worsened by hypothermia, so patients and any blood products they receive should be actively warmed.

British Committee for Standards in Haematology, Blood Transfusion Task Force. Guidelines for the use of fresh-frozen plasma, cryoprecipitate and cryosupernatant. *Br J Haematol* 2004; 126: 11–28.

Isbister JP. Blood transfusion. In Bersten AD, Soni N. *Oh's Intensive Care Manual*, 6th edn. Edinburgh: Butterworth-Heinemann, 2009; pp. 995–1010.

Question C24: Risk of acute kidney injury

Pharmacological strategies to reduce the risk of acute kidney injury in critically ill patients include:

A. *N*-acetyl-cysteine
B. Fenoldopam
C. Low-dose dopamine infusion
D. Vasopressin in preference to norepinephrine
E. Furosemide

Answer: TFFFF

Short explanation

Dopamine infusions and fenoldopam have not been shown to be nephroprotective in acute tubular necrosis or contrast-induced nephropathy. Furosemide does not improve outcome in renal failure in controlled trials. Vasopressin has not been shown to be superior to norepinephrine in trials.

Long explanation

Acute kidney injury (AKI) is a clinical syndrome with a spectrum of severity and multiple underlying aetiologies. Numerous trials have sought a pharmacological answer to modify the risk of patients developing AKI, but few have shown benefit.

Hypovolaemia and renal hypoperfusion are postulated as major contributing factors in AKI associated with sepsis, trauma and contrast-induced nephropathy. It follows, therefore, that judicious fluid resuscitation is of benefit in reducing AKI. Crystalloids are recommended as first-line fluid resuscitation fluids in the absence of bleeding, where blood products may be required. Colloids, particularly starches, have been shown to increase the incidence of renal impairment and should be avoided in the critically ill. There has been no difference in outcomes found between groups treated with human albumin solution versus saline solutions.

Maintaining an adequate perfusion to the kidney may also require the use of vasopressors and inotropes. No agent has been shown to be superior to another in reducing progression to AKI or renal failure. Low-dose dopamine infusions were popular in the 1990s, but have since been shown to be ineffective. Higher-dose dopamine infusions are associated with more adverse events such as arrhythmias. Fenoldopam is a dopamine A_1 agonist that did not show any nephroprotection in trials in septic patients. Furosemide reduces the metabolic requirements of the kidney; however, it is not nephroprotective, nor does it halt progression to renal failure. High-dose furosemide is associated with ototoxicity. *N*-acetyl-cysteine infusions may be of benefit in reducing the incidence of contrast-induced nephropathy, but are not useful in other causes of AKI.

KDIGO clinical practice guideline for acute kidney injury. *Kidney International Supplements* 2012; 2 (1): 8–27.

Waldmann C, Soni N, Rhodes A. *Oxford Desk Reference: Critical Care*. Oxford: Oxford University Press, 2008; pp. 312–15.

Question C25: ECG monitoring

Regarding 12-lead ECG monitoring:

A. Each lead combines the electrical signals from two or more electrodes
B. The leads display electrical signals in different directions across the heart
C. Leads I, II and III compare the arms and the left leg with a fourth reference electrode
D. The chest leads use a combined reference electrode from leads aVR, aVL and aVF
E. Leads aVR, aVL and aVF correspond to the signals from the limb electrodes

Answer: TTFTT

Short explanation

ECG leads display the voltage differences between two or more electrodes. The different leads display voltages in different vectors to provide information about different areas of the heart. Leads I, II and III display voltage differences between the three pairs of limb electrodes, whereas leads aVR, aVL and aVF display the signals from the limb electrodes to a composite of the other two. The precordial leads use a combined reference electrode from leads aVR, aVL and aVF.

Long explanation

Electrocardiography (ECG) is both an important part of standard monitoring in ICU (3-lead ECG) and a crucial diagnostic tool (12-lead ECG). The principles underlying both forms of ECG monitoring are the same. Cardiac electrical activity, in the form of depolarisation, originates in the sinoatrial node of the right atrium, spreads over the atria and passes via the atrioventricular node and Purkinjee fibres to the ventricles. Depolarisation causes a net change in electrical potential of around 100 mV, but attenuation and impedance by tissues reduces the signal received by ECG electrodes to 1–2 mV.

Leads are the displays of electrical voltage differences over time between two or more electrodes, although the term may be confused with the wires connecting the electrode to the machine. Each lead displays the voltage produced by the heart in various vectors, to allow examination of different parts of the heart. There are three standard leads, I, II and III, which are common to both 3-lead and 12-lead ECG monitoring. They are bipolar leads, in that the voltage difference between two electrodes is displayed. Lead I is the voltage difference between the left and right arms, lead II between left arm and left leg, and lead III between left leg and right arm.

The other leads are unipolar, which means they display the voltage difference between one electrode and a composite electrode formed by combining the signal from several electrodes. The augmented limb leads display the voltage difference between a limb electrode and the composite of the other two: so, for example, lead aVL uses the left arm electrode and the composite of the right arm and left foot electrodes. The chest leads V_1 to V_6 use the precordial electrodes and a composite of the three augmented limb leads.

Davis PD, Kenny GNC. *Basic Physics and Measurement in Anaesthesia*, 5th edn. London: Elsevier, 2005.

Question C26: Advanced Trauma Life Support

Concerning the Advanced Trauma Life Support (ATLS) style of assessment and management of a patient with multiple injuries, which of the following are correct?

A. The primary survey should be completed within the first 24 hours of admission to hospital
B. A brief history of the patient's allergies, medical history, medications, last meal and events surrounding the incident should be sought
C. Large-volume external haemorrhage should be dealt with before assessing the airway and cervical spine
D. Life-threatening chest injuries should be assessed and excluded or managed in the primary survey
E. If the patient is combative, the cervical collar and stabilisation can be removed safely

Answer: FTFTF

Short explanation

The primary survey should be carried out on first presentation to the emergency department and is designed to be completed within the first hour. The airway should always be assessed and established before management of the circulation. Combative patients may need a general anaesthetic to enable safe immobilisation of the cervical spine.

Long explanation

Management of the trauma patient has become an integral role for all critical care clinicians. Recent changes in the UK have resulted in the establishment of major trauma centres. However, patients with multiple injuries can and will continue to present to emergency departments in all hospitals. The ATLS approach to patients is now accepted worldwide as the gold standard of trauma care, allowing the standard of care to be consistent. The approach allows clinically trained staff to approach the patient in a systematic way, ensuring that life-threatening injuries are identified and dealt with earlier than less serious ones.

The airway, along with cervical spine control, is the priority. Rapid sequence induction with manual inline stabilisation should be considered for patients with a compromised airway. Front-of-neck airway access may be required if there is anatomical distortion or swelling. Life-threatening chest injuries such as airway obstruction, tension pneumothorax, massive haemothorax, open pneumothorax, flail segments with pulmonary contusion and cardiac tamponade should be excluded early. If there is suspicion or confirmation of these injuries, then appropriate management, for example chest-drain insertion, should be instigated immediately.

The circulation should be assessed at the same time as obtaining wide-bore intravenous access and sending bloods for cross-matching. Intravenous crystalloid boluses should be administered to all patients with evidence of hypovolaemia, remembering that hypotension is a late sign of shock in young fit patients. In a shocked patient, haemorrhage may be external or internal (intra-abdominal or from long-bone fractures) and should be stopped as early as possible by direct pressure, by splinting, or by emergency surgery such as damage-control laparotomy.

Committee on Trauma of the American College of Surgeons. *Advanced Trauma Life Support (ATLS) Manual*, 9th edn. Chicago, IL: ACS, 2012.

Question C27: Risk of electrocution

Regarding the risk of electrocution, which of the following are correct?

A. A current of 5 mA will cause ventricular fibrillation if applied directly to the myocardium
B. Direct current is less likely to cause ventricular fibrillation than alternating current
C. The muscles present the highest impedance to current flow when current is applied to the patient
D. As current frequency increases above 50 Hz the risk of ventricular fibrillation increases linearly
E. Microshock can occur when external ECG leads are applied to the chest

Answer: TTFFF

Short explanation

The skin presents the highest impedance to current flow when current is applied to a patient. The most lethal current frequency is 50 Hz. Microshock occurs when internal equipment comes into direct contact with the heart.

Long explanation

The risk of electrocution is potentially high in the operating theatre or intensive care unit, in view of the amount of electrical equipment used in close proximity to the patient. There are stringent safety requirements designed to reduce this risk and so there is a low reported incidence of patient harm from electrocution.

Current applied to the patient will flow through the patient if he or she is earthed. Different sizes of externally applied current will have different effects on the patient. 1 mA will cause tingling, 5 mA will cause pain, 15 mA will cause tonic muscle contraction and pain, 50 mA will cause tonic contraction of respiratory muscles and respiratory arrest, and 75–100 mA will cause ventricular fibrillation. The damage caused is also proportional to the duration of current application, the current pathway and the type of current. The direct current required to cause ventricular fibrillation is much higher than the alternating current. Mains current frequency (50 Hz) is the most lethal, and current frequencies much higher than this cause heating only.

The skin presents the highest impedance to flow. This impedance can be lowered if the skin is wet with sweat or inflamed. Microshock occurs when intracardiac equipment, such as a central line, comes into direct contact with the heart. In this situation current of only 100 μA will trigger ventricular fibrillation. This equipment must have almost undetectable current leakage in order to prevent harm to the patient.

Al-Shaikh B, Stacey S. *Essentials of Anaesthetic Equipment*, 3rd edn. London: Elsevier Churchill Livingstone, 2007; pp. 216–7.
Davis PD, Kenny GNC. *Basic Physics and Measurement in Anaesthesia*, 5th edn. London: Elsevier, 2005.

Question C28: Hand hygiene

Regarding hand hygiene:

A. Alcohol gel is effective against *Clostridium difficile* spores
B. Alcohol gels are not virucidal
C. The palms and thumbs are often missed areas when hand washing
D. Up to 40% of healthcare-associated infections (HCAIs) are prevented by adequate hand hygiene
E. Some alcohol gels are ineffective after repeated applications

Answer: FFFTT

Short explanation

Alcohol gels are virucidal but not effective against *Clostridium difficile* spores. The backs of the hands and the thumbs are often missed when hand washing.

Long explanation

Adequate hand hygiene is one of the most important preventive strategies against healthcare-associated infections (HCAIs). Up to 40% of HCAIs can be prevented by adequate hand hygiene. Hand hygiene can be achieved by hand washing with either soap or antibacterial formulations, or by the use of alcohol gels on socially clean hands.

In general there is no evidence to support the use of antibacterial hand-washing agents over soap for general decontamination of the hands. Antibacterial hand-washing agents should be used when preparing for sterile procedures to reduce the bacterial load on the hands, as gloves still allow some bacterial translocation.

Alcohol gels are bactericidal, fungicidal and virucidal but are not effective against *Clostridium difficile* spores and are not recommended in some outbreaks, such as norovirus. Some alcohol gels are ineffective after 10 applications, and therefore periodic hand washing throughout a shift is recommended.

Hand-washing technique is also important, as the backs of the hands, tips of the fingers, web spaces and thumbs are commonly missed areas. The wearing of rings and false nails is associated with a reduction in the effectiveness of hand hygiene and has been associated with transmission of infection.

Inweregbu K, Dave J, Pittard A. Nosocomial Infections. *Contin Educ Anaesth Crit Care Pain* 2005; 5: 14–17.
Loveday HP, Wilson JA, Pratt RJ, *et al.* epic3: national evidence based guidelines for preventing healthcare-associated infections in NHS hospitals in England. *J Hosp Infect* 2014; 86 (Suppl 1): S1–70.

Question C29: Hyponatraemia

Causes of hyponatraemia include:

A. Citalopram
B. Small-cell lung cancer
C. Conn's syndrome

D. Bacterial meningitis
E. Hyperthyroidism

Answer: TTFTF

Short explanation

Selective serotonin reuptake inhibitors (SSRIs) can cause hyponatraemia due to the syndrome of inappropriate antidiuretic hormone secretion (SIADH). Small-cell lung cancer can secrete ADH, resulting in hyponatraemia. Conn's syndrome is primary mineralocorticoid excess, leading to hypokalaemia, and does not cause hyponatraemia. Bacterial meningitis can result in SIADH. Hypothyroidism can cause hyponatraemia.

Long explanation

Hyponatraemia is one of the commonest electrolyte disturbances seen in hospital inpatients, particularly in critically ill adults. Most cases of hyponatraemia are mild (130–135 mmol/l) and they often resolve spontaneously when the patient's health improves or when the cause is removed. Severe cases of hyponatraemia (< 125 mmol/l) require urgent intervention, particularly if there are neurological signs (e.g. seizures) or if the sodium fall has been rapid.

The cause of hyponatraemia should be sought and treated if possible. Hyponatraemia is often seen in renal, hepatic and cardiac failure as part of the disease process, but there are some specific causes which should be excluded, such as drug-induced hyponatraemia. There are a number of commonly prescribed medications that can either be a primary cause or contribute to the development of hyponatraemia. Many of these drugs cause the syndrome of inappropriate antidiuretic hormone secretion (SIADH) or potentiate the action of ADH. Examples include selective serotonin reuptake inhibitors (SSRIs) and tricyclic antidepressants (TCAs) such as amitryptilline.

There are other causes of SIADH. Some cancers secrete ADH, particularly small-cell lung cancer. Central nervous system disorders are another cause of SIADH. This can include traumatic brain injury, CNS tumours, CNS bleeds and CNS infections such as meningitis. There are also many endocrine causes of hyponatraemia. Addison's disease or hypoadrenalism can cause hyponatraemia due to reduced potassium excretion and sodium reabsorption in the distal tubule.

Conn's syndrome is usually caused by a mineralocorticoid-producing adenoma and leads to excessive potassium losses and sodium retention in the distal tubule. The cause of hyponatraemia in patients with hypothyroidism is not fully understood but is likely to be a combination of both inappropriate ADH production and a reduction in the glomerular filtration rate (GFR).

Khan A, Nair S, Waldron J, Davies M, Heald A. Hypothyroidism and hyponatraemia: diagnostic relevance of ADH measurement. *Endocrine Abstracts* 2008; 15: 364.

Kumar S, Berl T. Sodium. *Lancet* 1998; 352: 220–8.

Thompson CJ. Hyponatraemia: new associations and new treatments. *Eur J Endocrinol* 2010; 162: S1–3.

Question C30: Peripheral tissue perfusion measurement

The following are direct measures of peripheral tissue perfusion:

A. Serum lactate levels
B. Central venous oxygen saturations ($ScvO_2$)
C. Capillary refill time (CRT)

D. Forearm-to-finger skin temperature gradient
E. Near-infrared spectroscopy (NIRS)

Answer: FFTTT

Short explanation

Serum lactate levels and $ScvO_2$ are commonly measured in the critically ill as indicators of tissue perfusion, but in fact reflect the mismatch between tissue oxygen delivery and demand and may be affected by other factors (e.g. increased lactate in hepatic failure). CRT, skin temperature gradients and NIRS are direct measures of peripheral perfusion.

Long explanation

A major goal in the monitoring of haemodynamic parameters in critical care is to detect tissue and organ hypoperfusion and hypoxia, and monitor the effects of treatment. Standard, universal monitoring (blood pressure, heart rate, pulse oximetry etc.) do not reflect tissue and organ perfusion, and therapeutic measures aimed at improving such parameters, for example vasoconstrictors for blood pressure, may worsen tissue hypoxia and metabolic acidosis.

Serum lactate levels are commonly measured in critical care and used as a guide for resuscitation. Elevated lactate levels are usually a result of tissue oxygen demands exceeding supply, either locally or globally. Serum lactate may also be raised in hepatic dysfunction, lymphoma, ethanol poisoning or use of drugs such as metformin, and as such it is an indirect measure of tissue perfusion. Similarly with $ScvO_2$ levels, which are reduced in states of relative tissue hypoperfusion, but may be normal or raised in septic shock due to shunting.

Direct measures of tissue perfusion may be based on clinical examination, body temperature gradients or optical measures. Clinical techniques include skin temperature, mottling or capillary refill time (CRT), which has been validated as a sensitive method of identifying early severe infections in children and predicting organ failure in adults (CRT > 4.5 s). Temperature gradients may be measured from ambient to skin, forearm to finger, or central to toe.

Optical monitoring of peripheral perfusion may use pulse oximetry or near-infrared spectroscopy (NIRS). Two absorption signals are detected by the pulse oximeter, static and pulsatile. The static component is due to absorption of light by bone, skin, venous blood, interstitial fluid and other tissues and is constant over time and usually discarded to arrive at the pulse oximetry reading. The pulsatile component is due to absorption by haemoglobin in arterial blood and varies with the cardiac cycle. The relative proportions of the two components are used to derive the peripheral perfusion index (PPI) by some pulse oximeters. NIRS uses the same principles of tissue absorption of electromagnetic radiation as pulse oximetry but has greater tissue penetration. Levels of haemoglobin, oxygen saturation and cytochrome aa3 redox state are monitored, and venous and arterial occlusion tests may also be employed. Correlation with other measures of perfusion has been shown to be good, but clinical validation of NIRS remains at an early stage.

Lima A, Bakker J. Noninvasive monitoring of peripheral perfusion. *Intensive Care Med* 2005; 31: 1316–26.

Rady M, Rivers E, Nowak R. Resuscitation of the critically Ill in the ED: responses of blood pressure, heart rate, shock index, central venous oxygen saturation, and lactate. *Am J Emerg Med* 1996; 14: 218–25.

Van Genderen ME, Van Bommel J, Lima A. Monitoring peripheral perfusion in critically ill patients at the bedside. *Curr Opin Crit Care* 2012; 18: 273–9.

Question C31: Echocardiography

With regards to the use of echocardiography on the intensive care unit, which of the following are correct?

A. Transducers are often made of PZT-5 crystals
B. Transoesophageal echocardiography uses higher-frequency transducers than transthoracic
C. A pericardial collection with a diameter > 1 cm is likely to be significant if cardiac tamponade is suspected
D. Transthoracic echocardiography is the investigation of choice for suspected endocarditis
E. Transthoracic echocardiography gives the best results in a ventilated patient

Answer: TTTFF

Short explanation

Transoesophageal echocardiography is the gold-standard investigation for suspected bacterial endocarditis, because of its superior resolution. Transthoracic echocardiography is often technically challenging in ventilated patients, because hyperinflation of the lung prevents passage of ultrasound beams through to the heart.

Long explanation

The use of echocardiography in the ICU has increased in recent years. Current training recommendations advise that intensive care trainees should consider undertaking a recognised training programme to acquire the skills to perform diagnostic transthoracic and transabdominal echocardiography. The technical skills are relatively easy to learn, but in order to be competent trainees need to perform many examinations and submit a logbook over a 2-year period.

There is some theoretical knowledge also required. Ultrasound generation is from a piezoelectric crystal which acts as a transducer. Higher-frequency ultrasound has higher resolution but penetrates tissues less deeply. Transoesophageal echocardiography is of a higher frequency to achieve higher-resolution images, as the ultrasound has a shorter distance to travel to the heart.

Echocardiography can be employed on the ICU for a variety of reasons. These include preload assessment in shocked patients, assessment of myocardial function, investigation of suspected cardiac tamponade, visualisation of right atrial, ventricular or pulmonary artery thrombus, assessment of valvular disease, diagnosis of left ventricular outflow tract obstruction, diagnosis of aortic dissection, and in trauma for assessment of thoracic or intra-abdominal injuries.

In a ventilated patient hyperinflation of the lungs, excessive PEEP or intrathoracic surgery can impair transthoracic image interpretation, and for this reason the preferred method in an intubated patient would be transoesophageal echocardiography.

Roscoe A, Strang T. Echocardiography in intensive care. *Contin Educ Anaesth Crit Care Pain* 2008; 8: 46–9.

Question C32: Tracheal drug administration

In the absence of intravenous access, these drugs should be administered tracheally, in the doses specified:

A. Epinephrine 3 mg
B. Atropine 3 mg
C. Bicarbonate 50 ml 8.4%

D. Amiodarone 300 mg
E. Naloxone 800 μg

Answer: FFFFF

Short explanation

The tracheal route of drug administration is no longer recommended even in the absence of intravenous access. A preferred method is intraosseous access. Amiodarone and bicarbonate are not suitable for tracheal administration in any case.

Long explanation

The endotracheal route is no longer recommended for drug administration. Instead, intraosseous (IO) access is preferred if intravenous (IV) access is not possible. This is because of unpredictable plasma concentrations when drugs are given via a tracheal tube, which means that the tracheal dose of most drugs is unknown and may be 3–10 times the IV dose. Some animal studies also suggest that the lower concentrations of epinephrine achieved when it is given via the trachea may produce transient β-adrenergic effects, which will cause hypotension and lower coronary artery perfusion pressure.

This advice is particularly relevant now that the use of supraglottic airways in resuscitation is increasing. Drug delivery via a supraglottic airway device is even less reliable and should not be done.

If IV access is difficult or impossible, IO access should be considered in both adults and children. There is evidence that IO injection of drugs achieves adequate plasma concentrations in a time similar to injection through a central venous catheter. Modern IO devices are simple and quick to use and have made this the second-line route of drug administration.

Drugs that used to be administered via tracheal tubes include epinephrine, atropine, lignocaine and naloxone. Calcium salts and bicarbonate are not suitable for administration at all via the tracheal route.

Deakin CD, Nolan JP, Soar J, *et al*. European Resuscitation Council Guidelines for Resuscitation 2010. Section 4: Adult advanced life support. *Resuscitation* 2010; 81: 1305–52.

Resuscitation Council (UK). Advanced life support algorithm. In *Advanced Life Support*, 6th edn. London: Resuscitation Council, 2011; Chapter 6.

Question C33: Abdominal compartment syndrome

Regarding intra-abdominal pressure monitoring, which of the following are correct?

A. The standard way of monitoring intra-abdominal pressure is via an intravesical catheter
B. An intra-abdominal pressure of < 20 mmHg is normal
C. Intra-abdominal compartment syndrome rarely requires surgical intervention
D. Following laparotomy, primary closure of the wound should always be attempted
E. Increased functional residual capacity leads to gas trapping in abdominal compartment syndrome

Answer: TFFFF

Short explanation

Normal intra-abdominal pressure should be < 12 mmHg. Abdominal compartment syndrome is defined as pressure > 20 mmHg. Surgical intervention is not infrequently required to decompress the abdomen. If the surgeon is struggling to close a laparotomy wound, then delayed closure should be considered. Functional residual capacity is reduced in abdominal compartment syndrome.

Long explanation

Abdominal compartment syndrome has long been recognised as a serious cause of morbidity in patients who are critically unwell. It most commonly occurs in patients with primary abdominal pathology such as haemorrhage, abdominal surgery, peritonitis and large hernia repairs. It can also occur in patients who have pathology elsewhere, such as burns or sepsis, and have received massive fluid resuscitation.

The balance between abdominal volume, compliance and pressure is complicated. Abdominal pressure is more affected by short-term changes in abdominal volume, such as following laparotomy. Normal intra-abdominal pressure is around 6 mmHg, and pressure greater than 12 mmHg is classed as intra-abdominal hypertension. Abdominal compartment syndrome is defined as a pressure of greater than 20 mmHg. Renal vein compression and reduction in systemic blood pressure leads to impaired renal function. Cardiac preload is reduced due to reduced venous return. The mechanical effects on the lungs include diaphragmatic splinting, reduced functional residual capacity, reduced compliance and high airway pressures.

Measurement of the abdominal compartment pressure should be undertaken in patients who are suspected of having compartment syndrome. An intravesical foley catheter is inserted and 50 ml of sterile fluid is instilled into the bladder. The pressure can be measured with a pressure transducer or by manometry (the level of the symphysis pubis is taken as zero). Management involves optimisation of cardiovascular and respiratory parameters in addition to renal support if required. Simple measures such as nasogastric decompression and prokinetics can be undertaken. Surgical decompression is often performed, but the exact timing depends on individual patient factors. If during a primary operation the surgeon is struggling to close the wound, then the compartment pressures should be measured during closure and consideration given to delaying closure.

Malbrain M, Cheatham M, Kirkpatrick A, *et al*. Results from the International Conference of Experts on Intra-abdominal Hypertension and Abdominal Compartment Syndrome. I. Definitions. *Intensive Care Med* 2006; 32: 1722–32.

Cheatham M, Malbrain M, Kirkpatrick A, *et al*. Results from the International Conference of Experts on Intra-abdominal Hypertension and Abdominal Compartment Syndrome. II. Recommendations. *Intensive Care Med* 2007; 33: 951–62.

Question C34: Hyperkalaemia

The following are ECG changes associated with hyperkalaemia:

A. Peaked P waves
B. Shortened PR interval
C. Widened QRS complexes
D. Peaked, inverted T waves
E. U waves

Answer: FFTFF

Short explanation

Hyperkalaemia often causes characteristic ECG changes. Mild hyperkalaemia is associated with tall, peaked T waves. Moderate hyperkalaemia is associated with small P waves, prolonged PR interval, widened QRS complexes and peaked T waves. Severe hyperkalaemia is associated with absent P waves, broad QRS complexes, progressing to sine wave pattern, ventricular fibrillation and asystole. U waves are associated with hypokalaemia.

Long explanation

Hyperkalaemia is a life-threatening emergency. Patients with hyperkalaemia are at great risk of fatal arrhythmias if not treated promptly. As serum potassium levels increase, there are often characteristic ECG changes which aid diagnosis. Some patients may have a normal ECG despite significant hyperkalaemia (e.g. long-term dialysis patients). Absence of ECG changes should not preclude prompt treatment.

The first ECG changes seen in mild hyperkalaemia (serum K^+ 5.5–6.5 mmol/l) are tall, peaked T waves, which may exceed the height of the preceding QRS complex. Moderate hyperkalaemia (serum K^+ 6.5–8.0 mmol/l) is associated with reduced size P waves, prolongation of the PR interval, widened QRS complexes and increasingly peaked T waves. Severe hyperkalaemia (serum $K^+ > 8.0$ mmol/l) is associated with absent P waves and broad QRS complexes, progressing to a sine wave pattern of activity, finally progressing to ventricular fibrillation and asystole.

Treatment of hyperkalaemia focuses initially on reducing the susceptibility of the myocardium to the increased potassium concentration, by administering calcium chloride or calcium gluconate. The next step is to attempt to move the potassium from the extracellular fluid to the intracellular fluid, using insulin and dextrose and nebulised salbutamol. The third step is to reduce the total amount of potassium in the body, by haemodialysis or haemofiltration, or by increasing its excretion by the kidney (using loop diuretics). Potassium absorption from the gastrointestinal tract may be reduced with the use of resins such as calcium resonium or sodium polystyrene sulfonate. Treatment of the underlying cause of the hyperkalaemia is also required.

Ahee P, Crowe AV. The management of hyperkalaemia in the emergency department. *Emergency Medicine Journal* 2000; 17: 188–91.

Webster A, Brady W, Morris F. Recognising signs of danger: ECG changes resulting from an abnormal serum potassium concentration. *Emerg Med J* 2002; 19: 74–7.

Question C35: Aminoglycoside antibiotics

Regarding the aminoglycoside antibiotics:

A. Peak levels correlate with toxicity
B. Trough levels correlate with toxicity
C. They are bacteriostatic
D. They exhibit good streptococcal cover
E. They exhibit no anaerobic activity

Answer: FTFFT

Short explanation

Aminoglycoside antibiotics are bactericidal, with no anaerobic cover and poor streptococcal cover. Trough levels correlate with toxicity.

Long explanation

The aminoglycoside antibiotics include gentamicin, tobramycin, amikacin and streptomycin. They are bactericidal antibiotics that block protein synthesis by binding to the bacterial 30S ribosomal RNA subunit. They also inhibit bacterial ribosomal translocation and disrupt the integrity of the bacterial cell membrane. They are active against Gram-negative bacilli but also *Enterococcus* and *Staphylococcus*, including MRSA. They only have limited cover for streptococci. They act synergistically with β-lactams and vancomycin but have no independent anaerobic activity.

They may produce nephro- and ototoxicity in a dose-dependent fashion. Peak levels correlate with efficacy, trough levels with toxicity. The risk is increased in renal failure and with the co-administration of loop diuretics. They may also cause muscle weakness due to a decrease in prejunctional release of acetylcholine.

Peck TE, Hill SA, Williams M. Antimicrobials. In *Pharmacology for Anaesthesia and Intensive Care*, 2nd edn. Cambridge: Cambridge University Press, 2006; pp. 311–35.

Question C36: Estimating the extent of burns

With regards to the calculation of the surface area of skin which is burnt, which of the following are correct?

A. The rule of nines is as useful in children as in adults
B. Calculations made on the first assessment are usually the most accurate
C. The area of a child's palm including the adducted fingers approximates 1% of body surface area
D. It is important to calculate the burnt area accurately
E. The whole of the anterior of the trunk in an adult approximates 9% of body surface area

Answer: FFTTF

Short explanation

The rule of nines is notoriously inaccurate in children. Calculations made on first assessment commonly underestimate the burnt area. The whole of the anterior of the trunk in an adult approximates 18% of body surface area.

Long explanation

There have been many proposed ways of accurately calculating the area of a patient's body surface area which is burnt. It has long been agreed that early accurate calculation is vital to ensure that fluid resuscitation and further treatment is appropriately administered. Adult patients with more than 15% burns, and children with more than 10%, should be referred to a regional burns centre. All patients with inhalational injury should also be referred. Most patients are assessed in the emergency department, often without the expertise of burn specialists.

Ways to assess burn area must be not only accurate but also quick and easy to apply. The Wallace 'rule of nines' has been used in the past. Areas of the body are divided up into areas of 9% or 18%. This is not accurate in children. The palmar surface method involves using the area of the patient's palm (including the adducted fingers). The size of the palm can be used to estimate 1% of the body surface area. It is good for small burns (< 15%) and large burns (> 85%, where the unburnt areas can be estimated) but not accurate for medium-sized burns. The Lund and Browder chart is probably the most accurate way of estimating burn area in children. It allows for variation in body shape with age.

Hettiaratchy S, Papini R. Initial management of a major burn: II – assessment and resuscitation. *BMJ* 2004; 329: 101–3.

Question C37: Trauma scoring systems

Regarding trauma scoring systems:

A. The Trauma Injury Severity Score (TRISS) is used for triage in the field
B. The Injury Severity Score (ISS) is a purely anatomical injury score
C. The Revised Trauma Score (RTS) uses GCS, respiratory rate and systolic BP only
D. An Abbreviated Injury Score (AIS) of 6 is unsurvivable
E. Major trauma is defined as ISS > 15

Answer: FTTTT

Short explanation

AIS classifies injuries to body regions from 1 (minor) to 6 (unsurvivable). The ISS is the sum of squares of the three highest AIS, and hence anatomical; a score of 16 or above is classed as major trauma, with mortality > 10%. The RTS uses only GCS, systolic BP and respiratory rate, and is combined with ISS to make TRISS, which includes complex algorithms and is used to assess hospital performance.

Long explanation

There are many trauma scoring systems of varying complexity, for use in the prehospital setting, the emergency department and the ICU.

The Injury Severity Score (ISS) is an anatomical injury scale based on the Abbreviated Injury Scale (AIS). The AIS assigns an injury severity score from 1 (minor) to 6 (unsurvivable) for nine body regions; some of these are combined to make six body regions for the ISS: head and neck; face; chest; abdomen; extermities (including pelvis); external. The ISS is the sum of the squares of the three highest scores. ISS > 15 is defined as major trauma and is associated with > 10% mortality. ISS is a simple prehospital triage system, but it discounts many injuries (e.g. multiple injuries to the same region) and ignores age, premorbid health and physiological derangements.

The Revised Trauma Score (RTS) is a physiological system, using clinical findings from the prehospital setting. It assigns weighted scores to three parameters – Glasgow Coma Scale (GCS), systolic blood pressure and respiratory rate, but uses a complicated algorithm which precludes its easy use in the field. RTS is a simplification of the earlier Trauma Score, which also included capillary refill and work of breathing.

ISS and RTS have been combined to form the Trauma Injury Severity Score (TRISS), which also includes age and the presence of penetrating or blunt trauma. It is too complex for use in the field, but can be used in emergency departments and allows calculation of predicted mortality. It can be used for comparison of the performance of different medical centres.

A Severity Characterisation of Trauma (ASCOT) score was introduced to circumvent shortcomings with TRISS. It uses the more complicated Anatomic Profile in place of the ISS, with different algorithms, but little predictive advantage over TRISS. A further model has been suggested, combining ICD-based injury severity score with RTS, which seems to have excellent predictive power for mortality, length of stay etc., but has yet to be widely implemented.

Palazzo M. Severity of illness and likely outcome from critical illness. In Bersten AD, Soni N. *Oh's Intensive Care Manual*, 6th edn. Edinburgh: Butterworth-Heinemann, 2009, pp. 17–30.

Question C38: Invasive arterial blood pressure monitoring

The following are sources of inaccuracy in invasive arterial blood pressure measurement:

A. Flexible connection tubing
B. Transducer height not at the level of the patient's heart
C. Peripheral site of arterial cannulation
D. Long arterial cannulae
E. Small air bubbles in fluid column within the giving set

Answer: TTTTT

Short explanation

Distensible tubing and long or narrow arterial cannulae can lead to resonance. Peripheral arteries may have lower pressure than central arteries in some conditions (coarctation, sepsis, vasoconstrictor use). The transducer needs to be at the level of the heart to prevent over- and under-reading of blood pressure.

Long explanation

Invasive arterial blood pressure monitoring is common in critical care, allowing constant, accurate, beat-to-beat monitoring of blood pressure (BP), and easy blood sampling. A catheter is inserted into an artery (commonly radial, brachial, femoral or dorsalis pedis), which is connected to a pressure transducer by tubing containing saline or other fluid. Any changes in arterial pressure over time are transmitted by the column of fluid to a flexible membrane in the pressure transducer. Perturbations of the flexible membrane are transduced into an electrical signal from which the arterial pressure waveform is displayed.

Two major sources of error are resonance and damping. Resonance occurs when oscillations in the column of fluid are magnified by parts of the measurement apparatus that have the same resonant frequency. To minimise the risk of this, short, wide, arterial cannulae should be used, connected to short, stiff tubing. Long cannulae or easily distensible tubing may have resonant frequencies below 40 Hz, causing inaccuracies.

Damping is the dissipation of energy leading to reductions in the amplitude of resonance of a system. A degree of damping is required to avoid prolonged measurement times; the compromise giving the quickest response with minimal oscillations is termed optimal damping. Over-damping leads to a flattened trace, with under-reading of systolic BP and over-reading of diastolic BP. Common causes of damping include air bubbles or blood clots in the column of fluid and kinking of the arterial cannula. Prevention of blood clotting may be achieved by the use of heparinised saline flushes.

Other sources of error include inappropriate transducer height and site of arterial cannulation. The transducer should be at the height of the patient's heart, or the effect of gravity on the column of fluid will be added to or subtracted from the BP reading. Peripheral arteries may have different pressures than central arteries, especially in conditions such as coarctation of the aorta, peripheral vascular disease and septic shock, and with the use of high levels of vasoconstrictors, all of which can lead to underestimation of the central BP.

Davis PD, Kenny GNC. *Basic Physics and Measurement in Anaesthesia*, 5th edn. London: Elsevier, 2005.

Question C39: ICU delirium

With regards to the management of patients with delirium, which of the following are correct?

A. Patients who remain unsedated while intubated have been shown to have a lower incidence of delirium
B. There is strong evidence for the use of atypical antipsychotics in the treatment of delirium
C. Haloperidol is useful as a first-line treatment for delirium
D. Benzodiazepines should be avoided in the treatment of delirium
E. Sedation breaks should be attempted regularly

Answer: TFTTT

Short explanation

In one published study from an ICU, patients did not receive any sedation despite being intubated, and the incidence of delirium was lower. The evidence for pharmacological management of delirium is not particularly strong. Haloperidol is of use in the management of patients with delirium, whereas benzodiazepines increase the risk of delirium. Sedation breaks have been shown to reduce delirium.

Long explanation

At present there is little strong evidence to support the routine use of any particular pharmacological agents in either prevention or treatment of delirium in ICU patients. There is relatively good evidence to suggest that the use of benzodiazepines increases the risk of delirium, and they should not be employed as treatment of the condition unless absolutely necessary to prevent patient harm. The mainstay of pharmacological treatment for delirium are antipsychotic agents such as haloperidol. Haloperidol is recommended as first-line in the UK, despite this being an off-licence indication for its use. Side effects of haloperidol include extrapyramidal symptoms, prolonged QT interval and neuroleptic malignant syndrome.

The use of atypical antipsychotics has also been studied. Olanzapine and quetiapine are the most commonly used. The results of studies comparing these drugs with haloperidol for both the prevention and treatment of delirium have been conflicting. However, one study did demonstrate a faster resolution of symptoms in patients receiving quetiapine compared to haloperidol. A study looking at the effect of rivastigmine, an anticholinesterase inhibitor, was halted early for safety reasons, and the drug is not recommended for use in ICU patients with delirium.

Non-pharmacological methods can be used to prevent and possibly treat delirium. Many of these methods are simple, cheap and easy to employ by all ICU staff. They include providing activities for cognitive stimulation, early mobilisation, regularly orientating the patients, promoting sleep and optimising communication by providing hearing aids and spectacles. Medical interventions such as providing effective analgesia, administering oxygen, fluid resuscitation, correcting electrolyte abnormalities, treating sepsis and providing alcohol withdrawal treatment can also help to prevent delirium. Avoidance of delirium-promoting medications such as anticholinergics can be achieved by daily review of the drug charts. The Awake and Breathing trial demonstrated the benefit of daily sedation holds in ventilated patients.

Alce T, Page V, Vizcaychipi M. Delirium uncovered. *J Intensive Care Soc* 2013; 14: 53–9.

Girard T, Jackson J, Pandharipande P, *et al.* Delirium as a predictor of long-term cognitive impairment in survivors of critical illness. *Crit Care Med* 2010; 38: 1513–20.

Ouimet S, Kavanagh B, Gottfried S, Skrobik Y. Incidence, risk factors and consequences of ICU delirium. *Intensive Care Med* 2007; 33: 66–73.

Van Rompaey B, Elseviers M, Schuurmans M, *et al.* Risk factors for delirium in intensive care patients: a prospective cohort study. *Crit Care* 2009; 13: R77.

Question C40: Hypertensive crisis

Regarding hypertensive emergencies:

A. Around 10% of people with hypertension will develop a hypertensive crisis during their lifetime
B. During treatment of hypertensive emergencies the goal of pharmacological therapy is a normal blood pressure
C. Renal disease is the commonest cause of secondary malignant hypertension
D. Patients of Afro-Caribbean origin are at a higher risk of hypertensive crises than Caucasian patients
E. Short-acting intravenous antihypertensive agents should be used for patients with hypertensive crises and evidence of end-organ damage

Answer: FFTTT

Short explanation

Around 1% of patients with hypertension will develop a hypertensive crisis. Most patients with hypertensive emergencies have previously been diagnosed with hypertension. The goal of pharmacological therapy is to reduce the blood pressure slowly to the patient's own baseline normal blood pressure over 24–48 hours.

Long explanation

The definition of hypertensive emergencies is currently under debate. The most recent literature suggests that sudden increases in systolic or diastolic blood pressure associated with end-organ damage can be described as hypertensive crises or emergencies. Malignant hypertension was a term previously used to describe acute elevation in blood pressure associated with encephalopathy and/or acute nephropathy. It is now no longer used, and this clinical presentation should be termed 'hypertensive emergency'. Other clinical presentations which fit under the umbrella term of hypertensive emergency include dissecting aortic aneurysm, eclampsia and hypertensive encephalopathy.

Most patients presenting with a hypertensive emergency will already be known hypertensive patients. Often the blood pressure control has been inadequate previously. Hypertensive emergencies are commoner in the elderly, in men and in Afro-Caribbean populations. The commonest secondary cause of hypertensive emergencies is renal parenchymal disease. Patients will present in a variety of ways with headache, visual disturbance, seizures, coma, angina, acute left ventricular failure or oliguria. The patient's normal blood pressure values should be sought and the blood pressure gradually reduced over a period of 24–48 hours. Intravenous antihypertensives should be reserved for the intensive care unit. Short-acting titratable agents such as labetolol or nitrate are recommended.

Varon J, Marik P. Clinical review: the management of hypertensive crises. *Crit Care* 2003; 7: 374–84.

Question C41: Cervical spine injuries

Regarding cervical spine injuries in the unconscious trauma patient:

A. All patients should have cervical spine immobilisation until radiological clearance is complete
B. Good-quality three-view plain radiographs (lateral, anterior–posterior and open-mouth views) will exclude cervical spine injuries
C. Magnetic resonance imaging is required to exclude ligamentous injuries
D. In the absence of distracting injuries, clinical examination and passive movement is sufficient to clear the cervical spine
E. Multi-plane helical CT scans reviewed by a consultant radiologist are sufficient to exclude all significant cervical spine injuries

Answer: FFFTF

Short explanation

Unconscious trauma patients cannot have 100% reliable C-spine clearance due to the possibility of clinically significant ligamentous injury. However, a combination of plain x-ray and high-resolution CT and review of those images by a trained radiologist will identify the overwhelming majority of unstable injuries. This should be weighed against the risks of prolonged C-spine immobilisation. MRI identifies soft tissue injuries, but is not necessary. Conscious, sober and otherwise uninjured patients can safely have their C-spine cleared clinically without the need to obtain radiological imaging.

Long explanation

The fully conscious, sober, cooperative trauma patient with no neck pain or tenderness or distracting injuries is highly unlikely to have a cervical spine injury. In this situation clinical examination and active movement of the neck from side to side, then flexion and extension, without pain is sufficient to clear the cervical spine of injury.

The fully conscious, sober, cooperative trauma patient with neck pain or tenderness but no distracting injuries should have three-view plain radiography (lateral, anterior–posterior and open-mouth) with CT for areas which are of concern or poorly imaged with plain radiography. If normal, then absence of subluxation on flexion and extension lateral radiographs is sufficient to clear the cervical spine.

Unconscious patients who are expected to be unsedated and cooperative within a short period of time (e.g. isolated lower limb injuries requiring operative fixation) can have their cervical spine protection maintained until the above clinical and/or radiological clearance procedure can be performed.

For all other patients, high-resolution CT images of the whole cervical spine are the gold-standard radiological investigation required for cervical spine clearance. The images obtained should be promptly reviewed by a consultant radiologist. The risk of missing an unstable cervical spine injury with high-resolution CT has been estimated at between 0.5% and 0.015%. This risk should be weighed against the risks of prolonged maintainance of cervical spine immobilisation.

Magnetic resonance imaging is very sensitive for soft tissue injuries but has a false-positive rate of up to 33%, and so its use should be restricted to patients with a high clinical suspicion of neurological or ligamentous damage.

Committee on Trauma of the American College of Surgeons. *Advanced Trauma Life Support (ATLS) Manual*, 9th edn. Chicago, IL: ACS, 2012.

Morris C, Guha A, Farquhar I. Evaluation for spinal injuries among unconscious victims of blunt polytrauma: a management guideline for intensive care. London: Intensive Care Society, 2005.

Question C42: Glasgow Coma Scale

On the Glasgow Coma Scale (GCS) in traumatic brain injury:

A. Abnormal flexion to pain scores 3 on the motor scale
B. Unintelligible sounds scores 2 on the verbal scale
C. Localising to painful stimulus scores 5 on the motor scale
D. Spontaneous eye opening scores 5 on the eye-response scale
E. Abnormal extension to pain scores more than abnormal flexion on the motor scale

Answer: TTFFF

Short explanation

Localising to painful stimulus scores 4 on the motor scale. The maximum score on the eye-response scale is 4 (spontaneous eye opening). On the motor scale, abnormal flexion to pain scores 3 and abnormal extension is a score of 2.

Long explanation

The Glasgow Coma Scale (GCS) was introduced in 1974 as a neurological scoring tool, to assess level of consciousness after head injury. Its role has since expanded, and it is widely used in the prehospital environment, emergency departments, critical care and general wards. While GCS as a tool has the greatest validity in head injury patients, its application to wider patient groups is appropriate. It forms part of many critical illness severity scoring systems (e.g. APACHE, SAPS, SOFA) and can be used to stratify risk following insults such as brain injury and subarachnoid haemorrhage.

The orginal GCS was a 14-point scale, but the Modified GCS, which added an extra motor category to produce a 15-point scale, is now almost universal.. The standard GCS cannot be used in young children, but several versions exist that are adapted for different age groups.

GCS is the total of three scores, for eye response, verbal response and motor response. The best response in each category should be recorded. Each category has a minimum score of 1, and so the lowest possible GCS is 3/15. Scoring is as follows:

Eye response	Spontaneous opening	4
	Open in response to voice	3
	Open in response to pain	2
	Do not open	1
Verbal response	Oriented, coherent speech	5
	Confused speech	4
	Inappropriate words	3
	Unintelligible sounds	2
	No response	1
Motor response	Obeys commands	6
	Withdraws from painful stimulus	5
	Localises to painful stimulus	4
	Abnormal flexion to pain	3
	Abnormal extension to pain	2
	No response to pain	1

Painful stimuli should be peripheral (upper limb) to allow withdrawal, but central stimuli may also be used for clarification. The motor category is the best discriminator of severity of brain injury.

Teasdale G, Murray G, Parker L, Jennett B. Adding up the Glasgow Coma Score. *Acta Neurochir Suppl* 1979; 28: 13–16.

Question C43: Hypercalcaemia

With regards to the assessment and management of severe hypercalcaemia, which of the following are correct?

A. Hypercalcaemic crisis is most commonly caused by primary hyperparathyroidism
B. Digoxin is the drug of choice for arrhythmias associated with hypercalcaemia
C. Malignant hypercalcaemia does not develop into a hypercalcaemic crisis
D. Acute kidney injury and anuria occur when calcium levels are > 4 mmol/l
E. Renal replacement therapy may be required if intravenous fluid resuscitation is unsuccessful

Answer: TFFTT

Short explanation

An increased sensitivity to digitalis and associated toxicity is well recognised in patients who are hypercalcaemic. Malignant hypercalcaemia is a less common cause of hypercalcaemic crisis but can occur.

Long explanation

Hypercalcaemia is usually a chronic condition managed in primary care. Patients present with vague symptoms such as lethargy, polydipsia, abdominal pains and constipation. The commonest cause for hypercalcaemia is hyperparathyroidism caused by either parathyroid adenoma or gland hyperplasia. The usual treatment involves encouraging oral rehydration followed by referral to an endocrinologist and surgeon for definitive parathyroidectomy. Other causes include malignancy such as myeloma, breast cancer, prostate cancer and lung cancer.

Once the calcium level rises above 3 mmol/l the patient is often unable to take in adequate oral rehydration. Intravenous fluid should be administered, and furosemide can also be given to promote a diuresis and reduce total body calcium levels. Hypercalcaemic crisis develops when the calcium level reaches a critical level (usually > 4 mmol/l). At this point two organs are at risk: firstly the kidneys, because oliguria and anuria can develop, leading to renal failure; and secondly the brain, as drowsiness and coma will develop if the calcium remains untreated.

In addition to intravenous fluid resuscitation, bisphosphonates can be administered. The advice of the local endocrinologist should be sought, as care is required in patients with renal impairment. Pamidronate or zoledronate are the recommended drugs. Renal replacement therapy may be required, and calcium-free or low-calcium dialysate should be used. Treatment may also require aggressive potassium and magnesium replacement, as these are often low and will fall further once rehydration is commenced. Corticosteroids can also be given to help lower the calcium levels, and this is particularly effective in patients with myeloma.

Ziegler R. Hypercalcemic crisis. *J Am Soc Nephrol* 2001; 12 (Suppl 1): S3–9.
Ramrakha P, Moore K. Endocrine emergencies. In *Oxford Handbook of Acute Medicine*, 3rd edn. Oxford: Oxford University Press, 2010; pp. 515–72.

Question C44: Epiglottitis in adults

In adult epiglottitis, which of the following are correct?

A. A small proportion of patients require admission to intensive care
B. MEWS score is a poor predictor of clinical outcome
C. Lateral neck x-ray can be helpful in diagnosis
D. The presence of stridor is the strongest predictor of the need for airway intervention
E. Positive blood cultures for *Haemophilus influenzae* type B are usually obtained

Answer: FFTTF

Short explanation

Up to 75% of adult patients with epiglottitis will require ICU admission. A low MEWS score (< 1) is a reasonable predictor of good clinical outcome. A high MEWS score (> 5) is a worrying sign. Negative blood cultures are the norm, and the causative organism is rarely identified.

Long explanation

The incidence of epiglottitis in children has steadily declined since mass vaccination against *Haemophilus influenza* type B (Hib) became routine in developed countries throughout the 1980s and 1990s. Epiglottitis is increasingly seen in adults, however, with an incidence of around 1–4 per 100,000 per year. Mortality varies but has been shown to be as high as 7–20%. Adult cases are less likely to have Hib identified as a causative organism, as blood cultures, throat swabs and sputum cultures are commonly negative. It is thought that other organisms such as group A β-haemolytic streptococci and viral pathogens are responsible for a significant number of adults cases.

Many adults will present with non-specific symptoms of upper respiratory tract infection and sore throat. Unfortunately, this results in patients presenting late in the course of the illness once airway obstruction is imminent. Flexible laryngoscopy by a specialist is the best way to diagnose the condition but may not be readily available. Lateral neck x-ray will often demonstrate the 'thumb sign', where the swollen and enlarged epiglottis is visible as a thumb-shaped shadow.

Airway intervention is not without risk, although some clinicians would advocate early intubation to avoid failed attempts once the patient is in extremis. Senior anaesthetic and ENT advice and skills should be actively sought in any scenario where epiglottitis is suspected and airway intervention is being considered. Medical Early Warning Scores (MEWS) or other early warning scores are useful in the identification of the high-risk patient but are not reliable indicators of specific airway problems. Stridor remains the strongest predictor of need for airway intervention. Unfortunately, this often occurs late and also predicts difficult intubation.

The mortality in patients who are managed in a critical care environment with timely interventions is low. In addition, the length of time on ICU is usually less than 2 days, but this is extended in those who require airway intervention. It is important to bear in the mind the risk of further airway complications, such as epiglottic abscess and retropharyngeal abscess. These complications can occur a few days after first presentation, once the initial infection appears to be improving. Surgical intervention may be required in these cases.

Ames W, Ward V, Tranter R, Street M. Adult epiglottitis: an under-recognized, life-threatening condition. *Br J Anaesth* 2000; 85: 795–7.

Lam P, Choi Y, Wong T, Lau C. Adult acute epiglottitis: predictors for airway intervention and intensive care unit admission. *Hong Kong J Emerg Med* 2009; 16: 198–207.

Question C45: Community-acquired pneumonia

A 35-year-old man with no significant medical history is diagnosed with community-acquired pneumonia (CAP). The following are likely causative organisms:

A. *Klebsiella pneumoniae*
B. *Streptococcus pneumoniae*
C. Methicillin-resistant *Staphylococcus aureus* (MRSA)
D. *Pseudomonas aeruginosa*
E. *Escherichia coli*

Answer: FTFFF

Short explanation

The commonest causative organisms in CAP are *Streptococcus pneumoniae, Haemophilus influenzae, Legionella, Staphylococcus aureus* (MSSA), *Mycoplasma pneumoniae, Chlamydia* and influenza A and B. *Klebsiella, Pseudomonas, E. coli* and MRSA are causes of hospital-acquired pneumonia.

Long explanation

Community-acquired pneumonia has an annual incidence of 0.5–1.1%, with 22–42% requiring admission to hospital and 1.2–10% of these requiring ICU admission. Mortality is related to severity. The mortality rate for patients managed in the community is < 1%; for those admitted to hospital it is 5–14%, and for those requiring ICU admission it is > 30%.

The causative organisms are predominantly bacteria, although around 13% of cases are viral. The commonest bacteria are *Streptococcus pneumoniae, Haemophilus influenzae, Legionella* species, *Staphylococcus aureus, Mycoplasma pneumoniae* and *Chlamydia* species. Many cases (> 30%) have no identifiable organism.

Treatment is initially empirical, while organisms are identified, and based on local microbiological guidelines. Commonly chosen antibiotics include amoxicillin or benzylpenicillin with clarithromycin. Patients with penicillin hypersensitivity should be treated with doxycycline, levofloxacin or a cephalosporin.

Lim W, Baudouin S, George R. BTS guidelines for the management of community acquired pneumonia in adults: update 2009. *Thorax* 2009; 64: ii1–55.

Question C46: Precordial thump

According to the Advanced Life Support guidelines, the precordial thump:

A. Should be used only if the cardiac arrest is both witnessed and monitored
B. Is more effective for VF than for VT
C. Has been shown to induce sinus rhythm from asystole
D. Has been shown to induce VF from sinus rhythm
E. Should not be used post cardiac surgery

Answer: FFTTT

Short explanation

The precordial thump is more effective for VT than for VF. It is only likely to be effective at a witnessed, monitored arrest, and should not delay defibrillation.

Long explanation

The precordial thump is performed by using the ulnar edge of a clenched fist brought down sharply onto the lower half of the sternum from a height of approximately 20 cm. It should not be used after sternotomy or cardiac surgery, as sternal fracture is a recognised complication.

A precordial thump is more effective for pulseless VT than for VF, and may conversely induce VF from VT or PEA. Very rarely it will induce a ROSC (return of spontaneous circulation) from asystole. This is most commonly seen in P-wave asystole, where the thump acts in a similar manner to percussion pacing. It is extremely unlikely to work in this circumstance, however, and external pacing is recommended. Current guidelines state that a precordial thump is only appropriate in the context of the first few seconds of a monitored, witnessed arrest, when it will not delay defibrillation if it fails.

Australian Resuscitation Council, New Zealand Resus Council. Guideline 11.3: precordial thump and fist pacing. http://www.resus.org.au/policy/guidelines/section_11/precordial_thump.htm (accessed June 2014).

Resuscitation Council (UK). Advanced life support algorithm. In *Advanced Life Support*, 6th edn. London: Resuscitation Council, 2011; Chapter 6.

Question C47: Spontaneous pneumothorax

Regarding spontaneous primary pneumothorax:

A. A posteroanterior (PA) chest x-ray in expiration is the diagnostic test of choice
B. A large pneumothorax is defined as one with an interpleural distance of > 2 cm at any point
C. Small pneumothoraces are managed conservatively
D. The prognosis is better than for secondary spontaneous pneumothoraces
E. Needle decompression is as effective as large-bore chest-drain insertion

Answer: FFFTT

Short explanation

PA chest films are done in inspiration; definitive diagnosis is by CT. A large pneumothorax is defined as one with an interpleural distance of > 2 cm at the level of the hilum. Conservative management versus intervention is decided on symptoms.

Long explanation

Spontaneous pneumothorax may be either primary or secondary. The former is usually better tolerated, regardless of the size of the pneumothorax, and is associated with less morbidity and mortality. Severity of symptoms relates to the degree of underlying lung disease and the size of the pneumothorax. Severe symptoms and signs of respiratory distress suggest a tension pneumothorax.

Diagnosis of a simple pneumothorax is generally by a standard erect PA chest x-ray in inspiration. This may miss small pneumothoraces. CT scanning is recommended for uncertain or complex cases. It will also define the size of the pneumothorax more accurately. The differentiation between a large and a small pneumothorax is the presence of a visible rim of > 2 cm between the lung margin and the chest wall (interpleural distance) at the level of the hilum.

Management of a pneumothorax is predominantly based on clinical features and degree of respiratory compromise rather than the size of the pneumothorax, although this has an impact on the rate of resolution. Small, asymptomatic spontaneous primary pneumothoraces may be managed conservatively. Initial management of symptomatic or larger pneumothoraces includes administration of oxygen followed by drainage of the pneumothorax. All patients should be admitted for 24 hours' observation even if well post drainage. Needle (14–16G) aspiration is as effective as large-bore (> 20Fr) chest drains, and may be associated with reduced morbidity and length of stay. If needle aspiration is unsuccessful a small-bore (< 14Fr) chest drain is recommended. Large-bore chest drains are not needed for simple pneumothoraces. If there is failure of the lung to re-expand or persistent air leak the patient should be referred to thoracic surgery.

British Thoracic Society Pleural Disease Guideline Group. BTS pleural disease guideline. *Thorax* 2010; 65 (Suppl 2).

Question C48: Seasonal and pandemic influenza

Regarding seasonal and pandemic influenza:

A. Influenza B is responsible for most pandemic cases of flu
B. Influenza A is less virulent than influenza B
C. Oral amantadine is the second-line treatment for pandemic flu
D. Oral oseltamivir is the first-line treatment for seasonal flu
E. Viral shedding occurs as soon as the patient is symptomatic

Answer: FFFFF

Short explanation

Influenza A usually causes a more severe illness than influenza B, and is responsible for pandemics. Oral oseltamivir is the first-line treatment for pandemic flu; seasonal flu is resistant to oseltamivir. Amantadine is ineffective against H1N1 pandemic flu. Viral shedding can occur before symptoms are apparent.

Long explanation

There are two types of influenza virus of clinical significance: influenza A and influenza B. Influenza A usually causes a more severe illness than influenza B. Both virus types may result in seasonal epidemics, but only influenza A viruses have the ability to cause a pandemic. Seasonal epidemics occur due to antigenic drift (minor random changes in the antigenic characteristics of the hemagglutinin and neuraminidase glycoproteins of the influenza viruses). Pandemics occur with antigenic shift – a major change in the surface glycoproteins of the virus as a result of reassortment of genes between different influenza viruses, or through direct transmission of an animal virus to humans. This is the reason that pandemic flu predominantly affects young people, who lack prior exposure to other strains of the virus.

Person-to-person transmission occurs primarily through droplet spread from coughing, sneezing or exposure to secretions during mechanical ventilation or intubation. The incubation period is 24–48 hours, but viral shedding can occur before symptoms are apparent. The duration of viral shedding is usually 5 days, but this may be prolonged in children, in the immunocompromised, and in critically ill patients. The duration of viral shedding may be reduced by antiviral medications.

Management of patients with influenza is largely supportive, with lung-protective ventilation where necessary, careful fluid management and renal replacement therapy as required. Antiviral treatment should be initiated as soon as possible, preferably within 48 hours, particularly in high-risk patients. Neuraminidase inhibitors (oseltamivir and zanamivir) are active against the pandemic H1N1 influenza A strain. Zanamivir should be used in the rare cases of oseltamivir resistance or where the enteral route is contraindicated. Adamantanes (amantadine and rimantadine) have no activity against the influenza A H1N1 pandemic strain but are effective for seasonal H1N1 influenza strains, which are 100% resistant to oseltamivir.

Health Protection Agency. Critical care management of adults with influenza with particular reference to H1N1 (2009). Version 3 (2011). http://www.hpa.org.uk/webc/HPAwebFile/HPAweb_C/1287148502205 (accessed June 2014).

Rello J, Pop-Vicas A. Clinical review: primary influenza viral pneumonia. *Crit Care* 2009; 13: 235.

Question C49: Ingestion of chemicals

In patients who have ingested strong acid or alkali solutions:

A. Gastric damage is greater with acidic solutions than with alkali
B. A nasogastric tube should be used to remove residual chemical
C. The risk of squamous cell cancer of the oesophagus is increased
D. Late stricture formation will be reduced by steroid administration
E. Upper gastrointestinal endoscopy should not be performed within the first 24 hours

Answer: TFTFF

Short explanation

Nasogastric tubes are contraindicated, and endoscopy should be performed in the first 24 hours. Steroids do not alter the risk of oesophageal stricture.

Long explanation

Ingestion of chemicals in adults is much more likely to be deliberate than it is in children. For this reason, injury is generally more severe, because the patient does not attempt to expectorate the substance. The severity of the damage depends on:

- the corrosive properties of the ingested substance
- the amount, concentration and physical form (solid or liquid) of the agent
- the duration of contact with the mucosa

Alkali ingestions typically damage the oesophagus more than the stomach or duodenum, and acids cause more severe gastric injury. Laryngeal and tracheobronchial injury may occur with aspiration of any substance. Acid ingestion usually has a worse prognosis. The severity of injury is usually classified in a manner similar to that of thermal burns, as first-, second- or third-degree burns.

Clinical features depend on the severity of the injury and the development of complications such as mediastinitis, peritonitis or chemical pneumonitis. Respiratory distress should be investigated promptly, as laryngeal damage may necessitate urgent tracheostomy rather than intubation.

Upper gastrointestinal endoscopy should be performed during the first 24 hours to assess the degree of damage. Endoscopy should be performed earlier in some circumstances, such as button battery ingestion, where mucosal damage may occur within 4 hours.

Other treatment for the inflammatory response to injury and complications is supportive. In severe injury, extensive surgery (e.g. oesophagectomy) may be required.

Emetics and neutralising agents are contraindicated, as they may increase the damage. Nasogastric tubes should be avoided, because they may cause retching or further damage weakened tissue.

Late complications include oesophageal stricture and an increased risk of squamous cell carcinoma of the stomach. Steroids do not decrease the risk of stricture.

Contini S, Scarpignato C. Caustic injury of the upper gastrointestinal tract: a comprehensive review. *World J Gastroenterol* 2013; 19: 3918–30.

Triadafilopoulos G. Caustic oesophageal injury in adults. *UpToDate* 2012. http://www.uptodate.com (accessed June 2014).

Question C50: Acute stroke

The following are appropriate initial management steps for patients with acute stroke:

A. CT brain for all patients with suspected acute stroke within 1 hour
B. Thrombolysis with alteplase if haemorrhage is excluded
C. Aspirin 300 mg unless the patient has a history of dyspepsia with aspirin
D. Glucose control to between 4 and 11 mmol/l
E. Urgent control of blood pressure if > 185/110

Answer: FTFTF

Short explanation

Urgent CT brain is required for patients with reduced GCS, risk factors for haemorrhage or candidates for thrombolysis. Others should have a CT within 24 hours. Thrombolysis is recommended for confirmed ischaemic stroke in hospitals with access to urgent CT and acute stroke teams. Patients with aspirin-related dyspepsia should be given a proton-pump inhibitor (PPI) as well as aspirin. Blood pressure control is only required in malignant hypertension, pre-eclampsia, aortic dissection, intracerebral haemorrhage or thrombolysis candidates.

Long explanation

Acute stroke is a major cause of mortality and morbidity. Prompt recognition and appropriate early management help to reduce mortality and levels of neurological deficit. Stroke is a rapidly developing disturbance of cerebral function of vascular origin lasting > 24 hours (or leading to death). If symptoms resolve within 24 hours, the event is known as a transient ischaemic attack (TIA). In the acute phase the two conditions are indistinguishable, and patients should all be treated as stroke.

An urgent CT brain scan (the next available slot, within 1 hour) is required for patients with risk factors for haemorrhage (anticoagulation, bleeding diathesis), reduced GCS, or signs suggestive of meningitis or intracerebral haemorrhage, and in patients under consideration for thrombolysis. Other patients should have a CT brain scan within 24 hours of presentation.

Thrombolysis using alteplase is recommended for all patients with ischaemic stroke (confirmed with imaging) in an appropriate setting. This means in hospitals with easy access to urgent imaging, stroke teams and level 2 care staff.

Aspirin 300 mg should be administered within 24 hours to all stroke patients who have had intracerebral haemorrhage excluded by imaging. Patients with dyspepsia related to aspirin should be co-administered a proton-pump inhibitor (PPI). Patients with intolerance of aspirin should receive an alternative antiplatelet agent, such as clopidogrel. Aspirin 300 mg should continue for 2 weeks.

Other supportive management includes supplemental oxygen to maintain saturations at > 94% and glucose control within the range 4–11 mmol/l. Hypertension should not be actively managed unless there is evidence of end-organ damage (encephalopathy, nephropathy, myocardial ischaemia), aortic dissection, pre-eclampsia or intracerebral haemorrhage. Patients being considered for thrombolysis should have their BP controlled if it exceeds 185/110.

National Institute for Health and Care Excellence. *CG68: Stroke: Diagnosis and Initial Management of Acute Stroke and Transient Ischaemic Attack (TIA)*. London: NICE, 2008. http://www.nice.org.uk/cg68 (accessed June 2014).

Question C51: Amniotic fluid embolism

Regarding a patient with suspected amniotic fluid embolus, which of the following are correct?

A. It only occurs during labour and delivery in the third trimester
B. Mortality is higher than 50%
C. Bronchospasm is the commonest cause of hypoxia
D. Inotropic support should not be delayed because of concerns over fetal toxicity or uterine hypoperfusion
E. Disseminated intravascular coagulation (DIC) and thrombocytopenia are hallmark signs of amniotic fluid embolism

Answer: FTFTF

Short explanation

Amniotic fluid embolus usually occurs during labour or delivery. Rare exceptions have been reported up 48 hours post-partum or during first- and second-trimester terminations. Ventilation/perfusion mismatch is the commonest cause of hypoxia. Bronchospasm occurs in around 15% of patients. Thrombocytopenia is unusual, whereas DIC is a hallmark sign of the condition.

Long explanation

Amniotic fluid embolism is a potentially devastating condition which continues to have a high mortality (60–80%). It was the seventh-commonest cause of overall maternal mortality in the UK between 2006 and 2008. Presentation is usually during labour or delivery but has been rarely reported during caesarean section or terminations in the first and second trimesters.

Initial presentation is usually that of maternal collapse with marked hypoxia and cardiovascular instability. Cardiac arrest can occur within minutes or may be the presenting feature. Rapid patient deterioration leading to death can occur quickly. The other cardinal symptoms are agitation, altered mental status and disseminated intravascular coagulation (DIC). Hypoxia is found in almost all patients and can be dramatic. It is thought to be due predominantly to raised pulmonary artery pressures and vasospasm in the pulmonary vasculature leading to ventilation/perfusion mismatching. Later left ventricular failure and resultant cardiogenic pulmonary oedema will contribute to hypoxia.

The precipitating factor is not entirely known. Early work suggested that fetal cells entering the maternal circulation resulted in obstruction of the pulmonary vasculature. However, more recent work has contradicted this, as fetal material has been found in the blood of pregnant women who do not suffer these consequences. An immunological basis for the condition is suspected, given the similarities between it and the profound and rapid deterioration seen in anaphylactic shock. Women who have drug allergies are at a slightly higher risk than those without. Arachidonic acid metabolites have been implicated in the inflammatory response seen.

Amniotic fluid embolus is a diagnosis of exclusion; sepsis, anaphylaxis, myocardial ischaemia and pulmonary embolism must all be considered as differentials. Management is entirely supportive. Oxygenation is key to prevent the permanent neurological sequelae seen in many survivors. If the woman has not yet delivered, then perimortem or expedited caesarean section should be considered to allow effective cardiovascular resuscitation of the mother. Inotropic support will often be required for vasoconstrictor effects and to improve left ventricular function. This should not be delayed because of concerns over fetal toxicity or placental hypoperfusion.

Almost all survivors of this condition will require intensive care. DIC should be corrected with clotting factors and red blood cells as required. Clinicians should be aware of the high risk of significant blood loss post delivery due to DIC. Standard drugs used to increase uterine tone should be readily available.

Moore J, Baldisseri M. Amniotic fluid embolism. *Crit Care Med* 2005; 33 (suppl): S279–85.

Question C52: Pulmonary artery catheter complications

The following are recognised complications of pulmonary artery (PA) catheters:

A. Air embolism
B. Complete heart block
C. Pulmonary infarction
D. Pneumothorax
E. Neuropathy

Answer: TTTTT

Short explanation

Complications of PA catheters may be related to central venous access, catheterisation or arterial occlusion. Central venous access complications include arterial puncture, haemothorax, pneumothorax and neuropathy. Catheterisation complications include valvular lesions and arrhythmias. Prolonged indwelling of PA catheters can lead to pulmonary embolism, pulmonary infarction and arterial trauma.

Long explanation

All medical procedures carry the risk of complications, the risk of which must be weighed against the benefits of the procedure itself. Multiple studies, RCTs and meta-analyses have been performed looking at the benefits of PA catheters, with no strong evidence that they improve outcomes. A large RCT (PAC-Man, published in 2005) failed to show any benefit of PA catheter use while finding a 10% complication rate. These complications were non-fatal but significant, leading to conclusions that PA catheters should be used with caution.

Complications may arise from the process of central venous cannulation, from passing the catheter into the pulmonary artery, from 'wedge pressure' measurements, or from prolonged indwelling of the catheter in the pulmonary artery.

Complications of central venous access include local haemorrhage, arterial puncture, haematomata, haemothorax, pneumothorax, air embolism and neurological damage (pain and neuropathy). A 2013 Cochrane review of PA catheters for adults in ICU estimated these risks at < 3.6%.

Complications of the process of passing the PA catheter from the superior vena cava through right atrium, tricuspid valve, right ventricle and pulmonary trunk to pulmonary artery include damage to any of these structures and arrhythmias, from ventricular ectopics to complete heart block. The 2013 Cochrane review estimated these risks to be 0.3–3.8%.

The process of measuring pulmonary capillary wedge pressure (an estimate of left atrial pressure) involves inflation of a balloon to occlude the pulmonary artery in which it resides. This procedure risks pulmonary artery embolus or rupture, and pulmonary infarction. PA catheters may stay in situ for many days, which increases the risk of bloodstream infection, migration of the catheter and venous thrombus. The 2013 Cochrane review estimated these risks to be 0.03–3%.

Harvey S, Harrison DA, Singer M, *et al*. Assessment of the clinical effectiveness of pulmonary artery catheters in management of patients in intensive care (PAC-Man): a randomised controlled trial. *Lancet* 2005; 366: 472–7.

Harvey S, Young D, Brampton W. Pulmonary artery catheters for adult patients in intensive care. *Cochrane Database Syst Rev* 2013; (2): CD003408.

Question C53: Delirium risk factors

With regards to the risk factors for delirium in patients on the intensive care unit, which of the following are correct?

A. Chronic alcohol dependence is not a risk factor for delirium
B. Use of benzodiazepines is associated with a reduced risk of delirium
C. Hearing impairment increases the risk of delirium
D. Anaemia increases the risk of delirium
E. Hypotension increases the risk of delirium

Answer: FFTTT

Short explanation

Risk factors for delirium include chronic alcohol dependence, use of benzodiazepines, visual and hearing impairment, anaemia and hypotension. Other risk factors include previous cognitive impairment, deranged electrolytes, sepsis, pain, renal and liver failure.

Long explanation

Delirium is common in patients on the ICU. The incidence is variable, depending on the tool used to assess patients, but can be as high as around 80%. Delirium is defined as an acute fluctuating disturbance of consciousness, attention, cognition and perception which develops over a short period of time (hours to days). There are many risk factors, including the patient's medical and social history, the presenting complaint and medications administered. A prior history of cognitive impairment, such as dementia, increases the risk of delirium, as do other neurological conditions such as depression, epilepsy, visual or hearing impairment and stroke. Older patients are more susceptible. Patients who are smokers, dependent on alcohol or malnourished are at a higher risk of delirium.

Most acute conditions will predispose to delirium, but certain factors increase the risk more than others. Sepsis, hyperthermia, hypoxia, pain and metabolic derangement (e.g. electrolyte abnormalities) all contribute to the incidence of delirium. It is important to note that there are a number of pharmacological agents, commonly prescribed in patients with acute illness, that increase the risk of delirium. Benzodiazepines, opiates and anticholinergics are the best-known of these. Avoidance of these agents is strongly encouraged in patients who are at risk of delirium, which includes most patients on the ICU.

Alce T, Page V, Vizcaychipi M. Delirium uncovered. *J Intensive Care Soc* 2013; 14: 53–9.

Girard T, Jackson J, Pandharipande P, *et al*. Delirium as a predictor of long-term cognitive impairment in survivors of critical illness. *Crit Care Med* 2010; 38: 1513–20.

Ouimet S, Kavanagh B, Gottfried S, Skrobik Y. Incidence, risk factors and consequences of ICU delirium. *Intensive Care Med* 2007; 33: 66–73.

Van Rompaey B, Elseviers M, Schuurmans M, *et al*. Risk factors for delirium in intensive care patients: a prospective cohort study. *Crit Care* 2009; 13: R77.

Question C54: Herpes simplex encephalitis

Regarding herpes simplex encephalitis:

A. It is most commonly caused by HSV-1
B. Treatment of choice is intravenous ganciclovir
C. It usually affects the frontal lobes
D. Untreated, mortality is up to 25%
E. It is characterised by a very high CSF protein level

Answer: TFTFF

Short explanation

HSV-1 encephalitis usually affects the frontal lobes. Treatment of choice is intravenous aciclovir. Untreated mortality is 70%, and CSF analysis usually shows a mildly elevated protein level.

Long explanation

Encephalitis is an infection or inflammation of the brain parenchyma, as opposed to meningitis, which affects the meninges and subarachnoid space. The clinical features that point to a diagnosis of encephalitis include focal neurological symptoms, speech disturbance, seizures, altered cognition or reduced conscious level. Encephalitis usually begins with flu-like symptoms, pyrexia, headaches and arthralgia.

There are numerous causes of encephalitis, including:

- infection, usually viral, e.g. HSV, CMV, West Nile virus, Japanese encephalitis, rabies
- post-infectious, immune-mediated inflammation days to weeks after an initial infection
- autoimmune, immune-mediated inflammation to a non-infectious cause such as malignancy
- chronic e.g. HIV-1, measles and rubella

Herpes simplex virus 1 (HSV-1) is the most common and serious cause of focal encephalitis and usually affects the temporal and frontal lobes. Diagnosis can be difficult: CT and MRI may show characteristic temporal lobe changes, and a finding of focal EEG abnormalities in this area is also suspicious. CSF will generally show a lymphocytosis with mildly elevated protein. CSF PCR may be positive in time.

Intravenous aciclovir for 14 days is the standard therapy. Untreated, HSV-1 encephalitis has a mortality of approximately 70%. Aciclovir can cause renal impairment, and therefore renal function should be monitored and hypovolaemia avoided. Seizures should be treated aggressively, and cerebral oedema may be treated with steroids, although there are no clinical trials to support this. Overall, mortality is 25%, but patients can also be left with significant disability in terms of cognitive dysfunction or seizures.

Cytomegalovirus (CMV) infection requires antiviral therapy with ganciclovir or valganciclovir.

Kennedy AM. Meningitis and encephalomyelitis. In Bersten AD, Soni N. *Oh's Intensive Care Manual*, 6th edn. Edinburgh: Butterworth-Heinemann, 2009; pp. 583–92.

Question C55: Indications for renal replacement therapy

Indications for renal replacement therapy on the intensive care unit include:

A. Serum potassium > 6.0 mmol/l in an anuric patient
B. Oliguria
C. Anuria
D. pH < 7.2 due to hypovolaemic shock
E. Urea > 20 mmol/l

Answer: FTTFF

Short explanation

Criteria for renal replacement therapy include a serum potassium > 6.5 mmol/l or rapidly rising and refractory to medical management; oliguria or anuria; uncompensated acidosis pH < 7.1 not due to tissue hypoperfusion; urea > 35 mmol/l.

Long explanation

There are numerous criteria for renal replacement therapy (RRT) in the intensive care unit, but evidence for when to commence treatment, or the intensity and duration of that treatment, is scant. The following are the most common indications for RRT, the presence of more than one increasing the requirement:

- serum potassium > 6.5 mmol/l or rapidly rising and refractory to medical management
- oliguria or anuria (in the presence of normal biochemistry, these are relative indications only, but they preclude the provision of adequate nutrition and make fluid balance very challenging in some conditions, e.g. left ventricular failure)
- uncompensated acidosis (pH < 7.1) not due to reversible tissue hypoperfusion, e.g. hypovolaemic shock
- urea > 35 mmol/l, or uraemic complications (encephalopathy, myopathy, pericarditis)
- creatinine > 400 μmol/l
- fluid overload unresponsive to diuretics
- core temperature > 40 °C
- overdose with a dialysable toxin, e.g. lithium, salicylates

The role of haemo(dia)filtration in the management of sepsis is an ongoing area of research. The general consensus is that where RRT is indicated it should be started early, as this prevents complications and may improve survival.

Bellomo R. Renal replacement therapy. In Bersten AD, Soni N. *Oh's Intensive Care Manual*, 6th edn. Edinburgh: Butterworth-Heinemann, 2009, pp. 515–21.

Waldmann C, Soni N, Rhodes A. *Oxford Desk Reference: Critical Care*. Oxford: Oxford University Press, 2008; pp. 64–5.

Question C56: Disseminated intravascular coagulation

Regarding disseminated intravascular coagulation (DIC):

A. Fibrin degradation products (FDPs) have a high diagnostic sensitivity
B. Gram-negative bacterial sepsis is more likely to induce DIC than Gram-positive bacterial sepsis
C. Fibrin degradation products (FDPs) have a high diagnostic specificity
D. Platelet count should be maintained > 100 × 10^9/l in a bleeding patient with DIC
E. Coagulation factor concentrates are an alternative to fresh frozen plasma in the treatment of DIC

Answer: TFFFF

Short explanation

FDPs have a high sensitivity but low specificity for DIC. FFP is preferred for the treatment of coagulation factor deficiency in DIC, and the platelet count should be kept above 50 × 10^9/l in the bleeding patient. The rate of DIC in severe sepsis is the same with Gram-negative and Gram-positive bacteria.

Long explanation

Disseminated intravascular coagulation (DIC) is not a disease entity in itself but occurs secondary to an underlying disorder. It is characterised by widespread activation of systemic intravascular coagulation, resulting in deposition of fibrin in the circulation and leading to compromised organ blood supply, organ dysfunction and failure. At the same time, the consumption of platelets and coagulation factors resulting from the ongoing coagulation may induce severe bleeding.

Sepsis is the most common cause of DIC, but there is no difference in the incidence of DIC in patients with Gram-negative or Gram-positive sepsis. Systemic infection by other microorganisms, e.g. viruses and parasites, may also lead to DIC. Components of the cell membrane or bacterial exotoxins are the triggers for activation of the coagulation cascade. DIC is also seen in trauma patients, where tissue factor release is responsible for coagulation activation. The picture in trauma may be confused by the co-existing coagulopathy seen in massive transfusion and in patients who are hypothermic and acidotic. Placental debris or amniotic fluid embolism may cause DIC in the obstetric patient.

Diagnosis of DIC is based on clinical picture and laboratory testing. A scoring system devised by the Subcommittee on DIC of the International Society of Thrombosis and Haemostasis as been validated as having a sensitivity and specificity of 95% for the diagnosis. Laboratory tests show a progressive fall in platelet numbers and fibrinogen and an increase in activated partial thromboplastin time (APTT) and prothrombin time (PT). Fibrin degradation products are found in DIC; they have a diagnostic sensitivity of 90–100% but a low specificity. Equally, fibrinogen also has a role as an acute-phase protein, so that a normal level does not exclude DIC and the trend is more useful.

Treatment of DIC should be directed at correction of the underlying condition, but supportive treatment for both thrombosis and haemorrhage will be required in most patients. Generally speaking, platelets should be replaced when the level is below 10–20 × 10^9/l in non-bleeding patients and 50 × 10^9/l in bleeding patients. Fresh frozen plasma (FFP) and cryoprecipitate are the preferred methods for replacing coagulation factors and fibrinogen as they contain all the coagulation factors and inhibitors deficient during active DIC. FFP and cryoprecipitate also lack traces of activated coagulation factors, which may be found in coagulation factor concentrates and exacerbate the coagulation disorder.

Franchini M, Giuseppe Lippi G, Manzato F. Recent acquisitions in the pathophysiology, diagnosis and treatment of disseminated intravascular coagulation. *Thromb J* 2006; 4: 4.

Levi M. Disseminated intravascular coagulation. *Crit Care Med* 2007; 35: 2191–5.

Question C57: Hypokalaemia

In hypokalaemia:

A. Peaked T waves are seen on the ECG
B. U waves are seen after the T waves on the ECG
C. The duration of the action potential and refractory period are reduced
D. Ventricular arrhythmias are more likely following myocardial infarction
E. Patients taking digoxin are relatively resistant to the effects of hypokalaemia

Answer: FTFTF

Short explanation

Peaked T waves are seen in hyperkalaemia, although giant U waves can be mistaken for peaked T waves in cases of severe hypokalaemia. The duration of the action potential and refractory period are increased. Hypokalaemia of any severity can result in arrhythmias in patients taking digoxin.

Long explanation

Hypokalaemia is a common electrolyte disturbance seen in hospital patients. There are many causes, including reduced intake of potassium (in food or fluids), vomiting and diarrhoea and diuretics or treatment for hyperkalaemia. In mild cases there are usually no ECG changes and the patient may be asymptomatic or feel weak and lethargic. As potassium levels fall, the resting membrane potential increases and repolarisation is delayed. This results in an increase in the duration of the action potential and refractory period, which is potentially arrhythmogenic.

The ECG changes that are seen are a reduction in the T-wave amplitude (T-wave flattening), depression of the ST segment and the appearance of U waves. U waves are small positive deflections seen after the T wave. They are seen best in leads V_2 and V_3. Giant U waves are sometimes seen in severe cases and can be mistaken for peaked T waves. They are differentiated from T waves by being broad-based, and there is apparent lengthening of the QT interval, which is really a QU interval. Peaked T waves in hyperkalaemia are usually narrow-based, with a prominent peak, and the QT interval is normal or decreased.

The risk of hypokalaemia is that ventricular arrhythmias can occur. This is more likely to occur in patients who have had a recent myocardial infarction. There is also a risk of prolongation of the QT interval and torsades de pointes. Patients taking digoxin are more sensitive to the effects of hypokalaemia, and ventricular arrhythmias are more likely to occur.

Alfonzo A, Isles C, Geddes C, Deighan C. Potassium disorders: clinical spectrum and emergency management. *Resuscitation* 2006; 70: 10–25.

Webster A, Brady W, Morris F. Recognising signs of danger: ECG changes resulting from an abnormal serum potassium concentration. *Emerg Med J* 2002; 19: 74–7.

Question C58: Jugular bulb oximetry

With regards to the measurement of jugular venous bulb oxygen saturation, which of the following are correct?

A. The jugular bulb is a dilatation of the internal jugular bulb just inside the skull
B. Jugular saturation is normally lower than central venous saturation
C. Continuous jugular bulb oxygen saturation monitoring accurately reflects tissue oxygenation in the injured brain
D. The internal jugular vein is cannulated in a retrograde manner to place the catheter
E. It should be considered for all patients with traumatic brain injury on the ICU

Answer: FTFTF

Short explanation

The jugular bulb is a dilatation of the internal jugular bulb just below the base of the skull. Jugular venous saturations reflect global cerebral tissue oxygenation but not regional differences that occur in the injured brain. Continuous monitoring is not always accurate, because of protein build-up on the catheter. It is only recommended as a second-line device to help treat raised ICP which is refractory to usual management.

Long explanation

Cerebral tissue oxygenation is very important in the management of patients with traumatic brain injury. It is difficult to directly measure cerebral tissue oxygenation even with invasive devices. One of the main problems of measuring global cerebral tissue oxygenation is that it does not reflect the oxygenation in all parts of the brain, particularly in damaged areas of brain. Jugular bulb oximetry acts as a measure of overall cerebral tissue oxygen uptake and extraction, which is usually higher than other tissues. Normal saturations range from 55% to 71%.

Jugular venous saturation is dependent on three factors: arterial oxygen saturation, cerebral blood flow and cerebral metabolic rate. If there is a change in any of these parameters in the normal brain, then autoregulation ensures that oxygenation of cerebral tissue is maintained. In the injured brain, autoregulation may fail, leading to tissue hypoxia.

The catheter is inserted in the same manner as a central venous catheter but directed in a retrograde direction towards the brain. Correct placement can be confirmed with a lateral x-ray. Continuous monitoring and blood sampling is possible. However, regular calibration is required and protein material can build up on the catheter, resulting in inaccurate results. As with any invasive device, there are potential complications – particularly with a device inserted close to the brain. For this reason, jugular bulb oximetry is recommended only as a means of cerebral monitoring in patients with refractory raised intracranial pressure, to guide further treatment. Newer non-invasive methods of measuring cerebral tissue oxygenation, such as near-infrared spectroscopy (NIRS), are being developed and used as an alternative to jugular bulb oximetry.

Pattinson K, Wynne-Jones G, Imray C. Monitoring intracranial pressure, perfusion and metabolism. *Contin Educ Anaes Crit Care Pain* 2005; 5: 130–3.

Question C59: Burns management

Which of these statements correctly describe the management of burn injury?

A. Fluid resuscitation should be commenced as early as possible even in the absence of shock
B. Prophylactic antibiotics should be administered to prevent ventilator-associated pneumonia
C. Early institution of enteral nutrition is recommended in major burns
D. Escharotomy is not usually required in full-thickness burns, because swelling is rarely a problem
E. Referral to a regional burns centre is advised for adults with 8% burns and inhalational injury

Answer: TFTFT

Short explanation

Prophylactic antibiotics are not recommended in patients with burns as the risk of developing resistant organisms is high. Escharotomy is often performed for patients with full-thickness and/or circumferential burns to release pressure from swelling.

Long explanation

The mortality from burns remains high and is around 13% of hospitalised patients with burns. Major risk factors, which increase mortality, are older age, significant comorbidity, more than 40% burns and inhalational injury. The management of major burns can be complicated and in general should be undertaken in a regional burns unit where protocols have been designed to achieve good patient outcomes. However, patients present to hospitals all over the country with burns, and initial management is commonly commenced in the emergency department. The initial management can make a big difference to long-term outcome.

Fluid resuscitation should be started in adults with over 15% body-surface-area burns, or over 10% burns with inhalational injury. Colloids should be avoided, and crystalloids such as Hartmann's solution or Ringer's lactate are recommended. The Parkland formula (4 ml per kg per % burn) is used to calculate the total volume of fluid required in the first 24 hours (from the time of the burn). Half of this should be administered in the first 8 hours, and the second half in the following 16 hours. Maintenance fluid is required in addition to this. Fluid therapy should be targeted at 0.5 ml per kg per hour of urine output, and patients may require further fluid boluses.

Burns patients are at great risk of infection (even in minor burns), but antibiotics should be administered only in proven infections and with microbiology advice. The risk of resistant organisms is high if antibiotics are administered prophylactically. Patients with major burns will mount an enormous systemic inflammatory response, and therefore a high temperature does not always signify infection, particularly in the first 24 hours. Early nutrition is advised to counteract the catabolic state and muscle wasting seen in major burns patients.

Bishop S, Maguire S. Anaesthesia and intensive care for major burns. *Contin Educ Anaesth Crit Care Pain* 2012; 12: 118–22.

Question C60: Carbon monoxide poisoning

Concerning the management of carbon monoxide poisoning, which of the following are correct?

A. Carbon monoxide in the blood is made up of endogenously produced and exogenously inhaled carbon monoxide
B. Carboxyhaemoglobin levels > 10% are invariably fatal

C. Patients with chronic obstructive pulmonary disease are protected from the toxic effects of carbon monoxide
D. Carbon monoxide binds less avidly to cardiac myoglobin than to haemoglobin
E. The relationship between inspired levels of carbon monoxide and arterial carboxyhaemoglobin levels is linear

Answer: TFFFT

Short explanation

Carboxyhaemoglobin levels between 15% and 20% are well tolerated in humans, and this appears to be the threshold above which symptoms start to become apparent. Patients with respiratory and cardiovascular comorbidities are more at risk of carbon monoxide toxicity. Carbon monoxide binds even more avidly to cardiac myoglobin.

Long explanation

Carbon monoxide poisoning remains an all-too-common cause of death due to faulty gas appliances and poor ventilation in domestic and industrial areas. Carbon monoxide is a colourless odourless gas which is not naturally detected by humans. High levels go undetected until symptoms emerge, or until death. Mild symptoms are non-specific and include nausea, dizziness and fatigue. As carboxyhaemoglobin levels increase, the patient may experience breathlessness, tachycardia, hearing loss, convulsions and loss of consciousness. Smokers may have more severe symptoms, as their carboxyhaemoglobin levels are already raised.

Carbon monoxide binds to haemoglobin up to 250 times more readily than oxygen. Once bound, carboxyhaemoglobin is very stable and oxygen content of the blood is proportionally reduced. This leads to tissue hypoxia and acidosis once levels rise above 20%. The heart and brain are more vulnerable to the toxic effects because of their high metabolic rate. In addition to reduced oxygen delivery, carbon monoxide has direct toxic effects at the cellular levels, particularly inhibition of cytochrome oxidases.

Standard pulse oximetry will not detect carboxyhaemoglobin, and oxygen saturations will read inappropriately high. CO-oximetry on an arterial blood gas sample must be performed to confirm the diagnosis. The half-life of carboxyhaemoglobin is significantly reduced in the presence of high inspired fractions of oxygen. In patients with suspected or confirmed carbon monoxide poisoning, administration of 100% oxygen increases the rate of release of carbon monoxide from haemoglobin. Hyperbaric oxygen can speed this process even further but is often not readily available.

Bauer I, Pannen B. Bench-to-bedside review: carbon monoxide – from mitochondrial poisoning to therapeutic use. *Crit Care* 2009; 13: 220.

Question C61: Thrombolysis in STEMI

The following are absolute contraindications to thrombolysis in STEMI:

A. Significant closed head injury 5 months ago
B. Ischaemic stroke 6 weeks ago
C. 6 cm abdominal aortic aneurysm diagnosed 2 weeks ago
D. Cardiopulmonary resuscitation 3 hours ago
E. Intracranial meningioma

Answer: FTFFT

Short explanation

Thrombolysis should be offered to patients with STEMI within 12 hours of onset of symptoms if primary PCI cannot be delivered within the next 120 minutes. Closed head injury within 3 months is an absolute contraindication, as is suspected aortic dissection, but aortic aneurysm and CPR are not.

Long explanation

The key to management of patients presenting with acute ST-elevation myocardial infarction (STEMI) is early reperfusion: early focused treatment to reopen acutely occluded coronary arteries. Reperfusion is more effective the earlier it occurs, particularly within the first 3 hours of onset of symptoms. Reperfusion with primary percutaneous coronary intervention (PCI) is superior to thrombolytic therapy, with reduced mortality and lower rates of recurrent MI and intracerebral haemorrhage.

As access to primary PCI has improved, the use of thrombolytic agents (e.g. tenecteplase, alteplase) has declined, but it still has a place in the treatment of acute STEMI. Thrombolysis should be offered to patients with STEMI within 12 hours of onset of symptoms if primary PCI cannot be delivered within the next 120 minutes. Caution should be exercised in patients at risk of bleeding.

Absolute contraindications to thrombolysis include:

- intracranial malignancy
- intracranial vascular lesion
- previous intracerebral haemorrhage
- closed head injury within 3 months
- ischaemic stroke within 3 months
- active bleeding (excluding menses)
- bleeding diathesis
- aortic dissection

National Institute for Health and Care Excellence. *CG167: Myocardial Infarction with ST-Segment Elevation*. London: NICE, 2013. http://www.nice.org.uk/cg167 (accessed June 2014).

Question C62: Guillain–Barré syndrome

Regarding the investigation and management of Guillain–Barré syndrome (GBS):

A. Patients with a vital capacity < 15 ml/kg are likely to need intubation
B. Gastroparesis in GBS means that intubation using a rapid sequence induction (RSI) with suxamethonium is required
C. Intravenous immunoglobulin is more effective than plasma exchange
D. Corticosteroids are a useful early treatment
E. Miller–Fisher syndrome is a subtype of GBS characterised by autonomic instability

Answer: TFFFF

Short explanation

Patients with a vital capacity (VC) < 20 ml/kg should be admitted for observation to critical care; patients with VC < 15 ml/kg or bulbar palsy should be intubated. Suxamethonium should be avoided owing to the risk of hyperkalaemia. Plasma exchange is as effective as immunoglobulin, but may be less well tolerated in autonomic instability. Corticosteroids are ineffective and may delay recovery. Miller–Fisher syndrome is a subtype of GBS characterised by ophthalmoplegia, areflexia and bulbar palsy.

Long explanation

Guillain–Barré syndrome (GBS) is a rare neurological disorder characterised by ascending flaccid paralysis, areflexia and autonomic instability. The pathology is an autoimmune (IgG) demyelination of peripheral nerves, often triggered by a pathogen (commonly *Campylobacter jejuni*, CMV, EBV or *Mycoplasma pneumoniae*). Some subtypes have only motor or sensory components. Miller–Fisher syndrome (MFS) is a subtype of GBS characterised by ophthalmoplegia, areflexia and bulbar palsy. Patients are typically admitted to critical care for management of respiratory failure, pneumonia or cardiovascular instability. Overall mortality is around 5–10%, and 20% of survivors are left with long-term disability.

Patients with GBS should have regular spirometry (vital capacity) for monitoring of their disease progression. Other investigations should be performed to exclude other diseases (CNS imaging, lumbar puncture, microbiological cultures, antibodies etc.). Most GBS patients typically have elevated CSF protein and abnormal nerve conduction studies within a week of the onset of symptoms.

Patients with a VC < 20 ml/kg should be admitted to critical care for monitoring. Patients with respiratory failure, poor cough, bulbar palsy or VC < 15 ml/kg should be intubated. Suxamethonium should be avoided as there is a risk of severe, life-threatening hyperkalaemia in patients with demyelination or paralysis. Cardiovascular instability is common, with bradycardia and labile blood pressure. Cardiac pacing is sometimes required.

Definitive treatment of GBS involves plasma exchange or intravenous immunoglobulins. These treatments are equally effective, but patients with cardiovascular instability may not tolerate plasma exchange. Corticosteroids are ineffective in the treatment of GBS and may delay recovery. General supportive measures are important in patients with paralysis, including DVT prophylaxis, physiotherapy, analgesia, feeding and psychological support.

Hughes R, Swan A, Van Doorn P. Corticosteroids for Guillain-Barré syndrome. *Cochrane Database Syst Rev* 2010; (4): CD001446.

Yuki N, Hartung HP. Guillain-Barré syndrome. *N Engl J Med* 2012; 366: 2294–304.

Question C63: Venous thromboprophylaxis

With regards to the prevention and management of venous thromboembolism in critical care patients, which of the following are correct?

A. Mechanical thromboprophylaxis has benefits similar to those obtained with pharmacological methods in preventing PE
B. Factor Xa levels need not be routinely monitored in patients receiving low-molecular-weight heparin (LMWH)
C. Aspirin therapy should be considered in high-risk patients with contraindications to heparin therapy
D. Fondaparinux can be used as an alternative to LMWH in patients with a previous history of heparin-induced thrombocytopenia (HIT)
E. Patients recovering from major trauma are at the highest risk of venous thromboembolism

Answer: FTFTT

Short explanation

Mechanical thromboprophylaxis has no proven benefit in reducing the risk of death due to pulmonary embolism. Studies demonstrating benefits in reduction of DVT have not been confirmed in critical care patients. Aspirin is not recommended for use in critical care patients as a method of thromboprophylaxis because it has unproven benefits and significant side effects.

Long explanation

Thromboembolic disease is a major cause of mortality and morbidity in all hospital inpatients, particularly in critical care patients. Evidence suggests that the incidence of pulmonary embolism at post-mortem is as high as 27%. Asymptomatic deep venous thrombosis (DVT) is extremely common, and although many are of the calf veins, these can lead to embolic complications. Critical care patients have multiple risk factors such as immobility, sepsis, trauma, recent surgery, respiratory and cardiac failure, haemodialysis, central venous catheters and dehydration.

Graduated elastic stockings and intermittent compression devices (mechanical thromboprophylaxis) should be used in all patients who have contraindications to pharmacological thromboprophylaxis. However, there is no robust evidence to support their benefits, although it is reasonable to suggest that they can work in a synergistic manner with other interventions designed to reduce DVTs.

Aspirin is no longer recommended as pharmacological thromboprophylaxis, and the risks of bleeding outweigh any potential benefits, particularly in the critically ill who are at risk of gastric ulceration. Unfractionated heparin can be administered three times daily subcutaneously (5000 units) as thromboprophylaxis, but only in those patients who have contraindications to low-molecular-weight heparins (LMWH), which have a safer side-effect profile (namely, a lower risk of heparin-induced thrombocytopenia (HIT) and osteoporosis). Thromboprophylaxis with LMWH is indicated in all adult patients admitted to the intensive care unit unless there is a specific contraindication. The most limiting factor is renal impairment, where levels are unpredictable, and so this needs to be taken into consideration when prescribing for critical care patients. Warfarin is not indicated. Fondaparinux can be used where heparins are contraindicated, such as with a history of HIT. It is a synthetic anti-Xa agent.

Regular full blood counts should be performed on all patients receiving thromboprophylaxis to ensure that they are not developing thrombocytopenia. In addition, there are a number of relative contraindications to pharmacological thromboprophylaxis such as platelets $< 50 \times 10^9/l$, underlying coagulopathy (INR > 1.5), active bleeding, recent central neuraxial blockade or lumbar puncture and new cerebrovascular accident within the previous 2 weeks.

Hunt B, Retter A. *Venous Thromboprophylaxis in Critical Care*. Intensive Care Society Standards and Guidelines. London: ICS, 2008.

Question C64: Treatment of MRSA

Methicillin-resistant *Staphylococcus aureus* (MRSA) can be successfully treated with the following antibiotics:

A. Intravenous ceftazidime
B. Oral vancomycin
C. Intravenous teicoplanin
D. Intravenous linezolid
E. Intravenous rifampicin

Answer: FFTTT

Short explanation

The traditional treatment for MRSA is intravenous vancomycin. Oral vancomycin is not absorbed systemically. Cephalosporin treatment is a risk factor for MRSA acquisition.

Long explanation

Methicillin-resistant *Staphylococcus aureus* (MRSA) is a mainly nosocomial infection causing major morbidity and mortality. It is endemic in many hospitals in the developed world. The traditional treatment for MRSA is intravenous vancomycin. Oral vancomycin is not absorbed and is therefore reserved for the treatment of *Clostridium difficile* diarrhoea. Other drugs suitable for use in MRSA infections include teicoplanin, linezolid and rifampicin. Their use is generally under the direction of microbiologists. Cephalosporin treatment is a risk factor for MRSA acquisition, as is treatment with penicillins.

Empirical treatment for MRSA should be on the basis of high clinical suspicion. Risk factors for MRSA infection in the community include intravenous drug use, chronic disease, antibiotic therapy and recurrent hospitalisation. Risk factors for MRSA colonisation and infection in hospital include increasing age, length of stay, critical care admission, chronic disease, antibiotic therapy, presence of a wound and/or indwelling lines or catheters. Patients should be screened before or on admission to hospital, and patients colonised with MRSA should be isolated to reduce spread. Topical eradication therapy may then be used, although patients may remain colonised for up to 3 years. MRSA colonisation is a risk factor for systemic infection. The mortality rate for nosocomial MRSA pneumonia is 33%, and for MRSA bacteraemia it is 50%.

Haddadin AS, Fappiano SA, Lipsett PA. Methicillin resistant *Staphylococcus aureus* (MRSA) in the intensive care unit. *Postgrad Med J* 2002; 78: 385–92.

Question C65: Massive blood transfusion

Regarding massive blood transfusion:

A. It is defined as the replacement of the circulating volume in 4 hours
B. Hypothermia shifts the oxyhaemoglobin dissociation curve to the right
C. Blood giving sets should have 50-micron filters in situ
D. Platelets may be given through a blood giving set
E. Transfusion aims to keep haemoglobin > 10 g/dl with ongoing bleeding

Answer: FFFFF

Short explanation

Massive transfusion is the replacement of the circulating volume in 24 hours. Standard blood giving sets have filters of 170-micron size. Platelets should be given through a dedicated giving set. Hypothermia shifts the oxyhaemoglobin dissociation curve to the left. Transfusion is generally to symptoms or to keep haemoglobin > 7 g/dl.

Long explanation

Massive blood transfusion may be defined as:

- replacement of the circulating volume in 24 hours
- 4 units of blood in 1 hour with continuing blood loss
- loss of 50% of circulating blood volume within 3 hours

Transfusion triggers are difficult to use in massive haemorrhage, and there is emerging evidence that the fewer the blood products the patient receives, the better the outcome as long as oxygen delivery is maintained. There is increasing emphasis on hypotensive resuscitation and early damage-control surgery to limit transfusion requirements. In general, a previously healthy adult will tolerate a haemoglobin of > 7 g/dl. Coagulation factors in the form of fresh frozen plasma (FFP) and platelets should be given as soon as massive haemorrhage is diagnosed, as it is easier to prevent coagulopathy than to treat it once it is established.

Hypothermia is common with massive blood transfusion, as the patient is often undergoing treatment for major trauma or extensive surgery. Hypothermia shifts the oxyhaemoglobin dissociation curve to the left, reducing oxygen delivery to the tissues and worsening any coagulopathy. Meticulous care should be given to warming the patient and the blood products he or she is receiving.

Standard blood giving sets have filters of 170-micron size to remove microaggregates. Platelets should be given through a dedicated giving set, which has a smaller priming volume although the filter size is the same.

Isbister JP. Blood transfusion. In Bersten AD, Soni N. *Oh's Intensive Care Manual*, 6th edn. Edinburgh: Butterworth-Heinemann, 2009; pp. 995–1010.

Maxwell MJ, Wilson MJA. Complications of blood transfusion. *Contin Educ Anaesth Crit Care Pain* 2006; 6: 225–9.

Joint United Kingdom (UK) Blood Transfusion and Tissue Transplantation Services Professional Advisory Committee (JPAC). *Guidelines for the Blood Transfusion Services in the UK*, 8th edn. London: TSO, 2013. www.transfusionguidelines.org.uk/red-book (accessed June 2014).

Question C66: Acute pancreatitis

Regarding the management of severe acute pancreatitis (SAP):

A. Patients with a Glasgow score of 3 or more should be managed in a critical care unit
B. Enteral feeding should be avoided for the first 7 days
C. Empirical antibiotics should be prescribed
D. Endoscopic retrograde cholangiopancreatography (ERCP) should be considered in patients with SAP and jaundice
E. Necrotic pancreatic tissue should be surgically debrided as soon as possible

Answer: FFFTF

Short explanation

Patients with SAP should be admitted to critical care according to the severity of their illness. Scoring systems (Ranson, Glasgow, APACHE) may help identify patients requiring critical care. Early enteral feeding is thought to be beneficial, and antibiotics should only be used in cases of confirmed infected necrosis or sepsis. Gallstone pancreatitis may be effectively treated by ERCP. Delaying surgery for resection of necrotic pancreatic tissue has been shown to be beneficial.

Long explanation

Acute pancreatitis has a UK incidence of 10–40 cases per 100,000 population. Up to 20% of episodes of acute pancreatitis are classified as severe (SAP). SAP is defined as acute pancreatitis with evidence of local (infection, cyst formation) or systemic (organ dysfunction, SIRS) complications. The commonest causes are alcohol and gallstones, but may be due to trauma, drugs, malignancy or viral infections.

Patients typically present with severe epigastric pain and vomiting, and they may show signs of hypovolaemia or multi-organ dysfunction. Serum amylase is typically raised, although it may be normal; lipase levels are more sensitive and specific. Abdominal ultrasound should be performed (to identify gallstones and fluid collections), although abdominal CT (with contrast) is increasingly used. A diagnosis of acute pancreatitis may be made in patients with two of the following three features:

- severe, acute, epigastric pain
- serum lipase or amylase at least 3 × the upper limit of normal
- features typical of pancreatitis on CT, ultrasound or MRI

Many patients with SAP will require critical care admission, but this should be according to severity of illness. Scoring systems such as Ranson, Glasgow or APACHE may aid identification of appropriate patients for critical care admission. Management is typically supportive, with particular focus on adequate fluid resuscitation, analgesia and monitoring. Empirical antibiotics are not recommended unless there is evidence of infected necrosis (e.g. cultured in aspirated fluid) or systemic infection.

Enteral feeding has been shown to reduce mortality and should be attempted in all patients. Patients with SAP secondary to gallstone obstruction of the pancreatic and common bile ducts should undergo early endoscopic retrograde cholangiopancreatography (ERCP). Surgery should be performed for drainage of collections or resection of infected necrotic tissue. These procedures are high risk and should be delayed for at least 2–3 weeks if possible.

Banks PA, Bollen TL, Dervenis C, *et al.* Classification of acute pancreatitis – 2012: revision of the Atlanta classification and definitions by international consensus. *Gut* 2013; 62: 102–11.

Nathens AB, Curtis JR, Beale RJ, *et al.* Management of the critically ill patient with severe acute pancreatitis. *Crit Care Med* 2004; 32: 2524–36.

Question C67: Abdominal trauma

In cases of abdominal trauma, which of the following are correct?

A. Bleeding patients with coagulopathy at presentation have a higher mortality than those without coagulopathy
B. Patients with isolated abdominal trauma and evidence of significant haemorrhage should undergo CT scanning as the first-line radiological intervention
C. Aortic cross-clamping is of use in the exanguinating patient
D. Tranexamic acid should be administered in the bleeding trauma patient
E. Definitive repairs of bleeding organs should be undertaken as soon as possible after injury

Answer: TFTTF

Short explanation

Initially a FAST ultrasound scan can be performed in the unstable patient with suspected abdominal haemorrhage. If the patient is haemodynamically stable or if the FAST scan is positive then CT scan should be performed as soon as possible for diagnosis. Patients who are too unstable should go directly to the operating theatre. Damage-control surgery should be undertaken in the shocked patient, and complicated repairs should be delayed until the patient is stable.

Long explanation

Multiple organ failure and death occur commonly in patients with uncontrolled post-traumatic bleeding. With coordinated, appropriate and timely management, these complications can be avoided in many patients. It is not only the volume of blood loss which dictates outcome, but the presence or absence of deranged physiological parameters such as coagulopathy, acidosis, hypothermia and hypoperfusion.

Initial management of the patient presenting with a history of blunt abdominal trauma should be coordinated by a trauma team. Early identification and diagnosis of haemorrhage should be a priority. In the emergency department, FAST (focused assessment with sonography in trauma) scans can be performed quickly and safely, even in an unstable patient. If there is evidence of free fluid in the abdomen, then the patient should either undergo CT scanning, if deemed stable enough, or should be transferred directly to the operating theatre for bleeding control either surgically or using interventional radiology.

Unstable patients who are transferred to theatre should undergo 'damage-control surgery', which consists of three components. Firstly, an abbreviated resuscitative laparotomy for control of bleeding, the restitution of blood flow and the control of contamination should be performed. If the patient is exanguinating then aortic cross-clamping may be required to direct blood flow to the brain and heart. Abdominal packing and temporary closure should be undertaken. The second phase involves intensive care, focusing on rewarming, correction of acidosis and correction of coagulopathy. The third phase is the definitive surgical repair, which should occur only once target parameters have been reached. Sometimes, interventional radiology can be used instead of surgery to repair bleeding vessels.

Rossaint R, Bouillon B, Cerny V, *et al.* Management of bleeding following major trauma: an updated European guideline. *Crit Care* 2010; 14: R52.

Question C68: The femoral triangle

Concerning the femoral triangle:

A. The roof is formed by the fascia iliaca
B. The femoral artery enters the triangle between the medial and middle thirds of the inguinal ligament
C. The femoral vein lies medial to the femoral artery throughout the femoral triangle
D. The great saphenous vein empties into the femoral vein within the femoral triangle
E. The femoral nerve lies lateral to the femoral sheath

Answer: FFFTT

Short explanation

The fascia lata forms the roof of the femoral triangle. The femoral artery enters the femoral triangle at the midpoint of the inguinal ligament. The femoral nerve lies lateral, outside the femoral sheath. The femoral vein enters the femoral triangle deep to the artery, but moves medially as it ascends and receives the profunda femoris and saphenous veins.

Long explanation

The femoral triangle is a triangular space on the anterolateral upper thigh commonly used for arterial and venous access. It is bounded superiorly by the inguinal ligament, laterally by the medial border of sartorius and medially by the medial border of adductor longus. The floor is formed by adductor longus, pectineus and iliopsoas; the roof is formed by the fascia lata. Its contents include the femoral artery, the femoral vein and the femoral nerve along with branches and tributaries, lymphatics and lymph nodes.

The femoral artery, a continuation of the external iliac artery, enters the femoral triangle at the midpoint of the inguinal ligament and runs inferiorly to the apex of the triangle, where it enters the adductor canal. A major branch of the femoral artery – the profunda femoris, which supplies most of the thigh – arises within the femoral triangle.

The femoral vein enters the femoral triangle close to the apex, deep to the femoral artery. As it travels superiorly, it receives tributaries (profunda femoris and great saphenous veins) and comes to run medial to the femoral artery. It exits the femoral triangle medial to the midpoint of the inguinal ligament, becoming the external iliac vein. The femoral sheath encloses the femoral artery and vein along with some lymphatics and lymph nodes.

The femoral nerve is formed from the lumbar plexus (L2–4) and enters the femoral triangle lateral to the midpoint of the inguinal ligament, outside the femoral sheath. It divides into several muscular branches and exits the femoral triangle with the femoral artery in the adductor canal as the saphenous nerve.

Moore KL, Dalley AF, Agur AMR. *Clinically Oriented Anatomy*, 7th edn. Philadelphia, PA: Lippincott, Williams & Wilkins, 2013.

Question C69: Botulism

With respect to botulism:

A. Antibiotics should be given empirically on clinical grounds
B. Antitoxin treatment may result in anaphylaxis
C. It causes an ascending flaccid paralysis
D. It invalidates brainstem death testing
E. Sensory nerves are affected first

Answer: FTFTF

Short explanation

Antibiotics are ineffective for botulism, which causes a descending flaccid paralysis affecting cranial, respiratory and autonomic nerves. Sensory nerves are unaffected.

Long explanation

Botulism is an acute descending motor paralysis affecting cranial, respiratory and autonomic nerves. It is caused by an exotoxin released from the anaerobic spore-forming bacterium *Clostridium botulinum*. There are a number of genetically distinct bacteria in the group, with different toxins, three of which (A, B and E) affect humans particularly. Botulism is encountered worldwide, as the bacterium is present in soil, vegetables, fish and putrid food. It may also be spread via intravenous or subcutaneous drug use. The spores are very heat-resistant and grow well in canned food. The toxin is absorbed across mucous membranes and spreads via the bloodstream to irreversibly bind to cholinergic receptors. This blocks the neuromuscular junction, autonomic synapses and parasympathetic nerve terminals. Cranial nerves are particularly affected, but sensory neurons and adrenergic synapses remain unaffected.

Foodborne botulism usually starts 12–48 hours after ingestion of infected food. Clinical features include nausea, vomiting and abdominal distension followed by cranial nerve palsies and descending flaccid paralysis. Autonomic involvement may lead to hypotension, urinary retention, constipation and fixed dilated pupils. Cortical function and sensation are preserved. Wound botulism has a similar clinical picture without gastrointestinal symptoms.

Diagnosis is by mouse bioassay, cultures of wound/stool samples and neurophysiology. Nerve conduction tests show normal nerve velocity, reduced muscle action potentials with post-tetanic enhancement, and no post-tetanic exhaustion.

Management is supportive, with ventilatory support often required. Antibiotics are ineffective for the primary infection. Specific trivalent (A, B, E) equine antitoxin should be given on clinical grounds, because microbiological confirmation takes time. The antitoxin is not effective once the toxin has bound to the receptors. Treatment with antitoxin may result in anaphylaxis. Recovery requires formation of new nerve terminals, and therefore may take up to 6 months.

Treacher D. Botulism. In Waldmann C, Soni N, Rhodes A. *Oxford Desk Reference: Critical Care*. Oxford: Oxford University Press, 2008; pp. 380–1.
Wenham T, Cohen A. Botulism. *Contin Educ Anaesth Crit Care Pain* 2008; 8: 21–5.

Question C70: Paracetamol-induced acute liver failure

In a case of paracetamol-induced acute liver failure:

A. The liver injury is due to a direct toxic effect of paracetamol on hepatocytes
B. Activated charcoal should be administered if within 4 hours of overdose
C. *N*-acetyl-cysteine is ineffective if given by the oral route
D. Patients with pH < 7.3 after fluid resuscitation should be referred for transplant
E. Intravenous *N*-acetyl-cysteine causes adverse reactions in up to 20% of patients

Answer: FFFTT

Short explanation

A toxic metabolite, NAPQI, is responsible for hepatotoxicity in paracetamol (acetaminophen) overdose. Activated charcoal should be given within 2 hours of overdose. *N*-acetyl-cysteine is equally effective given by the oral route, and is routinely administered orally in the USA. Intravenous administration causes adverse reactions in up to 20% of patients. King's College Hospital London's liver transplant referral criteria include pH < 7.3 despite fluid resuscitation.

Long explanation

Paracetamol is the commonest cause of acute liver failure in several developed countries, including the UK and the USA. Paracetamol is metabolised in the liver via a number of different pathways. At normal therapeutic levels, over 90% of paracetamol is conjugated to sulphate and glucuronide groups, forming non-toxic metabolites excreted by the kidney. The remainder is hydroxylated by cytochrome P450 enzymes to *N*-acetyl-p-benzoquinoneimine (NAPQI). NAPQI is toxic, but is rapidly conjugated with glutathione to form a non-toxic product that is also excreted by the kidneys. In overdose, the glucuronide and sulphate conjugation pathways for paracetamol become saturated, and so increased levels of NAPQI result. As NAPQI levels increase, glutathione reserves become exhausted, meaning that NAPQI starts to accumulate within hepatocytes, where it causes necrosis and liver failure. Patients with low levels of glutathione (e.g. alcoholism, malnutrition) or high cytochrome P450 activity (due to enzyme-inducing drugs such as isoniazid) are at increased risk of paracetamol-induced acute liver failure.

Paracetamol levels should be tested in all cases of suspected overdose, and treatment commenced with reference to a nomogram of serum level and time since overdose. Gastric lavage is no longer recommended, but activated charcoal may be administered within 2 hours of ingestion in a patient with a secure airway.

N-acetyl-cysteine is the mainstay of treatment. It should be commenced as early as possible, but may be of benefit even if delayed by over 24 hours. *N*-acetyl-cysteine is an amino acid that is metabolised to glutathione in the liver, replenishing stores for conjugation to NAPQI. It is administered intravenously in the UK, but is equally effective given by mouth. Oral administration is routine in the USA and has a lower incidence of adverse reactions, which may occur in up to 23% of patients treated with IV *N*-acetyl-cysteine. Adverse reactions include anaphylaxis, bronchospasm, hypotension, nausea and vomiting.

The most widely used liver transplant referral criteria are those developed by King's College Hospital in London. A patient satisfies the criteria with *either*:

- arterial pH < 7.3 despite adequate fluid resuscitation

or all three of:

- INR > 6.5
- serum creatinine > 300 μmol/l or anuria
- encephalopathy grade 3 or 4

Bernal W, Auzinger G, Dhawan A, Wendon J. Acute liver failure. *Lancet*, 2010; 376: 190–201.

Trotter JF. Practical management of acute liver failure in the intensive care unit. *Curr Opin Crit Care* 2009; 15: 163–7.

Question C71: The obtunded trauma patient

With regards to the management of obtunded adult trauma patients, which of the following are correct?

A. Level 1 evidence exists to guide radiological investigations and subsequent management of potential cervical spine injury
B. Patients with low risk of cervical spine injury should undergo dynamic fluoroscopy
C. MRI is the gold-standard investigation with the highest sensitivity and specificity for bone and ligamentous injuries
D. CT scan alone has been reported to have a false-negative rate as high as 4% for cervical spine injury
E. MRI should be performed as early as possible in all patients with clinical signs of spinal cord pathology

Answer: FFFTT

Short explanation

Most guidelines are based on meta-analyses of retrospective observational studies, also known as level 2b evidence. Dynamic fluoroscopy is no longer recommended; it has been superseded by the widespread availability of CT. MRI is not as sensitive as

CT at detecting bony injury and has a false-positive rate of up to 40% for ligamentous injury.

Long explanation

The investigation of obtunded adult trauma patients with suspected cervical spine injury remains a controversial and difficult subject for critical care physicians. The decision to use or remove spinal immobilisation should be taken by the trauma team as a whole with the advice of specialist radiologists, neurosurgeons and orthopaedic surgeons. It often requires critical care doctors to balance the risks of a missed cervical spine injury (present in only 5% of blunt trauma victims, of which only a small proportion will require surgery) against the risks of hard-collar immobilisation. The risks of immobilisation are far from insignificant. Higher rates of ventilator-associated pneumonia and delirium, both of which increase mortality in critical care patients, have been reported.

The EAST guidelines for investigation of cervical spine injury in awake patients are well accepted and followed by institutions throughout the world. However, standard guidelines for the obtunded patient remain less well described. In the past, dynamic fluoroscopy was recommended, but its use has now been superseded by the 24-hour availability of CT in most hospitals in the developed world. Current controversy centres around whether CT alone is adequate, or whether MRI should be performed in addition to CT in obtunded patients. A recent review of various studies and meta-analyses has demonstrated a worst-case (i.e. pessimistic likelihood) operative fixing rate of 0.29% in patients who undergo MRI following a normal CT scan. It would, however, result in 4.3% of patients undergoing prolonged spinal immobilisation before they could be assessed once awake.

Whether a hospital decides to use CT alone or in combination with MRI remains a local decision. Suggested recommendations are that documentation of limb movement at presentation should be completed in all cases, whole-spine CT should be performed in all obtunded blunt trauma patients, MRI should be performed in all patients with clinical signs suggestive of spinal cord injury, images should be reported by senior radiologists with adequate trauma and musculoskeletal experience, and spinal immobilisation should be removed as soon as possible after admission.

Como JJ, Diaz JJ, Dunham CM, *et al.* Practice management guidelines for identification of cervical spine injuries following trauma: update from the Eastern Association for the Surgery of Trauma Practice Management Guidelines Committee. *J Trauma* 2009; 67: 651–9.

Plumb J, Morris C. Clinical review: spinal imaging for the adult obtunded blunt trauma patient: update from 2004. *Intensive Care Med* 2012; 38: 752–71.

Question C72: Vasculitis

Regarding vasculitides:

A. They can be secondary to infective, inflammatory or malignant conditions
B. Wegener's granulomatosis (WG) affects large arteries
C. Churg–Strauss syndrome (CSS) is associated with asthma
D. Negative ANCA serology effectively excludes primary vasculitis
E. Management is purely supportive

Answer: TFTFF

Short explanation

Vasculitides may be primary or secondary to endocarditis, autoimmune disease or malignancy. WG is a disease of small vessels. CSS is typically preceded by asthma and rhinitis. Many vasculitides are ANCA-negative. The main treatments are corticosteroids, with cyclophosphamide in severe disease.

Long explanation

Systemic vasculitides are a heterogeneous group of rare conditions, with an annual incidence of 2–10 per 100,000 population. Vasculitis can be difficult to diagnose and can cause multi-organ failure, and patients requiring ICU admission have a mortality rate of over 50%. The common pathological finding is inflammation of blood vessel walls causing necrosis or granuloma formation.

Vasculitides may be primary or secondary to another disease. Primary vasculitides are either idiopathic (e.g. WG, polyarteritis nodosa (PAN)) or immune-complex-mediated (Goodpasture's, Henoch–Schönlein purpura). Secondary vasculitides may be drug-related (e.g. hydralazine, penicillamine, carbimazole) or seen in autoimmune disease (rheumatoid arthritis, lupus), infections (bacterial endocarditis) or malignancy (lymphoma, leukaemia). Primary idiopathic vasculitides may be further classified according to the size of vessel typically affected:

- large vessels: giant-cell arteritis and Takayasu's arteritis
- medium vessels: PAN, Kawasaki disease
- small vessels: WG, CSS, microscopic polyangiitis (MPA)

Clinical features typically include systemic, non-specific features such as malaise, weight loss and fever. The lack of pathognomonic features can make vasculitis difficult to distinguish from infection, autoimmune disease or malignancy. Some diseases have typical presentations that make them easier to identify: PAN is often associated with hepatitis B, and CSS is commonly preceded by asthma and rhinitis by months or years. Presentation to ICU is often due to renal failure or respiratory failure from pulmonary haemorrhage.

Typical laboratory findings in vasculitis include raised ESR and CRP, normocytic anaemia and evidence of renal impairment. Chest radiography may reveal nodules, infiltrates or haemorrhage. WG is often c-anti-neutrophil cytoplasmic antibody (cANCA)-positive, while MPA is typically pANCA-positive, but a negative ANCA does not rule out vasculitis. Likewise, a positive ANCA is not diagnostic of vasculitis.

The mainstay of treatment is immunosuppression. Mild cases often require corticosteroids alone, but cases requiring ICU care should also be treated with cyclophosphamide. Plasma exchange, immunoglobulins and specific antibodies have also been tried, although evidence for their use is currently lacking.

Semple D, Keogh J, Forni L, Venn R. Clinical review: vasculitis on the intensive care unit. Part 1: diagnosis. *Crit Care* 2005; 9: 92–7.

Semple D, Keogh J, Forni L, Venn R. Clinical review: vasculitis on the intensive care unit. Part 2: treatment and prognosis. *Crit Care* 2005; 9: 193–7.

Question C73: Patient decision making

Which of the following statements about patient decision making are correct?

A. An advance decision to refuse treatment is legally binding in England and Wales
B. An advance decision to refuse life-sustaining procedures must be in writing, signed and witnessed
C. No-one can make medical decisions on behalf of another adult in England

D. Patients can nominate more than one lasting power of attorney
E. Patients can make advance decisions to insist upon all life-sustaining treatment

Answer: TTFTF

Short explanation

Since the Mental Capacity Act 2005, powers of attorney have been extended to include health and welfare decisions for an adult without capacity. This includes consenting for medical treatment. Advance decisions cannot insist upon futile or inappropriate treatment or unlawful procedures.

Long explanation

The legal issues surrounding emergency medical treatment and end-of-life care are complicated. It is not necessary to know the intricate details for every possible situation but it is important to have a general understanding of the principles which underpin the law. There are some key points to remember. Since the Mental Capacity Act 2005 took effect in 2007, there are some changes relevant to clinicians caring for patients who do not have capacity to make decisions on their own medical care.

If a patient has a nominated lasting power of attorney (LPA), the nominated person may be able to make decisions for the patient. This would only be relevant if the patient had, while competent, made a formal legal transfer of health decision-making authority. This involves a formal written witnessed statement. This statement does not routinely extend to refusing life-sustaining treatment unless it is explicitly stated. Patients may have more than one nominated LPA.

Advance decisions regarding medical treatment are important and have significant legal implications. Patients often make these statements in case of future mental incapacity so that their wishes are respected and followed. In general they are advance refusals of treatment. They should be made when the patient has capacity, and they can be written or verbal statements. Where it is a verbal conversation, this should be recorded contemporaneously in the patient's medical record. Patients can refuse any medical treatment, but where the treatment is life-sustaining then there are stricter rules as to how this is recorded. Individuals must clearly indicate that their decision is to apply even if life is at risk and death will predictably result. They must also put the decision in writing and have it signed and witnessed. Patients cannot insist upon unlawful, inappropriate or futile treatment but may indicate their wish to receive particular treatments. This should be taken into account when making medical decisions.

For difficult welfare or medical decisions on behalf of an incapacitated adult where there is no LPA or close associate, clinicians and other professionals can apply for an independent mental capacity advocate (IMCA). This person is a lay person who will help to decide what is in the best interests of the patient, in an unbiased manner. If there are disputes, then an application can be made to the Court of Protection, and this will involve legal advisors, who should be contacted at the earliest opportunity. It is important to remember that it is unlawful and unacceptable to force treatment upon a patient who has validly refused it in advance.

British Medical Association. *Guidance from the Ethics Department: Advance Decisions and Proxy Decision-Making in Medical Treatment and Research*. London: BMA, 2007.

Question C74: Raised intracranial pressure

In the management of raised intracranial pressure (ICP):

A. Glucocorticoids should be used to reduce oedema secondary to diffuse axonal injury (DAI)
B. Hypertonic saline is more effective than mannitol in treating raised ICP
C. ICP monitoring should be used in ventilated patients with open head injuries
D. Rebound intracranial hypertension is a risk with hyperventilation to a $PaCO_2$ of 4–4.5 kPa
E. Therapeutic hypothermia should be used as first-line therapy for raised ICP in sedated patients

Answer: FFFTF

Short explanation

Steroids are only effective for oedema associated with tumours or vascular malformations. There is no evidence of superiority of hypertonic saline over mannitol, and there may be a rebound pressure increase with sudden cessation of hyperventilation. ICP monitoring is useful in closed head injuries. Adequate sedation and neuromuscular paralysis should be the first-line management of raised ICP, combined with surgery if indicated.

Long explanation

Normal intracranial pressure (ICP) in supine adults is 5–15 mmHg. Raised ICP is commonly defined as > 20 mmHg and is a medical emergency.

The Monro–Kellie doctrine states that the total volume of the brain and its constituents inside the cranium is fixed, so an alteration in the volume of one component will lead to a change in pressure unless there is a compensatory change in one of the other constituents. The approximate volumes are brain tissue 85%, cerebrospinal fluid (CSF) 10% (150 ml), and blood 5% (50–75 ml). Blood volume is the fastest physiological regulator of ICP, followed by CSF displacement into the spinal canal.

Various therapies have been studied for the acute reduction of ICP following traumatic brain injury. Most strategies require the measurement of ICP, as clinical signs and radiological features develop late. ICP monitoring is useful in ventilated patients with closed head injuries.

Management of raised ICP includes adequate sedation and neuromuscular paralysis to avoid hypoxia, hypercapnia and ventilator dissynchrony. The patient's position should be optimised with 30° head-up tilt and a neutral head position. Hyperventilation to a $PaCO_2$ of 4–4.5 kPa will reduce ICP, but this should be gradually discontinued as rebound rises in pressure may occur with sudden cessation.

Pharmacological management includes osmolar therapy with either mannitol or hypertonic saline. Neither has been shown to be superior to the other to date, and use depends on local protocols, availability and central venous access. Furosemide may also be used, although hypovolaemia should be avoided. Steroids have only been shown to improve ICP in patients with oedema from tumours or vascular malformations. They have no place in the management of traumatic brain injury. Thiopental infusions may be used when other sedative regimens have failed, but there is little evidence of improved outcome.

Pyrexia worsens outcomes and should be aggressively treated. However, although therapeutic hypothermia reduces ICP there is no strong evidence of an improvement in outcome and there is an increased risk of pneumonia.

Trials of surgical management of refractory raised ICP with decompressive craniectomy are ongoing, although the DECRA trial in 2011 showed that decompressive craniectomy was associated with lower ICPs but worse outcomes.

Clayton TJ, Nelson RJ, Manara A. Reduction in mortality from severe head injury following the introduction of a protocol for intensive care management. *Br J Anaesth* 2004; 93: 761–7.

Cooper DJ, Rosenfeld JV, Murray L, *et al.* for the DECRA Trial Investigators and the Australian and New Zealand Intensive Care Society Clinical Trials Group. Decompressive craniectomy in diffuse traumatic brain injury. *N Engl J Med* 2011; 364: 1493–502.

Smith ER, Sepideh Amin-Hanjani S. Evaluation and management of elevated intracranial pressure in adults. *UpToDate* 2013. http://www.uptodate.com (accessed June 2014).

Question C75: Metabolic alkalosis

Causes of a metabolic alkalosis include:

A. Diuretics
B. Eating disorders
C. Corticosteroids
D. Conn's syndrome
E. Citrate haemofiltration

Answer: TTTTT

Short explanation

All of the above may lead to a metabolic alkalosis.

Long explanation

A metabolic alkalosis is defined as a serum pH > 7.45 with a base excess > 2 mmol/l caused by the loss of non-carbonic acid or a gain of base. It is usually found in the context of renal impairment or hypokalaemia, as the kidneys will normally correct an excess of bicarbonate by increasing chloride reabsorption.

The causes of metabolic alkalosis may be divided into chloride-responsive alkalosis (urine chloride < 20 mmol/l) and chloride-resistant alkalosis (urine chloride > 20 mmol/l). Chloride-responsive alkalosis is more common and includes thiazide and loop diuretic use, which leads to a hypochloraemic alkalosis; and eating disorders, particularly when associated with excessive vomiting and loss of gastric acid (also seen with high nasogastric tube output).

Chloride-resistant alkalosis is associated with primary hyperaldosteronism (Conn's syndrome), Cushing's syndrome and glucocorticoid use. This is due to aldosterone-induced hypokalaemia or excess glucocorticoid acting on the mineralocorticoid receptor with the same effect (sodium retention, potassium excretion). Potassium is exchanged for hydrogen ions in the renal tubule leading to net loss of acid. Rare inherited causes of chloride-resistant metabolic alkalosis include Bartter and Gitelman syndromes.

Metabolic alkalosis can also be associated with citrate administration, massive blood transfusion and certain types of haemofiltration. Severe potassium or magnesium deficiency may also precipitate a metabolic alkalosis.

Emmett M. Clinical manifestations and evaluation of metabolic alkalosis. *UptoDate* 2012. http://www.uptodate.com (accessed June 2014).

Power I, Kam P. Acid–base physiology. In *Priniciples of Physiology for the Anaesthetist*, 2nd edn. London: Hodder Arnold; pp. 251–68.

Question C76: Ethylene glycol poisoning

Regarding ethylene glycol poisoning:

A. Activated charcoal should be given within 1 hour of ingestion
B. A normal anion gap metabolic acidosis is usually seen
C. Fomepizole should be administered intravenously because of poor oral bioavailability
D. Ethylene glycol is metabolised by alcohol dehydrogenase to non-toxic metabolites
E. Haemodialysis is a useful treatment

Answer: FFFFT

Short explanation

Activated charcoal is not recommended for ethylene glycol poisoning. A high anion gap metabolic acidosis is the usual metabolic picture. Fomepizole is usually administered intravenously, but oral absorption is rapid and almost complete. Ethylene glycol is metabolised to toxic acid metabolites by alcohol dehydrogenase and aldehyde dehydrogenase.

Long explanation

Ethylene glycol is commonly implicated in cases of both accidental and non-accidental poisoning. It is a major component of antifreeze, which is readily available. Ingestion results in a high anion gap metabolic acidosis due to its metabolism by alcohol and aldehyde dehydrogenase in the liver to toxic acids. These acids include formic, glycolic and oxalic acids. These organic acids are usually excreted renally, but as acute kidney injury is a common complication of ethylene glycol poisoning, they often accumulate.

In addition to routine organ support and critical care, treatment includes bicarbonate administration for urine alkalinisation, ethanol administration and haemodialysis. Ethanol administration works by providing an alternative competitive substrate (ethanol) for alcohol dehydrogenase. This results in reduced metabolism of ethylene glycol to toxic metabolites. Unmetabolised ethylene glycol is then excreted by the kidneys. Administration of ethanol requires careful maintenance of correct plasma levels, which may be labour-intensive and difficult, particularly if the patient is on haemodialysis.

Urinary alkalinisation is used to increase excretion of acid metabolites, whereas haemodialysis will effectively clear unmetabolised ethylene glycol from the plasma. Haemodialysis is recommended for patients with severe or refractory acidosis, deteriorating vital signs or acute kidney injury.

A newer antidote is available in the form of fomepizole. This is an inhibitor of alcohol dehydrogenase and has been used in the treatment of ethylene glycol poisoning. It is non-toxic, it is metabolised via the hepatic route, and it can be administered intravenously or orally every 12 hours. Dosing regimens are available which are based on the remaining plasma alcohol concentration of the patient, and which can also compensate for patients on haemodialysis. It has been used extensively in France and the USA, with good outcomes.

Megarbane B, Borron S, Baud F. Current recommendations for treatment of severe toxic alcohol poisonings. *Intensive Care Med* 2005; 31: 189–95.

Question C77: Critical illness in pregnancy

In the management of a critically ill pregnant patient, which of the following are correct?

A. Sepsis is a rare cause of maternal death in the developed world
B. Antibiotics should be withheld until an organism is identified, to prevent fetal toxicity
C. Central venous oxygen saturations will be lower than in the non-pregnant patient
D. Group A *Streptococcus* infection is implicated in a large proportion of maternal deaths resulting from sepsis
E. Vasopressors should be administered to maintain acceptable systemic blood pressure following fluid resuscitation

Answer: FFTTT

Short explanation

Severe sepsis and septic shock are relatively rare in pregnancy, but when they occur the mortality and morbidity are high. Sepsis was the leading cause of direct maternal death in the UK between 2006 and 2008. Management should be the same as for the non-pregnant patient, and early goal-directed therapy should be commenced as soon as sepsis is suspected. Broad-spectrum antibiotics should be administered within the first hour after discussion with the local microbiologist.

Long explanation

Critical illness during pregnancy can occur for a variety of reasons. There are a number of pregnancy-specific conditions which may require critical care admission. These include eclampsia, haemorrhage and amniotic fluid embolism. Patients with pre-existing medical conditions such as myaesthenia gravis, valvular heart disease and renal disease can deteriorate during pregnancy. Cardiac disease remains the overall leading cause of maternal death in the UK. Pregnancy also predisposes women to certain diseases that can be more severe when they develop, including pneumonia, ARDS, pulmonary embolism and sepsis.

Sepsis is a leading cause of maternal death both in the UK and worldwide. Common sources of infection include pyelonephritis, chorioamnionitis, endometritis and pneumonia. Most severe infections occur post-partum, known as puerperal sepsis. The leading risk factor for this is caesarean section. The commonest organisms are *Escherichia coli*, enterococci and β-haemolytic *Streptococcus*. Group A *Streptococcus* caused 50% of maternal deaths due to sepsis between 2006 and 2008 in the UK.

Goal-directed therapy should be commenced as early as possible in patients with evidence of sepsis and organ dysfunction. Critical care teams will need to liaise closely with obstetric teams in order to provide the appropriate level of care, which may require transfer from labour suite to ICU. Antibiotics, fluid resuscitation, vasopressor administration and invasive monitoring should be made readily available There is no evidence to suggest that norepinephrine has effects on fetal wellbeing. Central venous pressure remains the same in pregnancy but venous saturations fall towards term, and so achieving goals of 70% may not be possible. For a patient in early pregnancy, tetracycline and quinolone antibiotics should be avoided.

Neligan P, Laffey J. Clinical review: special populations – critical illness and pregnancy. *Crit Care* 2011; 15: 227.

Question C78: Percutaneous tracheostomy

Complications of percutaneous tracheostomy placement:

A. Include tracheo-oesophageal fistula formation
B. Are reduced by use of standard operating procedures
C. Include erosion into subclavian veins
D. Make continuous capnography mandatory in ventilated patients
E. Are less common than with surgical tracheostomy placement

Answer: TTFTF

Short explanation

A late complication of percutanous tracheostomy placement is haemorrhage due to erosion into the brachiocephalic (innominate) vessels. Complication rates are similar to those seen with surgical tracheostomy placement.

Long explanation

Tracheostomies on intensive care are commonly performed percutaneously, a procedure which has a similar rate of complications to surgical tracheostomy and reduces the need for the patient to be transferred. The patient should be monitored with standard anaesthetic monitoring including capnography. Ultrasound examination of the neck prior to insertion may help identify aberrant blood vessels. Flexible bronchoscopy should be performed through the endotracheal tube to confirm tracheal puncture, wire direction and tracheostomy placement within the trachea. Ideally the tracheostomy is placed between the first and second or second and third tracheal rings. Placement caudal to this risks late erosion into the brachiocephalic (innominate) arteries.

Other late complications of tracheostomy include tracheal stenosis, tracheo-oesophageal fistula, and skin tethering/scarring. Early complications of tracheostomy are bleeding, airway loss, pneumothorax, tube misplacement or removal, surgical emphysema, mucous plugging and stomal infection.

The 4th National Audit Project of the Royal College of Anaesthetists and the Difficult Airway Society (2011) investigated major complications of airway management in the United Kingdom and identified common themes in the management of adverse airway incidents associated with tracheostomy placement and management. These included:

- the lack of an individual with advanced airway skills immediately available to deal with a potentially complex situation
- increasing levels of obesity making airway management more challenging and tube displacement more likely
- a need for procedures and protocols for patient interventions, e.g. rolling/moving to ensure tube safety
- lack of continuous capnography monitoring
- lack of difficult airway equipment
- lack of algorithms for the management of accidental decannulation of the trachea and a stepwise approach to management of the compromised airway

Cook T, Woodall N, Frerk C. *Major Complications of Airway Management in the United Kingdom*. 4th National Audit Project of The Royal College of Anaesthetists and The Difficult Airway Society. London: Royal College of Anaesthetists, 2011.

Regan K, Hunt K. Tracheostomy management. *Contin Educ Anaesth Crit Care Pain* 2008; 8: 31–5.

Question C79: Micronutrients and trace elements

With regards to the nutritional requirements of an adult patient, which of the following are correct?

A. Vitamin B_1 should be provided to prevent lactic acidosis
B. Vitamins A, E and C have antioxidant properties that may counteract cell damage in critically ill patients
C. Zinc deficiency results in delayed wound healing
D. Selenium supplementation in parenteral nutrition is not recommended
E. Copper deficiency can lead to arrhythmias and altered immunity

Answer: TTTFT

Short explanation

Selenium deficiency can result in an acute cardiomyopathy. Europeans and some people in Australasia have a background low selenium status due to reduced levels in the soil. This means that when these patients are critically ill and consequently hypermetabolic, selenium deficiency can develop quickly.

Long explanation

The provision of trace elements and micronutrients is an integral part of artificial nutrition. There are particular deficiencies which cause well-known syndromes in malnourished patients. Examples include ascorbic acid causing scurvy and B vitamin deficiencies causing Korsakoff syndrome and Wernicke's encephalopathy.

There are other less commonly known, but well-recognised, consequences of vitamin and mineral deficiencies. Vitamin B_1 is particularly important in critically ill patients to prevent lactic acidosis, and requirements in an adult would be around 100 mg/day. Selenium is an essential trace element, and deficiency is relatively common in malnourished or critically ill patients. Low levels of selenium lead to a higher sensitivity to oxidative stress, resulting in tissue damage. This appears to have a greater effect on the heart, where cardiomyopathy can develop in a relatively short time.

There has been a lot of interest in the antioxidant properties of micronutrients and whether supplementation can affect overall outcome and mortality of critically ill patients. The evidence for excessive 'supranormal' supplementation is conflicting, but malnourished patients should receive these micronutrients to prevent deficiencies. Those with proven antioxidant properties include vitamin A, β-carotene, vitamin E, vitamin C and selenium.

There is also some evidence that supplementation with certain micronutrients, namely vitamin A and manganese, can be dangerous, particularly in those patients with severe liver insufficiency or enzyme abnormalities.

Singer P, Berger M, Van den Berghe G, *et al.* ESPEN guidelines on parenteral nutrition: intensive care. *Clin Nutr* 2009; 28: 387–400.

Thibault R, Pichard C, Raynard B, Singer P. Nutrition. ESICM PACT Module. Update April 2010. http://pact.esicm.org/media/Nutrition%25;20Updated%25;20April%25;202010.pdf (accessed June 2014).

Question C80: Nasogastric feeding tube insertion

Concerning the insertion of a nasogastric (NG) feeding tube:

A. Prior to insertion, the tube length required should be estimated using the NEX measurement

B. When using a chest radiograph to confirm correct placement, the feeding tube should always be seen below the diaphragm
C. If no aspirate is obtainable then the tube should be flushed
D. A pH of aspirated contents of > 4 is a contraindication to feeding
E. On a chest radiograph a correctly placed NG tube should bisect the carina

Answer: TTFFT

Short explanation

If no aspirate is obtainable the NG tube should never be flushed, and the 'whoosh' test is no longer recommended. A small amount of air can be injected to unblock the tube if this is thought to be the problem. Feeding may be commenced if the pH of the aspirate is between 1 and 5.5 using pH indicator paper that is CE marked.

Long explanation

There have been a number of serious adverse incidents involving incorrectly placed nasogastric (NG) feeding tubes. Feeding via an incorrectly placed feeding tube can lead to serious patient harm, including, in a number of cases, death. Following these incidents the National Patient Safety Agency issued a national safety warning. Feeding via a misplaced feeding tube is now classed as a 'never event' in the UK, and all staff should take steps to avoid it happening. Most trusts now have training packages for all staff involved in the use of feeding tubes.

Before placement of a feeding tube, the decision should clearly documented in the patient notes. The feeding tube should be placed by an experienced operator. The resources to check correct placement should be immediately available. These include a feeding tube with visible external length markings, pH indicator paper which is CE marked and intended by the manufacturer to test human gastric aspirate, and the availability of a radiographer and x-ray facilities. If this is not possible then insertion should be postponed until these conditions can be met.

The feeding tube length should be estimated before insertion using the NEX measurement. This involves placing the exit port of the tube at the tip of the nose, extending the tube to the earlobe and then on to the xiphisternum, where the length can be read from the markings on the tube. The tube should be inserted to this length and then securely fixed at the nose.

Following insertion, the operator should attempt to aspirate fluid from the feeding tube. The pH must be between 1 and 5.5 for feeding to safely commence. If the pH is not in this range then an erect chest x-ray may be required. If no aspirate is obtainable initially then there are a few possible manoeuvres including left lateral position, gentle injection of 10–20 mL of air, advancing or withdrawing the tube by 10–20 cm. It is recommended to wait for 15–30 minutes before re-attempting aspiration. At no point should water be used to flush the tube or the 'whoosh test' (injecting a large quantity of air with a syringe while listening at the stomach with a stethoscope) be performed. If, after these measures, no aspirate is obtainable, a chest x-ray should be performed. A correctly placed NG tube should bisect the carina and descend below the diaphragm.

Lamont T, Beaumont C, Fayaz A, *et al.* Checking placement of nasogastric feeding tubes in adults (interpretation of x ray images): summary of a safety report from the National Patient Safety Agency. *BMJ* 2011; 342: d2586.

National Patient Safety Alert. Patient Safety Alert NPSA/2011/PSA002. Reducing the harm caused by misplaced nasogastric feeding tubes in adults, children and infants. March 2011. Supporting information. http://www.nrls.npsa.nhs.uk/EasySiteWeb/getresource.axd%3F;AssetID=129697%26; (accessed June 2014).

Question C81: Stress ulcer prophylaxis

With regards to stress ulceration prophylaxis in the critically ill patient, which of the following are correct?

A. There is strong evidence that stress ulcer prophylaxis reduces mortality in septic patients
B. Histamine H_2 receptor antagonists (H_2RAs) are superior to proton-pump inhibitors (PPIs) in preventing gastrointestinal ulceration in the critically ill patient
C. Upper gastrointestinal bleeding is reduced in patients taking stress ulcer prophylaxis
D. Sucralfate is not as effective as H_2RAs in preventing stress ulceration
E. Evidence suggests that higher rates of hospital-acquired and aspiration pneumonia are seen in patients taking acid-suppressive medication

Answer: FFTTT

Short explanation

Despite many large trials, the evidence for mortality reduction by stress ulcer prophylaxis remains weak. H_2RAs and PPIs are probably equally effective in preventing gastrointestinal ulceration.

Long explanation

Stress ulceration is known to be a problem in critically ill patients. Most commonly, it occurs in patients with severe sepsis and severe burns. Clinically significant sequelae include gastrointestinal bleeding and intestinal perforation. Stress ulceration can however occur without serious consequences. Rates of clinically significant gastrointestinal bleeding have been shown to be as low as 1% of all ICU patients.

Prevention of stress ulceration predominantly involves the generic care that all patients receive, and includes treatment of the underlying condition, cardiovascular optimisation and nutritional support. The theory is that by improving the blood supply to the gastrointestinal tract and preventing mucosal atrophy, stress ulceration is less likely to occur.

The introduction of stress ulcer prophylaxis medication such as histamine H_2 receptor antagonists (H_2RAs) and proton-pump inhibitors (PPIs) is still controversial. The evidence for clear benefit by a reduction in clinically significant gastrointestinal complications and mortality is seen by many as weak. Some studies have shown small improvements, but the numbers needed to treat are as high as 1000 in some trials. On the other hand, there have also been a number of clinical trials which have demonstrated an increase in the incidence of ventilator-associated pneumonia (VAP) in patients receiving these medications. There is little or no evidence directly comparing H_2RAs with PPIs, and so it is not clear whether either is more efficacious or safe than the other.

Herzig S, Howell M, Ngo L, Marcantonio E. Acid-suppressive medication use and the risk for hospital-acquired pneumonia. *JAMA* 2009; 301: 2120–8.

Kahn J, Doctor J, Rubenfeld G. Stress ulcer prophylaxis in mechanically ventilated patients: integrating evidence and judgement using a decision analysis. *Intensive Care Med* 2006; 32: 1151–8.

Marik P, Vasu T, Hirani A, Pachinburavan M. Stress ulcer prophylaxis in the new millennium: a systematic review and meta-analysis. *Crit Care Med* 2010; 38: 2222–8.

Rubulotta F, Gullo A, Iscra F. Recommendations for ulcer prophylaxis in the treatment of patients with severe sepsis and septic shock.: a dog chasing its tail? *Intensive Care Medicine* 2007; 33: 718–20.

Question C82: Transfusion-related acute lung injury

Transfusion-related acute lung injury (TRALI):

A. Is acute lung injury occurring within 12 hours of blood transfusion
B. Is more common than haemolytic reactions, HIV and hepatitis B and C transmission
C. Is more likely with platelets than with red blood cells
D. Has no specific treatment
E. Carries a higher mortality than other causes of acute lung injury (ALI)

Answer: FTTTF

Short explanation

TRALI is acute lung injury within 6 hours of transfusion. Incidence per unit transfused is 0.02–0.05% (acute haemolysis 0.015%, HBV 0.005%, HCV/HIV 0.00005%). Platelets and fresh frozen plasma (FFP) carry the greatest risk. Management is standard resuscitation with lung-protective ventilation. Mortality is around 10% (40–50% for other causes of ALI).

Long explanation

Transfusion-related acute lung injury (TRALI) is defined as acute lung injury (ALI) developing within 6 hours of blood product transfusion. Since its first description in 1983, it has emerged as the leading cause of mortality associated with transfusion, yet is relatively under-diagnosed. This is particularly true in critical care medicine, where patients have multiple risk factors for ALI. In fact its incidence is reported to be 0.02–0.05% per transfused unit, in comparison with acute haemolysis (0.015%), hepatitis B (0.005%), hepatitis C or HIV transmission (both 0.00005%).

The pathogenesis of TRALI is still to be fully elucidated, but it is thought to involve antileucocyte antibodies from prior exposure of donors to allogenic antibodies during pregnancy or blood transfusion. This leads to complement activation, microaggregation of neutrophils in the lung parenchyma with interstitial oedema and acute respiratory failure subsequently developing. All plasma-containing products have been implicated in the development of TRALI, but fresh frozen plasma (FFP), red blood cells (RBCs) and pooled platelets (from multiple donors) have been shown to be particularly high risk.

Clinical features of TRALI are those of ALI (dyspnoea, respiratory failure and bilateral infiltrates on chest radiography), commonly with associated hypotension and fever. For a diagnosis of TRALI, the ALI must occur within 1–6 hours of blood product transfusion (symptoms often start within the first hour), and the patient should have no pre-existing ALI.

There are currently no specific treatments for TRALI, and management is therefore supportive. Around 72% of patients require mechanical ventilation with protective ventilatory strategies. Hypotensive patients should be fluid resuscitated and occasionally require vasopressor infusions to maintain blood pressure. Corticosteroids have been used, but as yet there is no evidence to support or preclude them. TRALI carries a much lower mortality rate (10%) than ALI of other aetiologies (40–50%).

Moore SB. Transfusion-related acute lung injury (TRALI): clinical presentation, treatment, and prognosis. *Crit Care Med* 2006; 34 (5 suppl): S114–17.

Question C83: Red cell transfusion

Regarding the guidelines for red cell transfusion in adult critically ill patients:

A. The default target Hb range should be > 9 g/dl
B. A transfusion threshold of ≤ 7 g/dl should be the default unless specific factors are present
C. Anaemic patients with stable angina should have Hb maintained > 10 g/dl
D. In patients who are weaning from the ventilator, Hb should be maintained > 9 g/dl
E. In patients with subarachnoid haemorrhage the target Hb should be 8–10 g/dl

Answer: FTFFT

Short explanation

The default target Hb range should be 7–9 g/dl for all critically ill patients unless specific factors are present that modify clinical decision making. Patients with stable angina or those who are weaning do not require a different Hb range. Targeting a higher Hb range should not be undertaken to assist weaning.

Long explanation

Over recent years, there has been considerable research aimed at defining optimal haemoglobin (Hb) levels and transfusion triggers in critically ill patients. There are rare but serious risks associated with blood transfusion, including blood mismatching, immunological reactions and transmission of infections. The short- and long-term effects on morbidity and mortality from blood transfusion are still not fully understood.

Clinical trials in intensive care patients, cardiac surgery patients and patients with fractured neck of femur have failed to demonstrate any outcome benefits of liberal transfusion policies, and have shown that restrictive policies do not result in worse outcomes. Some research has shown improved outcomes in those patients in the restrictive groups. These and other research publications have helped change practice to reduce the transfusion thresholds in critically ill patients, who on average receive 2–4 units of blood per ICU admission.

The default target Hb range should be 7–9 g/dl for all critically ill patients unless specific factors are present which modify clinical decision making. Patients with stable angina or those who are weaning do not require a different Hb range. Targeting a higher Hb range should not be undertaken to assist weaning.

British Committee for Standards in Haematology. Guidelines on the management of anaemia and red cell transfusion in adult critically ill patients. *Br J Haematol* 2013; 160: 445–64.

Carson J, Terrin M, Noveck H, *et al.* Liberal or restrictive transfusion in high-risk patients after hip surgery. *N Engl J Med* 2011; 365: 2453–62.

Hajjar L, Vincent J, Galas F, *et al.* Transfusion requirements after cardiac surgery: the TRACS randomized controlled trial. *JAMA* 2010; 304: 1559–67.

Hébert P, Wells G, Blajchman M, *et al.* A multicenter, randomized, controlled clinical trial of transfusion requirements in critical care. Transfusion Requirements in Critical Care Investigators, Canadian Critical Care Trials Group. *N Engl J Med* 1999; 340, 409–17.

Question C84: Chronic kidney disease

With regard to chronic kidney disease (CKD):

A. The commonest cause of CKD is hypertension
B. The combined use of an angiotensin-converting enzyme (ACE) inhibitor and an angiotensin II blocking agent is recommended to slow the progression to end-stage renal failure
C. Platelet transfusion is effective as a means of improving coagulation in patients prior to surgery
D. The free drug fraction of highly protein-bound drugs is decreased with CKD
E. Maximum doses of local anaesthetics are unchanged in CKD

Answer: FFFFF

Short explanation

The commonest cause of CKD is diabetes mellitus. There is no evidence to support the use of ACE inhibitors and angiotensin II blocking agents in combination to prevent end-stage renal failure. The free drug fraction is increased, and maximum doses of local anaesthetic are reduced by 25%. Platelet transfusion will not improve coagulation.

Long explanation

Chronic kidney disease (CKD) is defined as abnormalities of kidney structure or function, present for > 3 months and with implications for health. CKD is classified based on cause, glomerular filtraton rate (GFR) category and albuminuria category.

The commonest cause of chronic renal impairment is diabetes mellitus, followed by hypertension, glomerulonephritis and polycystic kidney disease. 20% of cases are of unknown origin.

KDIGO guidelines suggest an ACE inhibitor or angiotensin II blocking agent in all patients with progressive CKD, but there is no evidence currently supporting the use of both agents.

CKD has a number of systemic effects, including:

- **Cardiovascular system**: Hypertension, accelerated atherosclerosis, valvular heart disease and rarely uraemic pericarditis.
- **Respiratory system**: Pulmonary oedema from fluid overload, increased susceptibility to infection.
- **Haematological**: Most patients with CKD are anaemic. Coagulation is impaired, particularly platelet function. This is probably due to inadequate vascular endothelial release of a von Willebrand factor/factor VIII complex, leading to decreased adhesiveness and aggregation. This is not helped by platelet transfusion but may respond to desmopressin or cryoprecipitate.
- **Gastrointestinal system**: Anorexia, nausea, vomiting and malnutrition. Increased incidence of peptic ulceration.
- **Nervous system**: Peripheral and autonomic neuropathy, dementia and acute neurological changes related to dialysis.
- **Immunological**: CKD inhibits cell-mediated immunity and humoral defence mechanisms, rendering patients more susceptible to infection.
- **Pharmacokinetics**: Hypoalbuminaemia and acidosis increase free drug availability of highly protein-bound drugs and requires dose reduction. Local anaesthetic duration of action is reduced, and the maximum dose should be reduced by 25% because of reduced protein binding and a lower seizure threshold. Other effects include reduced metabolism or excretion of some drugs and a higher volume of distribution.

Kidney Disease: Improving Global Outcomes (KDIGO) CKD Work Group. KDIGO 2012 clinical practice guideline for the evaluation and management of chronic kidney disease. *Kidney Int* 2013; 3 (Suppl): 1–150.
Milner Q. Pathophysiology of chronic renal failure. *Contin Educ Anaesth Crit Care Pain* 2003; 3: 130–3.

Question C85: Drug metabolism in critical illness

Which of the following statements correctly describe the metabolism of drugs in critically ill patients?

A. Non-renal metabolism of vancomycin remains unaltered in patients with acute kidney injury (AKI)
B. Uraemic molecules present due to AKI may prevent the normal hepatic metabolism of drugs
C. Renal replacement therapy ensures that metabolism of renally excreted drugs is maintained
D. Hyper- and hypothermia can prevent drug metabolism by means of enzyme dysfunction and reduced activity
E. Patients who have thyroid dysfunction will be particularly sensitive to the effects of sedative agents

Answer: FTFTF

Short explanation

Non-renal metabolism of many drugs, including vancomycin, is also reduced in AKI. Renal replacement therapy does not appear to replace normal drug metabolism in AKI. Patients with hyperthyroidism may be relatively resistant to sedative medication because of their high metabolic rate. Those with hypothyroidism will be more sensitive to sedative medication.

Long explanation

The pharmacokinetics of drugs used in critically ill patients should be considered when prescribing on the intensive care unit. Absorption via the oral route can be considerably reduced or slowed because of gut dysfunction. This may be a primary reason for intensive care or secondary to a variety of pathologies such as sepsis, cardiac failure or electrolyte disturbance. Distribution is affected by age, fluid balance and plasma protein levels. In particular, albumin is usually low in critically ill patients, which can lead to higher free drug levels. This is not reversed by administration of albumin replacement.

Metabolism and excretion are affected by a variety of mechanisms such as acute kidney injury (AKI), hepatic failure, low cardiac output, hypoxia, co-administration of inducing and inhibiting drugs, age and diabetes mellitus. It is not surprising that renally excreted drugs and metabolites will accumulate in AKI. However, it is important to note that non-renal metabolism of drugs is also affected in AKI, including hepatic metabolism. This may be due to the presence of uraemic molecules, altered tissue blood flow and altered protein binding. Cytochrome P450 enzyme activity is also altered in AKI. Transporters which are present in some tissues to facilitate drug uptake or removal can be affected by AKI. For some drugs, such as vancomycin, the increasing duration of renal replacement therapy leads to a decline in non-renal clearance. Hyperthermia can inhibit cytochrome P450 enzymes, such as quinine in patients with malaria and fever.

Park G. Molecular mechanisms of drug metabolism in the critically ill. *Br J Anaesth* 1996; 77: 32–49.
Vilay A, Churchwell M, Mueller B. Clinical review: drug metabolism and nonrenal clearance in acute kidney injury. *Crit Care* 2008; 12: 235.

Question C86: Surgical site infection

Regarding surgical site infection:

A. Colonisation with methicillin-sensitive *Staphylococcus aureus* (MSSA) increases the risk of postoperative wound infection
B. Blood sugar should be kept at 4–6 mmol/l to reduce surgical site infection
C. Blood transfusion is associated with a higher incidence of surgical site infection
D. Oxycodone should be used in preference to morphine to reduce postoperative infection
E. Povidone–iodine is as effective as 2% chlorhexidine in preventing infections

Answer: TFTTF

Short explanation

While the ideal blood sugar range is 4–6 mmol/l to reduce surgical site infection, the risk of hypoglycaemia means that current recommendations are to keep blood sugar < 10 mmol/l. Povidone–iodine solutions are not as effective as 2% chlorhexidine at preventing surgical site infections.

Long explanation

Surgical site infection occurs in up to 16% of patients postoperatively . Variables conferring susceptibility to postoperative infection (including surgical site, respiratory, urinary tract and line infection) may be classified into non-modifiable and modifiable factors. Non-modifiable factors include patient age, comorbidities (e.g. diabetes mellitus), smoking, malnutrition, surgical site and type of surgery. Modifiable perioperative variables include antibiotic prophylaxis, hand hygiene, invasive lines, hypothermia, perioperative glycaemic control, volume status, blood transfusion and postoperative analgesia.

Antibiotic prophylaxis reduces the bacterial inoculum at the time of surgery provided the minimum inhibitory concentration of the antibiotic agent at tissue level is exceeded for the duration of the surgery from incision to wound closure. The infection rate is lowest when antibiotics are administered within 30 minutes of incision, with the incidence of infection increasing with administration after incision or > 60 minutes before.

The ideal blood sugar range is 4–6 mmol/l, but the risk of hypoglycaemia means that current recommendations are to keep blood sugar < 10 mmol/l.

Patients should be actively warmed unless hypothermia is required for surgery, as even a 2 °C drop in core temperature is associated with increased risk of perioperative infection.

Hand hygiene, aseptic technique and the use of 2% chlorhexidine where appropriate all reduce the risk of infection.

The mode of analgesia may be of importance in reducing postoperative infections. Regional anaesthesia is thought to be beneficial, as it improves vasodilatation and tissue oxygenation, reduces the stress response with improved analgesia, and may modify the inflammatory response. Morphine, fentanyl and remifentanil all have immunosuppressive properties, while oxycodone and buprenorphine have no effect on the immune system and tramadol may have immune-enhancing properties. While the choice of analgesia has not been shown to be an independent risk factor to date, it may be sensible to avoid certain agents in patients with a high risk of developing postoperative infections.

Goal-directed fluid therapy and the avoidance of blood transfusion where possible also reduce the risk of surgical site infection.

Gifford C, Christelis N, Cheng A. Preventing postoperative infection: the anaesthetist's role. *Contin Educ Anaesth Crit Care Pain* 2001; 11: 151–6.

National Institute for Health and Care Excellence. *CG74: Prevention and Treatment of Surgical Site Infection*. London: NICE, 2008. http://www.nice.org.uk/cg74 (accessed June 2014).

National Institute for Health and Care Excellence. *QS49: Surgical Site Infection*. London: NICE, 2013. http://www.nice.org.uk/qs49 (accessed June 2014).

Question C87: Selective decontamination of the digestive tract

Regarding selective decontamination of the digestive tract (SDD):

A. It is associated with a reduction in mortality
B. It increases the likelihood of infection with resistant bacteria
C. Topical therapy alone (selective oral decontamination) reduces ventilator-associated pneumonia
D. SDD does not affect fungal infections
E. SDD is a method of controlling exogenous infections in critical care patients

Answer: TFTFF

Short explanation

SDD is an enteral and parenteral antibiotic and antifungal protocol that aims to reduce mortality from endogenous infections in critically ill patients. Exogenous infections are those acquired without prior colonisation, and they should be prevented by good hygiene measures. Treatment with topical prophylaxis alone reduces respiratory infections but not mortality.

Long explanation

Selective decontamination of the digestive tract (SDD) is an enteral and parenteral antibiotic protocol that aims to reduce mortality from endogenous infections in critically ill patients. Endogenous infections may be classed as primary or secondary. Primary endogenous infections are those present on admission to critical care, while secondary endogenous infections are those acquired later as a result of prior colonisation. Exogenous infections are those acquired without prior colonisation, and they may be prevented by good hygiene measures. So far SDD has not been universally adopted, despite robust evidence, because of largely unfounded concerns regarding cost and the potential for an increase in antibiotic resistance.

The latest Cochrane review found that a combination of topical and systemic prophylactic antibiotics reduced respiratory tract infections and overall mortality in adult ICU patients. Treatment with topical prophylaxis alone (selective oral decontamination) reduced respiratory infections but not mortality. The risk of antibiotic resistance was only measurable in one trial, which did not show evidence of this.

D'Amico R, Pifferi S, Torri V, *et al*. Antibiotic prophylaxis to reduce respiratory tract infections and mortality in adults receiving intensive care. *Cochrane Database Syst Rev* 2009; (4): CD000022.

Zandstra DF, Van Saene HKF. Selective decontamination of the digestive tract (SDD). In Waldmann C, Soni N, Rhodes A. *Oxford Desk Reference: Critical Care*. Oxford: Oxford University Press, 2008; pp. 474–5.

Question C88: Post-traumatic stress disorder

Post-traumatic stress disorder (PTSD) in patients after intensive care:

A. Is reduced in incidence by a self-help recovery package given to patients on discharge
B. Is more common in patients with delusional memories
C. Occurs in up to 1 in 10 ICU patients
D. Should be assessed using validated screening tools
E. Should prompt psychiatric referral in all patients at risk

Answer: FTTTF

Short explanation

Studies have shown that PTSD is not reduced by a self-help recovery package given to patients on discharge. Patients with severe symptoms require psychiatric referral, but those with moderate symptoms may be managed expectantly.

Long explanation

Post-traumatic stress disorder (PTSD) is a psychological disorder precipitated by a traumatic event with a wide variety of symptoms specific to the individual. It occurs in up to 1 in 10 ICU patients. Severe PTSD will impair a patient's ability to lead a normal life.

Symptoms generally occur within 1 month of the event, but may be delayed by months or years. Patients experience flashbacks and nightmares, and feel isolated, irritable and guilty. They will try to avoid anything that reminds them of the traumatic event. Patients recalling delusional memories from their critical care admission are at much higher risk of PTSD and anxiety than patients whose memories are real. Patients with PTSD are generally unwilling to talk about what has happened to them. Insomnia is common, and concentration spans are often reduced, with a state of hyperarousal and continuous anxiety. Emotional numbing describes a state where the patient tries not to remember or feel anything at all. They may withdraw from their usual activities.

The course of the illness varies, from relapsing and remitting to constant. ICU patients should be screened for PTSD with validated tools such as the Impact of Event Scale, PTSS-10 or PTSS-14. Staff should be trained in assessing patients, and should be aware of warning signs. NICE guidelines suggest that patients with PTSD should be given literature on the symptoms of PTSD, but a study of using a self-help recovery package on discharge showed no impact on psychological symptoms, although physical rehabilitation improved. The role of ICU diaries has yet to be fully investigated, but they may improve the patient's understanding of what happened, ameliorate amnesia and refute delusional memories. Patients with moderate symptoms may be managed with regular follow-up, but severe symptoms require psychiatric evaluation.

Jones C, Griffiths RD. Critical care follow up. In Waldmann C, Soni N, Rhodes A. *Oxford Desk Reference: Critical Care*. Oxford: Oxford University Press, 2008; pp. 586–7.

Wake S, Kitchiner D Post-traumatic stress disorder after intensive care. *BMJ* 2013; 346: f3232.

Question C89: Organ donation

Concerning organ donation and transplantation:

A. Organ donation should be considered in every patient expected to die in ICU
B. Family members have no right to refuse to authorise donation if the patient is on the organ donor register (ODR)
C. Family members may authorise donation if there is no indication of the prior views of the patient
D. Donation after circulatory death (DCD) can be classified as controlled or uncontrolled
E. Organ donation coordinators may only be approached after authorisation for donation has been received

Answer: TFTTF

Short explanation

All ICU deaths should be considered for organ donation, and donation coordinators should be involved early. Consent is implied by the presence of a patient on the ODR, but familial assent must also be obtained. Patients not on the ODR may still donate with the consent of the family. DCD may be controlled (following withdrawal of life-sustaining treatment) or uncontrolled (organised after the unexpected death of a suitable patient).

Long explanation

All patients who are expected to die in ICU should have the possibility of organ donation considered. There are few contraindications to organ donation:

Absolute contraindications	
Infective neurodegenerative disease (e.g. variant Creutzfeldt–Jakob disease)	
AIDS/HIV disease (HIV infection alone is not a contraindication)	
Relative contraindications	
Age over 90 years	
Cancer	Disseminated cancer
	Treated cancer within 3 years (except skin and cervical cancer)
	Melanoma (unless locally excised > 5 years prior to donation)

Organ donation coordinators should be contacted once a patient has been recognised as a possible candidate for organ donation. The process of checking the organ donor register (ODR), discussing with the family and consent are greatly facilitated by the presence of donation coordinators.

Consent to organ donation is complex. If a patient is on the ODR, then this is taken as an indication of the wishes of the patient, but the family should still be approached for consent to proceed to organ donation. If the family objects despite the presence of the patient on the ODR, then organ retrieval cannot occur. For patients not on the ODR, then consent needs to be obtained from the patient's family. Patients with maintained capacity are able to consent to organ donation themselves, but this is very rare, owing to the nature of conditions leading to consideration of organ donation.

Donation after brain death (DBD) is becoming less common as road safety and care of traumatic brain injury improves. Live organ donation (kidney, partial liver) and donation after circulatory death (DCD) are becoming increasingly common to compensate. DCD may be controlled or uncontrolled. Controlled DCD occurs following withdrawal of life-sustaining treatment in critical care. Therapy is withdrawn once organ retrieval teams are available. Retrieval can only occur if the patient dies within a certain, organ-specific time following withdrawal. Uncontrolled DCD is uncommon, as it requires the summoning of retrieval teams after the patient has died unexpectedly.

National Institute for Health and Care Excellence. *CG135: Organ Donation for Transplantation.* London: NICE, 2011. http://www.nice.org.uk/cg135 (accessed June 2014).

Question C90: Central pontine myelinolysis

With regards to central pontine myelinolysis (CPM), which of the following are correct?

A. It is more commonly seen in patients with alcohol dependence
B. Rapid correction of acute hyponatraemia is the main cause
C. MRI is the imaging modality of choice for diagnosis
D. Microscopically there is degeneration of axons in the pons with preservation of oligodendrocytes
E. Parkinsonism, catatonia and movement disorders suggest extrapontine myelinolysis

Answer: TFTFT

Short explanation

Rapid correction of chronic hyponatraemia is believed to be the main cause of CPM. Correction of acute hyponatraemia has only been reported as a cause in a few patients. Oligodendrocytes appear to be more prone to apoptosis, and this may be due to osmotic stress triggering the apoptosis cascade.

Long explanation

Central pontine myelinolysis (CPM) is a condition which many clinicians fear when correcting hyponatraemia. Rapid correction of chronic hyponatraemia is believed to be the main cause of CPM. Correction of acute hyponatraemia has only been reported as a cause in a few patients. Unfortunately, despite close monitoring and avoidance of hypertonic saline, the sodium often rises faster than clinicians would like, particularly in severe hyponatraemia.

CPM was first described in the 1950s as a post-mortem diagnosis. A link between the syndrome and rapid correction of hyponatraemia was established in the 1980s. The usual clinical picture is of encephalopathy or seizures due to severe hyponatraemia followed by a period of recovery following correction. After a few days, the patient may deteriorate with neurological signs such as dysarthria, dysphagia, oculomotor abnormalities and flaccid quadriparesis which later becomes spastic. The 'locked in' syndrome can also occur with large lesions. CPM can also be accompanied by extrapontine myelinolysis (EPM), with features including catatonia, mutism, parkinsonism and dystonia.

CPM is unusual in patients who have no other comorbidities; usually patients are alcoholics or malnourished. It is rare in diabetic or renal dialysis patients, probably because there is a protective mechanism from the high levels of glucose or urea.

Pathologically, there is axon fibre preservation with loss of oligodendrocytes in the basis pontis of the pons. Rarely the lesion spreads to the medulla or the midbrain. The cause of the demyelination may be due to the triggering of apoptosis of oligodendrocytes brought about by over-activation of ion channels during the osmotic changes that occur when hyponatraemia is corrected. Slower correction of sodium levels can prevent the syndrome occurring, although the mortality of uncorrected severe hyponatraemia is also very high. Expert advice regarding correction of severe hyponatraemia should be sought, particularly in high-risk patients such as alcoholics.

Martin RJ. Central pontine and extrapontine myelinolysis: the osmotic demyelination syndromes. *J Neurol Neurosurg Psychiatry* 2004; 75: iii22–8.

Index

Printed in the United States
By Bookmasters